G

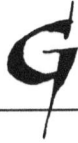

THE GEORGE GUND FOUNDATION
IMPRINT IN AFRICAN AMERICAN STUDIES

The George Gund Foundation has endowed
this imprint to advance understanding of
the history, culture, and current issues
of African Americans.

*The publisher and the
University of California Press Foundation
gratefully acknowledge the generous support of the
George Gund Foundation Imprint in
African American Studies.*

Death by Design

Death by Design

PRODUCING RACIAL HEALTH INEQUALITY
IN THE SHADOW OF THE CAPITOL

Sanyu A. Mojola

UNIVERSITY OF CALIFORNIA PRESS

University of California Press
Oakland, California

Library of Congress Cataloging-in-Publication Data

Names: Mojola, Sanyu A., author
Title: Death by design : producing racial health inequality in the shadow
    of the capitol / Sanyu A. Mojola.
Description: Oakland, California : University of California Press, [2025] |
    Includes bibliographical references and index.
Identifiers: LCCN 2025001832 (print) | LCCN 2025001833 (ebook) |
    ISBN 9780520303010 cloth | ISBN 9780520421165 paperback |
    ISBN 9780520972629 ebook
Subjects: LCSH: African Americans—Medical care—Moral and ethical
    aspects | Health and race—Washington (D.C.)—History
Classification: LCC RA448.5.B53 M65 2025 (print) | LCC RA448.5.B53 (ebook) |
    DDC 362.1089960753—dc23/eng/20250721
LC record available at https://lccn.loc.gov/2025001832
LC ebook record available at https://lccn.loc.gov/2025001833

GPSR Authorized Representative: Easy Access System Europe, Mustamäe tee
50, 10621 Tallinn, Estonia, gpsr.requests@easproject.com

34 33 32 31 30 29 28 27 26 25
10 9 8 7 6 5 4 3 2 1

CONTENTS

ILLUSTRATIONS

FIGURES

TABLES

Introduction

Herein lie buried many things which if read with patience may show the strange meaning of being Black here at the dawning of the ~~Twentieth~~ *Twenty-First* Century. This meaning is not without interest to you, Gentle Reader; for the problem of the ~~Twentieth~~ *Twenty-First* Century is the problem of the Color Line.

WILLIAM E. B. DU BOIS (1904:5) *[my edits]*

The health of the most socially advantaged group in a society indicates a level of health that should be possible for everyone.

PAULA BRAVEMAN ET AL (2010:S194)

UNEQUAL DEATH IN THE UNITED STATES

Let me start by stating the obvious. Until there is a pill for human immortality, 100% of Americans will die of something someday. However, while death can seem random at an individual level, from a population point of view, who gets sick, who dies, and when, how, and where death occurs is not random. It is highly predictable and unequal. For example, Americans may share a common citizenship; however, how long they can expect to live varies widely and predictably across the US. Figure 1 illustrates life expectancy at birth by state across the US in 2021.[1] It shows that people born in states like Hawaii, Massachusetts, Connecticut, New York, and New Jersey could expect to live about 79 or more years, while those born in states like Mississippi, West Virginia, and Alabama could expect to live about 70 to 72 years—a significant seven- to nine-year difference. What this map makes clear is that where you are born and where you live has something to do with how long you live. This suggests that there is something above and beyond individual genetics, decision-making, and

US Life expectancy by state
Life expectancy at birth as of 2021

70   80 years

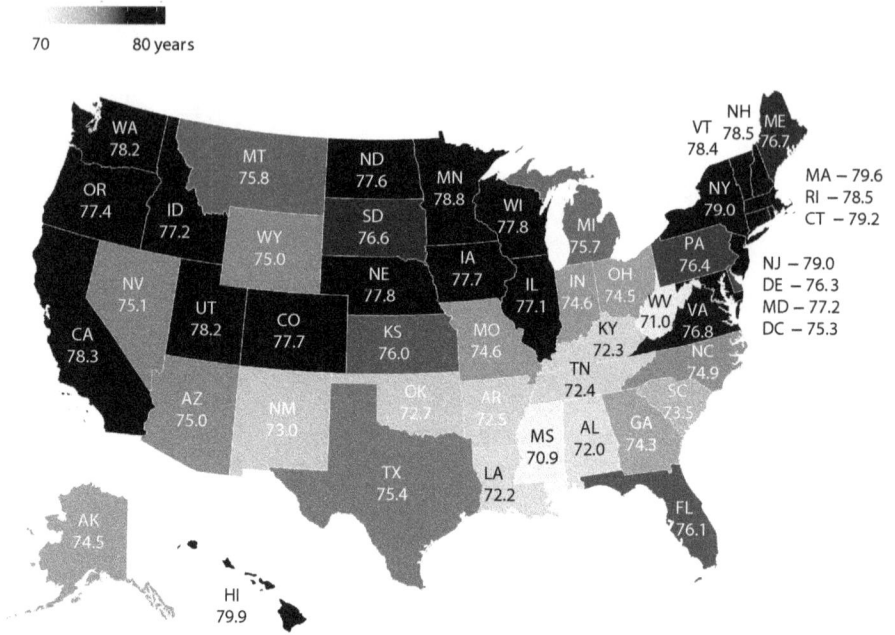

FIGURE 1. US life expectancy at birth by state, 2021. Data source: National Center for Health Statistics, National Vital Statistics System (Arias et al 2024).

personal responsibility that determines why some Americans are more likely to get sick, why some spend more years managing significant chronic illnesses, and why some will bury more family members at younger ages.

At the heart of this book is a story of the creation, design, and maintenance of America's unequal playing fields of life and death. Its basic assertion is that at a population level, a large part of the variability of death rates across states, counties, and neighborhoods is due to policy decisions that work together to create and sustain places that make groups of people more or less prone to early and/or chronic illness and premature death.[2] The book focuses on examining the paradigmatic Black-White gap in illness and death, and the story unfolds in the District of Columbia, the capital city, which has the nation's largest racial life-expectancy gap—whether compared to states, territories, counties, or the thirty most populous cities, such as New York City, Los Angeles, Chicago, Houston, Baltimore, or Detroit.[3] Black men and women born in Washington, DC, can expect to live a startling 18.01 years and 12.3 years less than their White men and women counterparts, respectively.[4]

I start from the city's founding in 1790 and continue until 2022, drawing on multiple sources, including archival and contemporary materials, US census and vital statistics data, and crime and disease surveillance data, along with life history and key informant interviews. I illustrate how the city's physical, social, and policy designs contributed to the production of multiple overlapping and interacting epidemics and the reproduction of racial inequality in illness and death throughout its history, despite dramatic social change. I focus more specifically on the last 60 years, examining HIV/AIDS, drug abuse, and homicide in depth, and more briefly examining COVID-19, the latest driver of the racial gap, as well as other causes of death. I describe the entangled histories of the city and Congress and show how policies were both deliberately and benignly designed and implemented by Republican and Democratic, White and and non-White actors. I show how these policies worked together to create—and importantly, recreate—disproportionate and premature illness and death for Black Americans across generations. By moving back and forth between the national and city stories, I will show that while DC's story is a product of its peculiar history and status as a federal city, it is also, in some ways, a microcosm of the national production of racial health inequality and what I am calling *death by design*.

In the rest of this chapter, I examine national trends in life expectancy by race and gender in order to place DC in context. I then discuss the theoretical framework and key concepts I will be using to examine why and how racial inequality in health is produced and persists. Finally, I discuss the case of Washington, DC, my data and methods, and the book outline.

Progress, Stalls, and Reversals in US Life Expectancy

Despite dramatic gains in several dimensions of social life such as basic civil rights, income, and educational access over the 20th and 21st centuries, Black-White health disparities remain some of the most intransigent and enduring markers of inequality in the United States.[5] A key measure of this is life expectancy. Figure 2 illustrates trends in US life expectancy between 1880 and 2022. Overall, there has been a remarkable improvement in life expectancy at birth between 1880 and 2022, especially during the first half of the 20th century. Life expectancy rose from a low of 30.8 years for Black people in 1904 and 39.8 years for White people in 1918 to a high of 75.6 years and 79.1 years in 2014 for Black and White people, respectively. Notably, as Elizabeth Wrigley-Field observed, peak Black life expectancy in 2014, was below White

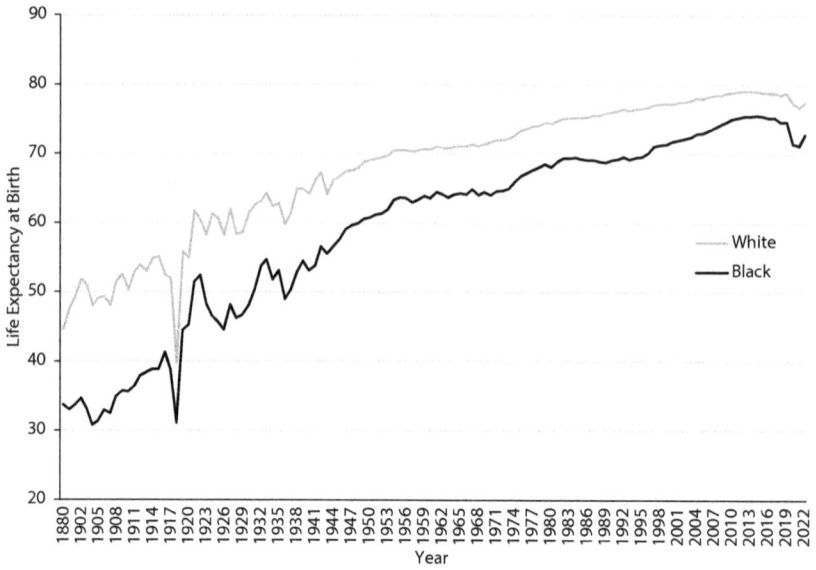

FIGURE 2. Trends in US life expectancy at birth by race, 1880–2022. Data source: National Center for Health Statistics.

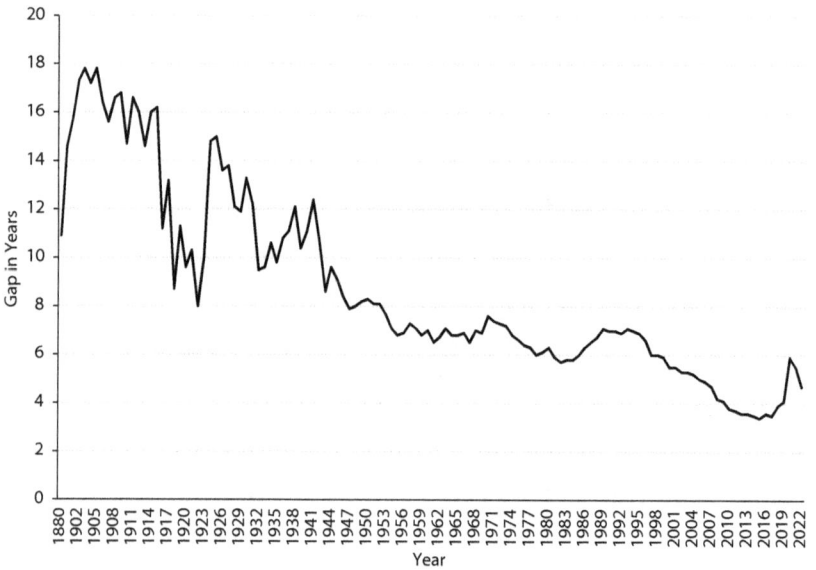

FIGURE 3. The Black/White gap in US life expectancy by race, 1880–2022. Data source: National Center for Health Statistics.

life expectancy in 1989, a 25 year difference in life expectancy gains.[6] Between 2014 and 2019, life expectancy stalled before dramatically declining to lows of 71.2 and 76.7 years for Black and White people, respectively, following the 2020–21 COVID-19 epidemic waves. The epidemic had returned US life expectancy back to levels last seen in 1997–98 for Black people and 1995–96 for White people, about 25 years of a reversal in gains.[7] By 2022, life expectancy had rebounded to 72.8 years for Black people (last seen in 2004) and 77.5 years for White people (last seen in 2002).

Figure 3 shows the Black-White life-expectancy gap between 1880 and 2022. As the figure illustrates, gap declines were greatest between 1905 and 1954, falling from 17.8 years to 7.1 years. The racial gap then fluctuated between 6.1 and 7.6 years between 1954 and 1980 before declining to a low of 3.4 years by 2015. The gap widened to 5.9 years during the COVID-19 epidemic and currently stands at 4.7 years (last seen in 2007). There is wide state variation around this average, with states that are close to or at equality in the northeast (such as Massachusetts and Rhode Island), and states with high gaps in the Midwest (such as Wisconsin and Illinois).[8]

Figure 4 illustrates life expectancy by race and gender (1880–2022). The figure makes clear the significance of gender in understanding US life expectancy. Black and White women began to have significantly longer life expectancy than their male counterparts from the mid-1940s onwards. However, there are race and gender disparities. Over the last 142 years, while White women have always had the highest life expectancy, Black men have always had the lowest life expectancy. White women also experienced the smallest reversal during COVID relative to other groups (about a 1.8 year loss between 2019 and 2021), while Black men experienced the largest reversal (White men lost 2.3 years, Black women lost 3.1 years, and Black men lost 3.7 years). In 2022, Black men's and women's life expectancies were 69.1 and 76.5 years, respectively, while White men's and women's life expectancies were 75.1 and 80.1 years, respectively.

Figure 5 illustrates the changing life-expectancy gap between Black and White men and between Black and White women over the last 142 years. The figure shows an overall decline in the gap but a growing gender divergence over time. Among women, the within-gender racial life-expectancy gap declined from 17.9 years in 1903 to 2.7 years in 2017. The post-COVID-19 gap in 2022 was 3.6 years. Among men, the within-gender gap declined from 17.8 years in 1903 to a low of 4.2 years in 2014, after which it rose. The 2022 gap was 6 years. In addition to wide state variation in the racial life expectancy gap noted above,

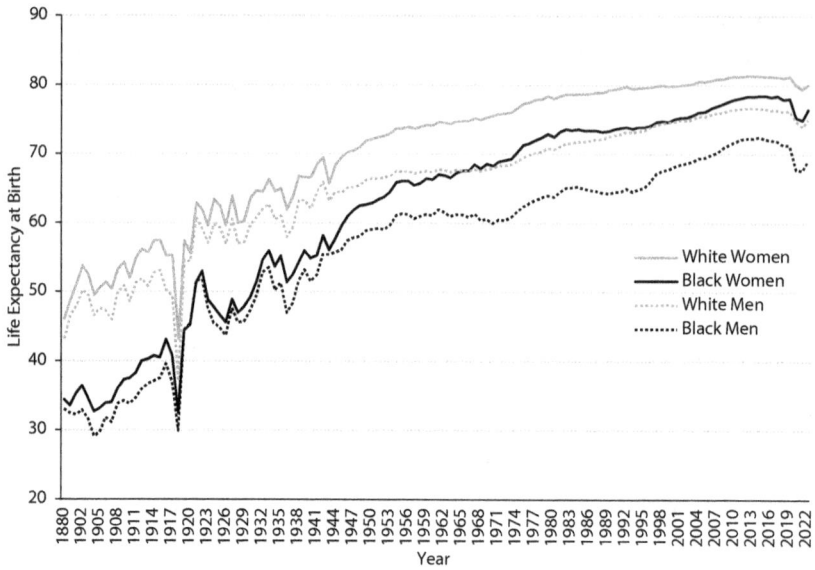

FIGURE 4. Trends in US life expectancy at birth by race and gender, 1880–2022. Data source: National Center for Health Statistics.

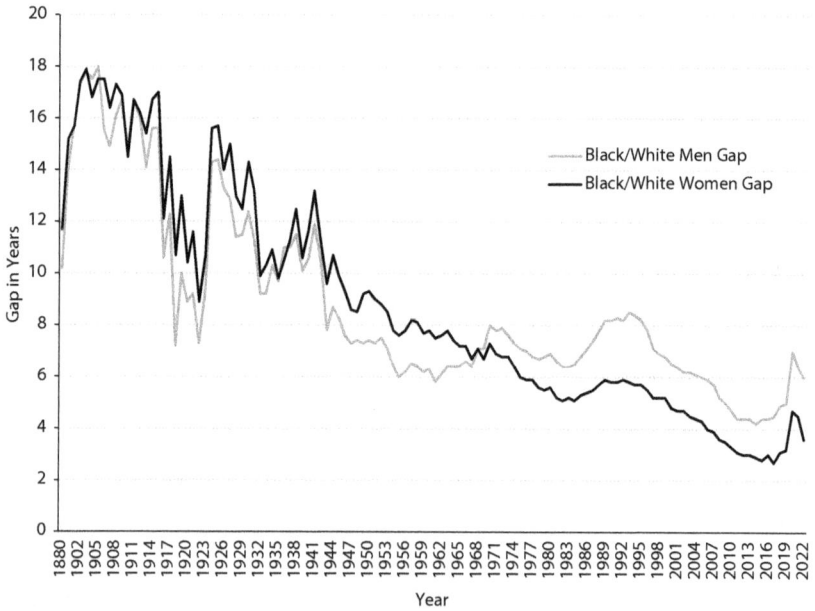

FIGURE 5. The US race/gender gap in life expectancy, 1880–2022. Data source: National Center for Health Statistics.

there is also wide county variation in the gap. The next highest counties follow-ing DC for women are Cambria, PA (10.3 years), New York, NY (9.5 years), and San Francisco (9.1 years); for men they are San Francisco (12.3 years), New York, NY (12.2 years), and Richmond City, VA (11.4 years).[9]

In light of the above, it is clear that DC's racial life-expectancy gap, at 18 years for men and 12 years for women, lies at the more extreme end of national trends. The gap approximates trends last seen nationally in 1903 for men and in 1938 for women. If, as argued by Braveman and colleagues in the opening epi-graph, the health of the most socially advantaged group should be possible for everyone, then Washington, DC, has a century's worth of gains to make.

Causes of Death

Nationally and in Washington, DC, the two biggest causes of death for Black and White people are heart disease and cancer.[10] However, in examining racially distinct contributions to the widening and narrowing of the Black-White life-expectancy gap, Anne Case and Angus Deaton attributed what they called deaths of despair (chronic liver diseases, drug and alcohol poison-ings, and suicide) to increases in middle-age White mortality,[11] while several studies attribute AIDS, homicide, unintentional injuries (including poison-ings), and infant mortality to Black contributions to the gap over the last 60 years.[12] Victor Fuchs, for example, found that HIV/AIDS and homicide rates had the largest differences between Black and White people, with Black peo-ple having a 7.5 times higher AIDS death rate and a 5.7 times higher homicide death rate.[13] A focus on epidemics is important because, as illustrated in Figures 2–5, epidemics such as influenza in 1918 and COVID-19 have the capacity to dramatically reverse several years of hard-won gains in life expect-ancy. Further, the intransigence of the racial health gap despite significant social change suggests something more structural, historical, and institution-alized about the mechanisms producing health inequality.

THEORETICAL FRAMEWORK: EXPLAINING
PERSISTENT RACIAL HEALTH INEQUALITY

1. Syndemic Zones

The nonrandom distribution of deaths underscores the now well understood and institutionalized idea that health is at least in part socially determined.[14]

However, this public health axiom wars with an ideology at the core of what it means to be American: that having "life, liberty, and the pursuit of happiness" means our lives and fates are in our hands, that we are the masters of our destiny, and that therefore our poor health outcomes are mostly the result of poor decisions, laziness, and/or lack of self-control or willpower. This entrenched victim-blaming approach aligns with the predominance of public health messaging aimed at encouraging individuals to practice good health habits, such as avoiding smoking and sugary drinks, eating fruits and vegetables, using a condom, engaging in physical activity, and so on. These are crucial but only partial explanations of health disparities from a population-level point of view. The COVID-19 epidemic brought special clarity to this point, as it gradually became clear that illnesses and deaths were neither purely random nor merely a function of individual preventive activities, such as handwashing, masking, and social distancing. Rather, it most affected people who lay at the intersections of the major systems of inequality in the US: social class or socioeconomic status (SES) (i.e., income, education, occupation, etc.), gender, race/ethnicity/nativity, and the expressions of these in places of work or residence (housing conditions, neighborhood, county, state).[15] In other words, the same social determinants that underlie a range of illnesses and premature deaths in the US.[16] But how exactly do these systems come to shape group- and individual-level health outcomes?

A broader conception of disease vulnerability acknowledges that it exists not only when individuals or groups engage in risky practices but also when people who may or *may not* engage in risky practices navigate their social lives in a disease risk environment. I use the definition for "risk environment" advanced by Tim Rhodes and colleagues:

> In its broadest sense, the "risk environment" comprises all risk factors exogenous to the individual [and] encourages a focus on the *social situations, structures* and *places* in which risk is produced rather than a reliance on a conception of risk as endogenous to individuals' cognitive decision-making and immediacy of interpersonal relations … We define the risk environment as the space—whether social or physical—in which a variety of factors exogenous to the individual interact to increase the chances of [disease] transmission.[17]

Situating individual disease outcomes in such a way, as I will show, enables a better understanding of the *production* of socially patterned disease outcomes—making some groups more vulnerable than others. It also sheds light on the institutionalized dimensions of social contexts that are likely to perpetuate generalized disease vulnerability from one generation to the next, regardless of the disease. This perspective suggests that a major driver of Black people's disproportionate and premature illness and death across time is not just a function of individual practices but also their higher likelihood of living in disease risk environments that make them vulnerable to a range of diseases.

Indeed, many of the diseases and causes of death disproportionately affecting African Americans cluster and interact with each other to exacerbate and create excess burdens of disease and death. The term *syndemic,* coined by medical anthropologist Merrill Singer, describes the clustering of two or more epidemics among particular populations where biological interactions or social synergies among the diseases further exacerbate vulnerability within the population. This disease clustering is often accompanied and driven by a clustering of economic and social disadvantages,[18] which I elaborate in the next section. There are several syndemics primarily affecting African Americans, including various combinations of tuberculosis, asthma, sexually transmitted infections, depression, substance abuse, domestic/street violence, homicide, and HIV/AIDS.[19] In addition to clustering, syndemics can also be amplified. The SAVA (substance abuse, violence, AIDS) syndemic,[20] for example, can be amplified by mental illness epidemics, as well as having additional marginalized or stigmatized identities, such a gender or sexual minority status.[21] Depression and stigma can lead to substance abuse, which then increases HIV risk.[22] The most recent example of syndemic amplification is the COVID-19 epidemic. It interacted with and exacerbated preexisting chronic disease epidemics, such as diabetes, heart disease, and kidney disease, forming a syndemic, which amplified death among people living with those diseases[23] and amplified the opioid overdose, domestic violence, homicide, and mental illness epidemics.[24]

Crucially, syndemics do not occur randomly but rather are clustered in particular places. For example, the hardest hit counties for HIV/AIDS were also the hardest hit counties for COVID-19. Both were predominantly minority-group counties.[25] Thus, people most subject to syndemics live in what I refer to in the book as *syndemic risk environments* or *syndemic zones* for shorthand. Building on these ideas and drawing from a range of scholars,[26] I will be working with a simple framework (Figure 6) in my examination of how syndemic zones are produced and reproduced.

Rather than beginning with individual-level practices, the framework instead asserts that syndemic zones stem from major systems of inequality

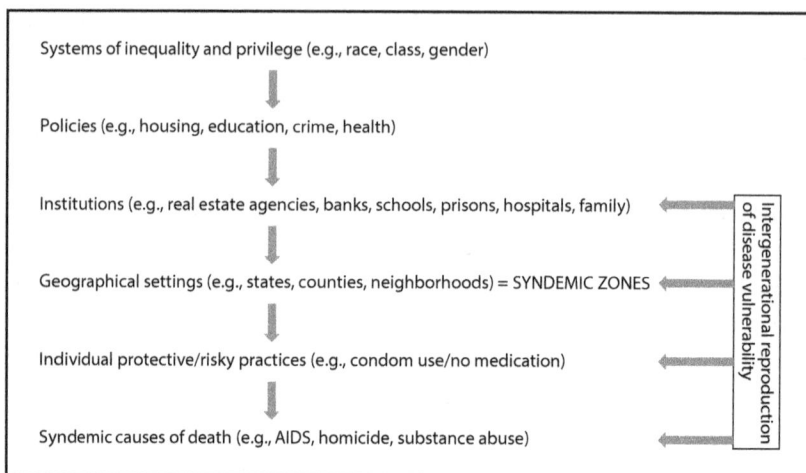

FIGURE 6. The Production of a Syndemic Zone.

and privilege, such as gender (or heteropatriarchy/structural sexism), social class/SES (classism), and race/ethnicity/nativity (or structural racism).[27] These systems are operationalized and expressed in a wide range of governmental and nongovernmental policies, laws, and regulations, across domains such as banking, education, housing, crime, and health, and exist at the federal, state, or local level. These policies work through institutions to favor, discriminate against, or act neutrally towards people along these gender/class/race lines. They often have their full effect in specific places—particular geographical jurisdictions such as states, counties, neighborhoods, and homes—and can produce syndemic zones. For example, county offices may implement zoning laws around the placement of environmental hazards; banks and real estate agencies may shape group-level disease vulnerability through structuring the level and frequency of exposure to these hazards by lending and steering policies enabling or undermining access to housing in safe neighborhoods; and hospitals can enable or undermine prevention and protection from illness or death through limited or ample access to quality health care based on insurance company policies.

Families are the primary institution in the early lives of most individuals. Tragically, combinations of disease vulnerabilities cluster among families living in syndemic zones, including unhealthy neighborhoods, poor schools, disease-burdened social networks, risky health practices through socialization, and biophysiological and epigenetic factors. This is reflected in the clustering of premature diseases and deaths within Black families relative to

White families, as illustrated in research by Debra Umberson and colleagues.[28] Mothers can also transmit disease or disease vulnerability to their children not just directly (e.g., in the womb, during labor, or while breastfeeding)[29] but also indirectly, through impacts on mothers' bodies such as chronic stress from living in unsafe neighborhoods and other debilitating life circumstances, which can lead to low birth weight and infant mortality.[30] Low birth weight can in turn lead to a lifetime of poor health outcomes for a child, such as insulin resistance, hypertension, and cardiovascular disease.[31] In these ways, families in syndemic zones, along with the institutions with jurisdiction over them, can reproduce disease vulnerability for the next generation. It is within this larger multilayered syndemic zone context that individuals engage in risky or protective practices that shape their health outcomes.

Once syndemic zones are established, people born into, growing up in, moving to, living in, or passing through such places are at greater risk of exposure to and acquisition of one or more disease or mortality causing processes. While for causes of death such as infectious disease or homicide, even a short exposure to a syndemic zone—being in the wrong place at the wrong time, so to speak—can result in illness or death, for syndemic zone residents, chronic diseases can also develop through repeated long-term exposures, leading to premature illness and/or death. Indeed, Bridget Goosby and colleagues noted that "by middle age, African American adults show numerous signs of accelerated aging . . . [and are] more likely to experience earlier onset of age-related chronic diseases and fatal chronic conditions."[32]

In this book, I draw on life history interviews to examine lived experiences of syndemic zone residents, as well as on archival and contemporary materials to examine the social production of syndemic zones and syndemics in Washington, DC, from its founding in 1790 until 2022, with a principal focus on the SAVA syndemic.[33] Specifically, I focus on substance abuse epidemics (1960–2016) with a focus on drugs (heroin and cocaine), violence with a focus on homicide epidemics (1960–2010), and the HIV/AIDS epidemic (1983–2022). I briefly discuss overlapping epidemics such as infant mortality, mental illness, and COVID-19.

2. Social Containment

At its core, the idea of syndemic zones expresses the fact that systems of inequality and privilege are anchored in the social organization of physical and social space and place[34] through social containment.[35] Here, I intend the term to encapsulate segregation—the physical separation of groups on the basis of a particular characteristic such as income/class or race—as well as what Charles Tilly called "opportunity hoarding" and what Max Weber described as "social closure"—both of which capture the clustering together of privileges by and for particular groups of people. Social containment thus characterizes how a dominant group creates and then maintains its status through gathering, consolidating, and entrenching privileges and resources, and then works through a variety of institutional mechanisms, such as laws, policies, and regulations, and through interpersonal mechanisms, such as discrimination, to exclude other groups from them. And critically, this occurs primarily, though not exclusively, through inclusion in and exclusion from space.[36] In a competition over resources, this can result in a zero-sum game, creating parallel processes of gathering and clustering inequalities. While there are many kinds of social containment, in this book, I primarily focus on class and racial containment, and to a lesser degree sexual containment.

Class Containment and Syndemic Zones. Socioeconomic status (SES), a major determinant of life expectancy in the US,[37] is anchored in space. The US is highly spatially and residentially classed. Sociologists Kendra Bischoff, Sean Reardon, and their colleagues found that between 1970 and 2009, fewer families lived in middle-income neighborhoods, while more families lived in higher- or lower-income neighborhoods, with some evidence of these trends continuing into the subsequent decade. They also found that within-race income gaps grew particularly sharply among Black families relative to White families.[38] This highlights growing economic inequality in the US as a whole and within racial minority groups in particular.[39] It also illustrates the intergenerational reproduction of those whom William Julius Wilson called "the truly disadvantaged."[40] Indeed, as Kathy Edin and colleagues demonstrated in their recent book *The Injustice of Place,* the poorest people are increasingly located in the poorest—typically rural—parts of America.[41] These parallel processes suggest that the production of advantaged neighborhoods with high life expectancy can simultaneously produce disadvantaged neighborhoods—spaces that cluster together social ills and concomitantly low life expectancy.

Class containment might occur intentionally, through numerous interlocking laws and regulations that favor middle class and affluent Americans while exploiting or shortchanging the poor, as comprehensively documented by Matt Desmond.[42] It may also result from the need for a city or state to site sewage treatment plants, hazardous waste and garbage dumps, commuter highways, and industrial facilities. These sites, which Steve Lerner described as "sacrifice zones,"[43] have the cheapest housing and/or contain populations perceived to have limited power to push back. As Lerner, Robert Bullard, and others have powerfully documented, residents of these spaces suffer from predictable ailments, such a variety of cancers and respiratory diseases.[44] Sacrifice zones thus give birth to syndemic zones. Sacrifice zones are contained through physical barriers, such as highways, bridges, railway tracks, and parks,[45] separating affluent, middle-income, and poor neighborhoods and people. In this way, processes of class containment also create, contain, and institutionalize syndemic zones and unequal life chances. Indeed, a large body of literature, crowned by Robert Sampson's *Great American City*, comprehensively demonstrates the significance of "neighborhood effects" on individual- and group-level health outcomes.[46]

The Intersection of Racial and Class Containment and Implications for Racial Health Inequality. The unique history of the US means that race, ethnicity, and nativity often serve as master social determinants of health because they cluster together a range of social and economic disadvantages[47] not just among people groups, but also, importantly, within particular spaces. Names such as "projects" and "ghettos" are shorthand for oppressive historical legacies that have produced predominantly Black places, in a process described by Douglas Massey and Nancy Denton as "American apartheid."[48] (While not the focus of this book, it is nonetheless important to note that the oppressive use of place to subjugate racial groups in the US has had its most devastating effect on Native Americans, who have the nation's lowest life expectancy and suffered the most from COVID-19).[49] The role of space in diminishing the health and life chances of Black people was famously and comprehensively documented by the father of American sociology, W. E. B. Dubois,[50] in his magisterial *The Philadelphia Negro: A Social Study*, first published in 1899.[51] This spatial role has persisted well into the 21st century; Black-White segregation has declined, but still remains high.[52] David Williams and Chiquita Collins have argued that racial residential segregation is a fundamental cause of racial health inequality,[53] and indeed, Arun Hendi estimated that nationally, within-county racial inequality accounted for more than 90% of the racial life-expectancy gap. He further found that segregation increased the men's gap by 16.3 years and the women's gap by 4.96 years.[54] Segregation profoundly influences SES, which in turn impacts health.[55] Williams and Collins, along with Zinzi Bailey, and Tyson Brown among many others, have argued that in addition to affecting SES, institutional racism and discrimination exert independent effects on Black Americans, constraining their ability to achieve better health outcomes. Racially contained Black neighborhoods are more likely to be characterized by some combination of poverty, substandard education, higher levels of violence, poor air quality because of location near pollutants such as highways or toxic dumps, more food deserts, and lower access to health-promoting neighborhood amenities.[56] They also have a higher proportion of health-demoting amenities. For example, Thomas LaVeist and John Wallace found that Black neighborhoods have a disproportionate number of liquor stores, even after controlling for SES, and this has been linked to historic government-sponsored zoning discrimination against Black people.[57] Additionally, a landmark 1987 report by the United Church of Christ, *Toxic Wastes and Race in the United States,* documented the disproportionate siting of hazardous waste in Black and other minority neighborhoods by federal and state governments as well as industry.[58] This highlights the role of policy in creating syndemic zones in marginalized class and racially contained spaces.

Wealthier Black people do not necessarily escape the health consequences exerted by systems of inequality through space. As many scholars, such as Joyce Ladner, Patricia Hill Collins, and Kimberle Crenshaw have argued, systems of inequality, such as race, class, and gender, intersect,[59] producing matrices of domination and oppression,[60] and these intersections have paradoxical effects on health outcomes. Several scholars have found that there is nonequivalence between the meaning and utility of class (as measured by education or income) across racial groups when considering health outcomes. For example, Paula Braveman and colleagues, along with other scholars, have demonstrated that infant mortality rates among White women who dropped out of high school were lower than those of college-educated Black women, a finding that has endured.[61] In addition to institutional discrimination in health care settings, worse health outcomes for more advantaged Black people may be in part because Black and White people live in very different residential and ecological contexts, regardless of income.[62] In their study of 170 US cities, Robert Sampson and William J. Wilson concluded that "the worst urban contexts in which whites reside are considerably better than the average context of Black communities."[63] Further, as Patrick Sharkey demonstrated, Black people tend to remain "stuck in place" across generations. He found that 75% of White children, compared to 9% of Black children, born between 1955 and 1970 "were raised in neighborhoods with less than 10% poverty." Further, "essentially no White children were raised in neighborhoods with at least 30% poverty, but three in ten African Americans were." These conditions had not improved for Black children born between 1985 and 2000.[64] Further, he estimated that "more than 70% of black children who are raised in the poorest quarter of American neighborhoods will continue to live in the poorest quarter of neighborhoods as adults [and] since the 1970s, more than half of black families have lived in the poorest quarter of neighborhoods *in consecutive generations*, compared to just 7% of white families."[65] Thus, in addition to intergenerational immobility among most Black families, the wealthiest Black children grow up with more poverty than their wealthy White counterparts.

This place-based disadvantage is evident in health outcomes. Schwandt and colleagues found that in 1990, "for most age groups, Black Americans living in the highest income US areas had substantially higher mortality rates than White Americans in the country's lowest income areas."[66] By 2018, they found that "much of the improvement" in mortality rates accounting for a narrowing racial life-expectancy gap occurred among Black people living in the poorest counties in America,[67] suggesting growing intraracial *equality* in health outcomes but also a relative loss in health advantage for wealthy Black Americans. In these ways, Black Americans do not derive the same advantages from class privilege with respect to health as White Americans. As I will illustrate, in DC, racial and class containment were intertwined and undergirded each other in sustaining privilege and producing both interracial and intraracial health inequality.

The Intersecting System of Gender and Sexuality. Within syndemic zones, disease vulnerability is also likely to be deeply shaped by gender dynamics, especially in the context of epidemics such as HIV/AIDS, drug abuse, and homicide. Like other systems of inequality, the system of gender is anchored in space[68] and exerts its influence on health through affecting individual gendered identities, beliefs, and practices, including how people navigate gendered space, how they interact and are interacted with in those spaces by others, and how localized institutions such as hospitals and clinics, drug economies, and criminal justice systems differentially treat people occupying particular gender categories.[69] Its main operating principle is heteropatriarchy—as it is principally geared towards privileging men and heterosexual people, and jostling for power is a key means through which this is enacted. Violence between men and against women, as well as women's sexual, reproductive, and household labors, anchored in space and often on unequal terms, undergirds the hetero-patriarchal system.[70] Gender also differentially shapes, constrains and guides how lives unfold as people age[71] in ways that protect against or amplify the negative consequences of gender on their health outcomes. Gender differences in death rates are a paradoxical and ironic result of all these dynamics; men may have more class privilege, but they die earlier than women; women's social and spatialized expectations and constraints as they age (e.g., disproportionate work within the home, caregiving that regularly puts them in the path of health care systems, and occupational discrimination from dangerous jobs) also limits spatial exposure to many forms of premature death, even while exposing them to more illness than men.[72]

Importantly, biological sex characteristics, such as hormones, chromosomes, and internal and external reproductive organs, shape differential susceptibility to illness and death. For example, there is more efficient male-to-female HIV transmission than vice versa due to vaginal physiology and seminal plasma dynamics,[73] and there are sex differences in drug addiction dynamics.[74] However, it is often the *entwinement* of sex with gender and the social meanings ascribed to the genders that produce profound differences in health outcomes.[75] Men's higher propensity to both commit and be victims of homicide is not just due to evolutionary or biological reasons but also to profoundly social, gendered lifestyles, socialization, contexts, and expectations of masculinity, especially in the transition into and through young adulthood.[76] Similarly, people who are transgender and/or gender nonconforming confront both sources of illness deriving from biological sex characteristics, such as reproductive organs, as well as those deriving from gender identity and presentation, such as stigma, dis-crimination and violence, the latter of which have significant impacts on their overall well-being and health-seeking behavior and outcomes.[77] Finally, gender interacts with sex and sexuality to produce HIV risk. This may arise from dif-ferences in individual bio-physiological and socio-physiological experiences of sexual identity, desire, and functioning, and power-laden negotiations within partnerships over practices such as monogamy and condom use. It may also arise from larger institutional factors such as the sexual economy and the con-tainment of sexuality within particular spaces, which together shape the avail-ability and distribution of partners, among other factors.[78]

Overall, the book shows how racial- and class-containment dynamics cre-ated and enabled racialized syndemic zones, which in turn concentrated the impact and exacerbated the spread of the SAVA syndemic in gendered ways in DC. It also illustrates how sexual containment—in the form of the closet, gayborhoods, and gay power politics—interacted with racial containment to shape racial inequality in HIV/AIDS outcomes.

3. Race, Institutions, and Embodied History

The persistence of racial health inequality is also due to the historic embeddedness of racism across a range of institutions that work together to reproduce disease vulnerability across generations despite dramatic social change.

The System of Race. Many aspects of the US racial system have changed since 1776 when the US was founded. One means of tracking this change is through shifting racial categories in the census. In the first US census in 1790, people occupying the category Black today would have been subcategorized as slaves or free; by 1890, the so-called one drop rule was operationalized through classifications based on Black blood quotient (octoroon—1/8, quadroon—1/4, mulatto—1/2, Black); by 1920, it was mulatto or Black. Then any amount of Black blood made one "colored"; between 1930 and 1960, the census category was "Negro." From 1970, "Black" was added to Negro; in 2000, "African American" was added; and in 2010 and 2020, additional categories allowed demographers to parse out "non-Hispanic Blacks" from "Hispanic Blacks," in order to estimate "Black or African American alone, non-Hispanic" populations.[79]

Michael Omi, Howard Winant, and other scholars of race in America have described this socially constructed nature of race as occurring through a process called racial formation, "the sociohistorical process by which racial categories are created, inhabited, transformed, and destroyed."[80] And racial categories matter greatly for life chances. As I will show in the case of DC, each category was associated with differential access to White society and all its privileges, including freedom of housing, freedom of mobility, and access to higher-income employment, among other things. (In this book, I retain the original categories as used in their historical time and otherwise interchangeably use Black or African American). But what held constant as categories changed was that the highest level of discrimination and the greatest limitations applied to people considered fully Black, reflecting the core idea underlying White supremacist ideology that Black people are inferior to White people. As the country has shifted from perceiving itself as biracial to more fully multiracial, and as the color line described by DuBois in the opening epigraph has shifted from de jure to de facto, Vilna Bashi Treitler and other scholars have shown the relational nature of the racial system. They argue that new immigrant groups have worked not to blur the Black-White distinction but instead to harden it as they assimilate more easily into White or honorary White categories over time, while those classified as Black anchor the racial stratification system.[81]

And as seen in Figures 2–5, inhabiting the Black category in the US is consequential for health. US immigrants from a range of racial/ethnic groups often have better health than their native-born counterparts; however, as Tod Hamilton and others have demonstrated, while first-generation Black immigrants fare better than their native-born counterparts, these effects disappear in the next generation as their children exhibit health outcomes similar to other native-born Black people.[82] Assimilation to US society means assimilation to its system of racial inequality and all it comes with. The resilience of the US racial system is also illustrated in the many reversals that occur whenever progress towards racial health equality is being achieved. Stalls and reversals exemplify the power of the underlying machinery of the racial system to maintain and reproduce unequal outcomes across generations. The perpetual intergenerational reassertion of race in determining life chances has led scholars such as Eduardo Bonilla-Silva, Joe Feagin, and others to view race and racism as more than an individual "bad apple" phenomenon and instead as one that is systemic and structural, requiring an examination of "the mechanisms and practices that reproduce White advantages"[83] and the ideology of colorblindness that has emerged to mask it.[84]

Racialized Institutions. In explaining why structural racism persists over time, Victor Ray highlighted the crucial role of racialized organizations in reproducing racial inequality.[85] Following this line, in this book, I take a system-wide approach[86] to examining the role of a range of institutions and the social containment principle in the reproduction of racial health inequality. Institutions have operating principles or logics that derive from systems of inequality. These are a combination of cultural schemas (coagulated and automated beliefs, assumptions, and stereotypes about people groups), rules, and resources (physical and symbolic) that are entrenched in institutional processes, procedures, policies, laws, and practices. Institutional logics shape organizational ways of "seeing," thinking about, and categorizing people, social problems, and solutions, as well as organizational ways of assigning resources and applying rules accordingly.[87] While individual actors within organizations make decisions, they do so within these default institutional tendencies. Effective operating principles can spread from one institution to another, creating redundancies that help to sustain systems geared towards perpetuating privilege or inequality.[88] Thus, the same institutional logic or principle, in this case social containment, can be seen operating across a range of institutions such as schools, neighborhoods, prisons, legal systems, health care settings, local and federal governments, and so on. As Barbara Reskin argued, a system-wide approach shows why social change in one institution or setting may be insufficient to overturn inequality in a particular domain because it is reinforced in other settings.[89] To use an example from the system of gender, progress in norms around equitable housework sharing may be undercut by inflexible workplace family policies, leading to an overall stall in gender equality in both the workplace and the home.[90]

As I will show in this book, a focus on systems, processes, laws, procedures, and policies—and not just on actors—illustrates clearly that the reproduction of racial health inequality in DC was not just due to racist White people; rather, it involved a broad range of actors including White and Black, Republican and Democratic, and ill- and well-intentioned individuals. I show how the institutional and systemic entrenchment[91] of an orienting racist and classist logic—social containment—meant that even well-intended efforts to tackle the range of epidemics disproportionately affecting African Americans were often frustrated. I will also show how, as Ellis Monk Jr. put it, "the dominated themselves are coerced and recruited to reproduce their own domination even as they attempt to resist being dominated."[92] The book will illustrate how, as a result of policy impasses, class containment undergirded racial containment as middle class and affluent African Americans pursued class strategies to secure their safety, health, and well-being. However, in the process, racial health inequality was perpetuated.

The Embodiment of History. Nancy Krieger described the "profound embodied connections that exist between people, politics, ecologies, and health," highlighting how we "embody . . . biologically the dynamic contexts in which our lives are enmeshed."[93] Krieger pointed out the recency of the dismantling of Jim Crow laws in 1965 and the fact that many African Americans alive today were born and grew up under those laws, and they are now living out the long-run health consequences of those laws and policies. Thus, the accelerated aging described by Goosby and colleagues was set in motion during a historical period when a thicket of discriminatory regulations and policies were explicitly and legally levied against African Americans across a range of institutions, such as schools, banks, workplaces, and health care settings. This points to the importance of not just understanding contemporary institutional drivers of racial health inequality but also deeply understanding the historical contexts that set in motion dynamics that are shaping current health outcomes.[94] As Krieger observed:

> The totality of people's lived experiences, shaped by their societies, lodge and manifest in their bodies, such that to understand the state of the people's health, one must start by grappling with their histories, in societal context, within and across generations ... Transgenerational societal inheritance of adverse or beneficial conditions of life (i.e., the social reproduction of inequities, not genetic or epigenetic inheritance) is plausibly the most powerful driver of differential health profiles of social groups across generations.[95]

As such, this book will locate the lives and health outcomes of people I interviewed within the city's historical trajectory, drawing on life history interviews, archival material, and histories of Washington, DC. Further, following in the footsteps of disease historians such as Charles Rosenberg, Keith Wailoo, Samuel Roberts, and James Colgrove,[96] I examine how the city and federal governments thought about and managed racialized epidemics in DC throughout its history. Through interpreting these histories and archives, the book makes visible the operating principles of the racial system, its patterns and continuities in laws, policies, practices, and procedures, and in particular, how the city's health crises were used to produce and reproduce racial containment and subsequent racial health inequality across generations.

4. Death by Design

The concept of *death by design* characterizes the central argument of this book: that persisting racial health inequality is the result of policy-designed social containment and the production and reproduction of syndemic zones. I show how these zones are the intended and unintended result of a web of interrelated policies, including land policies, transportation policies, housing policies, banking policies, educational policies, criminal justice policies, and health policies, among others. I show how policies enacted through institutions exerted interactive and cumulative effects throughout the course of people's lives and across generations, producing disproportionate illness and premature death among African Americans.

The idea that something is by design implies intentionality and culpability. The legal standard of mens rea (guilty mind/criminal intent) is perhaps the most obvious and makes it easy to assign blame. Indeed, one reading of disproportionate, multigenerational Black death is that it represents what Achille Mbembe has described as necropolitics, the state's "power and capacity to dictate who is able to live and who must die. To kill or to let live. . ."[97] Because from slavery, to mass incarceration, to siting hazardous waste in Black neighborhoods, to excessive police brutality, systemic racism makes Black life disposable, and disproportionate Black morbidity and social and physical death at the hands of the state remains routine and normalized. The layer below mens rea is design that creates, to borrow from Immanuel Kant, the "conditions of possibility" for certain outcomes. Here we can think of design that enables or discourages healthy and unhealthy practices, like the basket of fruit regularly placed in the breakroom or the zoning law–driven saturation of liquor stores in Black neighborhoods; in other words, design with predictable health effects that nonetheless leave plenty of room for choice. Here culpability can seem less clear. Finally, there is designed inertia and inaction that produces bad outcomes—like not maintaining public housing that eventually becomes a hazardous place to live. Related to this is how to think about causality. Causes of death can be direct, such as a bullet to the head, indirect, such as neglecting to inspect the electrical system in a building that catches on fire, or distal, such as placing a commuter highway near a public housing building (or vice versa), thereby contributing to residents' infant mortality or asthmatic children's deaths.

By calling attention to design, I also aim to preempt the blame game that inevitably ensues. Among some African Americans, there are persistent beliefs in "The Plan," and other conspiracy theories about the government's malfeasant intentions towards Black people.[98] Further, it is a political axiom that Democrats tend to blame structures, and Republicans tend to blame individuals. While it is clear that African Americans' distrust of the government and the medical system is grounded in historical and contemporary facts and lived realities, as comprehensively documented by Harriet Washington and Dorothy Roberts,[99] among others, and that both structures and individual actions matter for health outcomes, I will show that Republican and Democratic presidents and congressional representatives, as well as White and Black administrators, contributed to the narrowing and widening of the racial health gap, and that both institutional operating principles, such as racial containment, and individual risky practices contributed to illness and death. Actors are important for both reproducing inequality as well as dismantling it; however, narrowly focusing on actor intentions often distracts from careful attention to patterned workings of institutions and their operating principles, which persist long after a given set of politicians and administrators have left office. Further, while people's plans, motivations, and actions may change over time, "it"—racial containment—retains its original logic, and that is what requires close examination.

Attention to design and introducing a historical perspective also preempt the national forgetting that is revealed during political blame games. An analogy to a theater stage is useful here—once the stage (or structure) is set up, the stage hands (or relevant actors) disappear from view. The audience present during construction can see clearly how the stage was set up and by whom and why. Indeed, after the riots following the assassination of Martin Luther King Jr., the predominantly White presidential Kerner Commission, which produced a 424-page document that sold over two million copies, was able to bluntly albeit controversially state on its opening page:

> Segregation and poverty have created in the racial ghetto a destructive environment totally unknown to most white Americans. What white Americans have never fully understood—but what the Negro can never forget—is that white society is deeply implicated in the ghetto. White institutions created it, white institutions maintain it, and white society condones it.[100]

But all this appears to have disappeared from view for those in subsequent eras. As Mitch Duneier observed:

> The pernicious circular logic of the ghetto is evident. Isolation from mainstream society, as well as the decrepitude caused by overcrowding, produced notorious conditions, behaviors, and traits that could gradually be invoked to rationalize further negative attitudes and more extreme isolation. The consequences of ghettoization provided an apparent justification for the original condition.[101]

Thus, new generations simply enter into the world the show creates. They are then shocked at what they see and respond in a variety of circumscribed ways—hand-wringing, blame, punishment, charity, and piecemeal/patchwork solutions—all of which are easier than dismantling and rebuilding the stage to reset the initiating terms of condition. Zooming out and looking at designs enables us to see the mechanisms underlying the continued creation, maintenance, and condoning of syndemic zones that underlie racial health inequality, and what it might take to dismantle them.

SETTING, DATA, AND METHODS

Washington, DC: The Capital City, the Second City, and the Syndemic City

The nation's capital is a paradoxical place. It is an architecturally majestic city—with the National Mall lined by museums and monuments on each side, anchored by the Lincoln Memorial, the Washington Monument, and the Capitol Building. It is the nation's legal and political center and the seat of the most powerful nation on earth. It is a city where decisions affecting millions of Americans and global citizens are made on a daily basis. Washington's streets and lawns have hosted many of the nation's most important marches and protests, led by cascading generations of activists. Many of the nation's major agencies directed at improving and protecting American health are located in and around the city, such as the National Institutes of Health, the Department of Health and Human Services, the Food and Drug Administration, and the Environmental Protection Agency.

The city also has a proud African American heritage, not just as a culturally vibrant place, launching some of America's finest musicians, such as Duke Ellington, but also as a place with a rich educational history, with the first Black high school in the nation (Dunbar) and the prestigious, historically Black Howard University, and a rich civil rights history, as many Black DC residents have led national and local battles against racial inequality.[102] The city and its suburbs host a disproportionate number of the nation's Black middle class and elite, including the nation's first Black president and first lady, and some of the wealthiest Black neighborhoods in the country. In 2019, the DC metro area was second only to the New York City metro area in the number of Black-owned employer businesses.[103]

But there is another DC: In the words of locals, there is "a second city." This face of the city is most visible in its health outcomes, which have appeared in several "worst in the nation" news headlines over the past few decades. For example, it has several times been the "infant mortality capital"[104] and has had the "highest infant mortality rate of 25 rich world capitals."[105] It has, more than once, had the worst maternal mortality rate in the nation, most recently in 2018.[106] It has several times been designated the "murder capital of the nation."[107] Its lead pipe problem was said to be "20 to 30 times worse" than Flint (Flint, a Michigan city, allowed lead contamination into its water supply for a year and a half, affecting thousands of predominantly Black children).[108] DC's HIV/AIDS rate was 10 times that of the US as a whole, and it has been the HIV/AIDS capital of the nation.[109] And across these outcomes, African Americans have been disproportionately affected.

In sum, Washington, DC, is a syndemic city and an important site in which to examine the historical production and persistence of racial health inequality. As I will illustrate, in some ways, it is unique and stands on its own in the nation, as a federal capital city only partially constrained by democracy and often operating as a national-policy sandbox for Congress. In other ways, it is a microcosm of the US, with similar dynamics to those occurring in other parts of the country, albeit to a more extreme degree in DC.

Data and Methods

This study began as a small summer project in June and July of 2011, when the city's HIV epidemic was near its height. I conducted 37 life history interviews with African American men, women, and trans women aged 20–61 with a variety of sexual identities who were living with HIV. Between 2011 and 2023, I also conducted 10 in-depth key informant interviews with District government and public health officials, African American community leaders, and heads and staff of community-based organizations (including neighborhood churches, hospitals, and HIV prevention and AIDS service provision organizations).

By the end of summer 2011, it was clear to me that this was more than a summer project, as I realized that HIV/AIDS was just the latest of a series of worst-in-the-nation epidemics. It evolved from one purely focused on the city's contemporary HIV epidemic to a larger historical project examining multiple epidemics, starting from the city's founding in 1790 and continuing through to 2022. My methods shifted to reading and analysis of archival and contemporary primary and secondary sources, including newspapers, official federal and District reports, and academic and popular literature on Washington, DC. I also began to draw on longitudinal quantitative data, including census data, National Center for Health Statistics data, homicide data, and the city's HIV/AIDS surveillance data, among other sources.

Data analysis and writing proceeded by triangulating my various data sources to examine the (re)production of racial health inequality in Washington, DC, as well as to understand and locate my respondents' lives, choices, and health outcomes in the flow of the city's history. As such, the book regularly moves across levels of analysis, mixing primary archival material, quantitative data, individual narratives, and analysis of the city's political and institutional arrangements to fully unpack the story. (For narratives, I use pseudonyms and change minor identifying details to protect my interviewees' privacy). A detailed methodological note with more on my data, methods, sources, and theoretical and analytical approaches follows the conclusion chapter.

Book Outline

The book is organized into five parts. Part 1 examines the institutional creation and outworkings of social containment and how it undergirded the production and reproduction of syndemic zones and racial health inequality across three eras of the city's history. In the first era (Chapter 1), 1790–1890, I examine the racial organization and politics of city housing, with a focus on racialized and classed slum/alley dwellings, and examine their connection to health outcomes. In the second era (Chapter 2), 1890–1950, I show how racial containment reconstituted itself and reproduced racial health inequality through urban renewal and the construction of public housing. In the third era (Chapter 3), 1950–present, I show how "chocolate city, vanilla suburbs"[110] and "cappuccino city"[111] models of gentrification and racial containment exacerbated racial health inequality despite Black mayoral governance. Throughout Part 1, I highlight the role of multiple institutions and policies, as well as how health crises were used to further policy goals and reconstitute racial containment despite dramatic social change.

In Part 2, I examine the puzzle of disproportionate Black vulnerability to HIV and show how gendered sexuality intersected with racial containment to produce unequal health outcomes for Black people. By tracing the distinctive histories of gay, bisexual, and heterosexual men and women (including transgender women), I illuminate how racial containment structured partnerships and HIV risk and prevention in syndemic zones for each group. For

Black gay and bisexual men (Chapter 4), I show how sexual containment intersected with racial containment to produce racialized exclusion from gayborhoods and racially homogamous (same-race) sexual networks and its consequences for HIV risk. For Black heterosexual men and women (Chapter 5), I show how racial homogamy combined with other forms of racial containment, such as mass incarceration, to produce distortions in marriage markets that were consequential for HIV risk. I also show how transgender women were subject to the challenges of both sexual minority men as well as other heterosexual women, with the combination of stigma, partner shortage, and concurrency amplifying their HIV vulnerability.

In Part 3, I examine the role of racial containment in the production and reproduction of drug epidemic zones and how these zones in turn gave birth to spillover epidemics such as homicide and HIV/AIDS, creating syndemic zones. The section highlights the interaction of individual characteristics, social networks, city and federal government actions, and global geopolitical dynamics in shaping the rise and fall of the drug epidemics, and the homicide epidemics they gave birth to. Focusing specifically on the heroin–homicide–HIV syndemic (Chapter 6) and the crack–HIV–homicide syndemic (Chapters 7–9), I show how both syndemics depended on racialized residential containment, city sacrifice zones, the wider DMV (DC, Maryland, Virginia) metro area residents, as well as federal and local government complicity for their sustenance. I describe the amplifying role of the city's commercial sex industry (Chapter 8) as well as the racially differential approaches to drug treatment to quell epidemics (Chapters 6 and 8). Finally, I examine the crack-homicide syndemic and the lived experiences of individuals and families in syndemic zones. I highlight both the disproportionate suffering wrought by racialized containment of disadvantaged populations living in syndemic zones, as well as the multigenerational impact of these zones on the reproduction of racial health inequality (Chapter 9).

In Part 4, I examine mass incarceration—a more intense form of racial containment—and how it exacerbated racial health inequality in the community. In Chapter 10, I examine the War on Drugs in Washington, DC, and in particular in institutions such as the police, schools, and prisons. I examine policing procedures and practices and discuss how criminal justice created and thrived on intraracial division. I then discuss racial inequality in legislation and sentencing and the city's school-to-prison pipeline. In Chapter 11, I examine the prison syndemic—with a focus on its thriving drug and sexual economies, limited harm reduction, as well as the consequences for community syndemic amplification, as prisoners circulated back and forth from prison, shuttled by the structural pull of policies around drug addiction and parole law.

In Part 5, I examine the city's attempts to control the HIV/AIDS epidemic. Chapter 12 examines why racial inequality in AIDS mortality dramatically widened following the introduction of antiretroviral therapy, which prolongs the lives of people living with HIV. I describe how a pioneering city response stalled and then fractured along intersectional lines as a result of social containment. I describe racial inequality in the allocation of health care resources, the interaction of White gay and Black power politics, and intraracial dynamics of Black homophobia and indifference to poor Black people. In Chapter 13, I discuss the city budget crisis whose congressional resolution resulted in cutting programs for the Black poor, thus exacerbating the epidemic. I then examine the actions of the District's HIV/AIDS agency, describing the agency's scandals and failures as well as its spectacular success in controlling the epidemic. I highlight the enduring role of racial containment by showing the limits of technocratic expertise; bringing the epidemic under control made little difference to racial health inequality. In the Conclusion, I briefly summarize the book's contributions and discuss some ways forward. This is followed by a detailed methodological note.

Finally, at end of this chapter and the conclusion, as well as at the end of each Part's overview, there is an eclectic "starter" playlist drawing on multiple genres, including DC's home-grown go-go music, as a soundtrack to accompany readers' journey through the book. This is to acknowledge the fact that African Americans have been living and feeling through, thinking, expressing, and writing analytically about this book's topics.[112] In adding these voices, I am also acknowledging that this book is necessarily a "partial story."[113] A focus on institutional processes and dynamics and a focus on illness and death means there is not much in this book on the sheer enjoyment of living, resilience, resistance, and heroic everyday grassroots efforts to challenge and change racist structures and processes, and to great national effect, as the past century and a half has shown. These are the larger and surely more important stories of the African American experience. Nonetheless, while it is a partial story, I believe this book tells a necessary story. It is my hope that it contributes to the national effort towards crafting "a more perfect Union" and a city and country in which race no longer determines life chances.

· · ·

INTRODUCTION PLAYLIST

Louis Armstrong	(What Did I Do To Be So) Black and Blue (1937)
Mahalia Jackson	Move On Up a Little Higher (1947)
Sam Cooke	A Change Gonna Come (1963)
Marvin Gaye	What's Going On (1971)
Chuck Brown & The Soul Searchers	We the People (1972)
Grandmaster Flash & The Furious Five	The Message (1982)
Kirk Franklin	Revolution (1998)
Whitney Houston ft. Shirley Caesar and the Georgia Mass Choir	He's All Over Me and He's Keeping Me Alive (1996)
Rare Essence	Lock-It (1991)
Chuck Brown & The Soul Searchers	Bustin' Loose (1979)

Racial Containment and Health in Historical Context

Nations reel and stagger on their way; they make hideous mistakes; they commit frightful wrongs; they do great and beautiful things. And shall we not best guide humanity by telling the truth about all this, so far as the truth is ascertainable?

WILLIAM E. B. DU BOIS (1935:701)

In reality ... the bourgeoisie has only one method of solving the housing question ... that is to say, of settling it in such a way that the solution continually poses the question anew. ... No matter how different the reasons may be, the result is everywhere the same: the most scandalous alleys and lanes disappear to the accompaniment of lavish self-glorification by the bourgeoisie on account of this tremendous success, but—they appear again at once somewhere else. ... The breeding places of disease, the infamous holes and cellars ... are not abolished; they are merely shifted elsewhere!

FRIEDRICH ENGELS AND
CLEMENS PALME DUTT (1872:71, 74)

THIS PART EXAMINES HOW RACIAL health inequality in Washington, DC, was created and reproduced. I describe the role of racial containment in the creation and reproduction of Washington, DC's, syndemic zones, spaces creating disproportionate vulnerability to syndemic disease (through multiple overlapping and interacting epidemics) among African Americans, beginning from the early years of the city's founding. Specifically, I show how the city's health crises were built into and institutionalized in the making and remaking of Washington, DC, where racial containment reconstituted itself across three different eras—the tertiary and secondary segregation era (1790–1890), the primary segregation era (1890–1950), and the Chocolate City/Cappuccino City era (1960–present). As I will illustrate, the containment of Black people, and especially poor Black people, in particular city spaces was in effect also containing them in spaces where they were then subject to disproportionate illness and premature death. I also examine the role of Black intraracial dynamics in contributing to these trends—in living arrangements and livelihoods, in health outcomes, where data is available, and in the enactment of policies contributing to racial health inequality. Overall, following Du Bois's call in the epigraph, I show the persistent and direct connections between where Black people lived and their health outcomes, and I show how the mechanism of racial containment perpetuated racial health inequality across generations.

A TALE OF TWO CITIES

Many local DC observers, including the city government, have documented that the contemporary health profile of DC reveals a clear tale of two cities—

a White DC and a Black DC. Studies conducted in the 2010s and early 2020s have found that Black vulnerability to premature death starts early and continues throughout the life course. A 2016 Georgetown University report led by Christopher King and Brian Floyd documented that the Black infant mortality rate was 9.9/1,000 compared to 1.7/1,000 for White babies. Young men aged 15 to 34 accounted for 89% of homicides, and Black men were 10 times more likely to be victims than White men. At older ages, Black people died at twice the rate of White people from heart disease and six times more from diabetes. Finally, it reported that Black people comprised about half the city population but had three-quarters of the city's HIV/AIDS cases.[1] As of February 2022, when the city was 42% Black and 37% White[2], the city's COVID-19 portal showed that 77.7% of all COVID-19 deaths were among Black people, while only 8.8% were among White people.[3] Perhaps the most striking racial inequality relates to life expectancy at birth. A 2024 study found that while the city's White men could expect to live 86.1 years, its Black men could only expect to live 68.1 years, a life expectancy almost two decades shorter (18 years). White women could expect to live 89.4 years, compared to Black women who could only expect to live 77.1 years, a life expectancy just over a decade shorter (12.3 years).[4] Overall, these statistics illustrate Black DC residents' disproportionate vulnerability to syndemic disease and premature death.

Local city observers have noted that space is an important aspect of the city's disease outcomes.[5] Black people are not randomly distributed throughout the city, and neither is illness. An underlying mechanism linking space and illness is socioeconomic status (SES), a well-documented and fundamental cause of illness and premature death, and its mapping onto spatial residential patterning.[6] Many Black DC residents are among the nation's poorest, and the city has the some of the highest levels of income inequality.[7] A 2017 DC Fiscal Policy Institute study found that "households in the top 20% of income have 29 times more income than the bottom 20%. The bottom fifth of DC households had 2% of total DC income in 2016, while the top fifth had a staggering 56%."[8] In wealth terms, Black families have "81 times less wealth than White families."[9] A 2021 DC Policy Center study found that while only 5.1% of White residents live below the poverty line, a fifth (21.6%) of Black people do. Black Washingtonians' median household income was $49,652, compared to $149,734 among White Washingtonians.[10]

Importantly, these inequalities are not just expressed in bank accounts but also in space. Figure 7 shows a clear racial geography of wealth distribution in

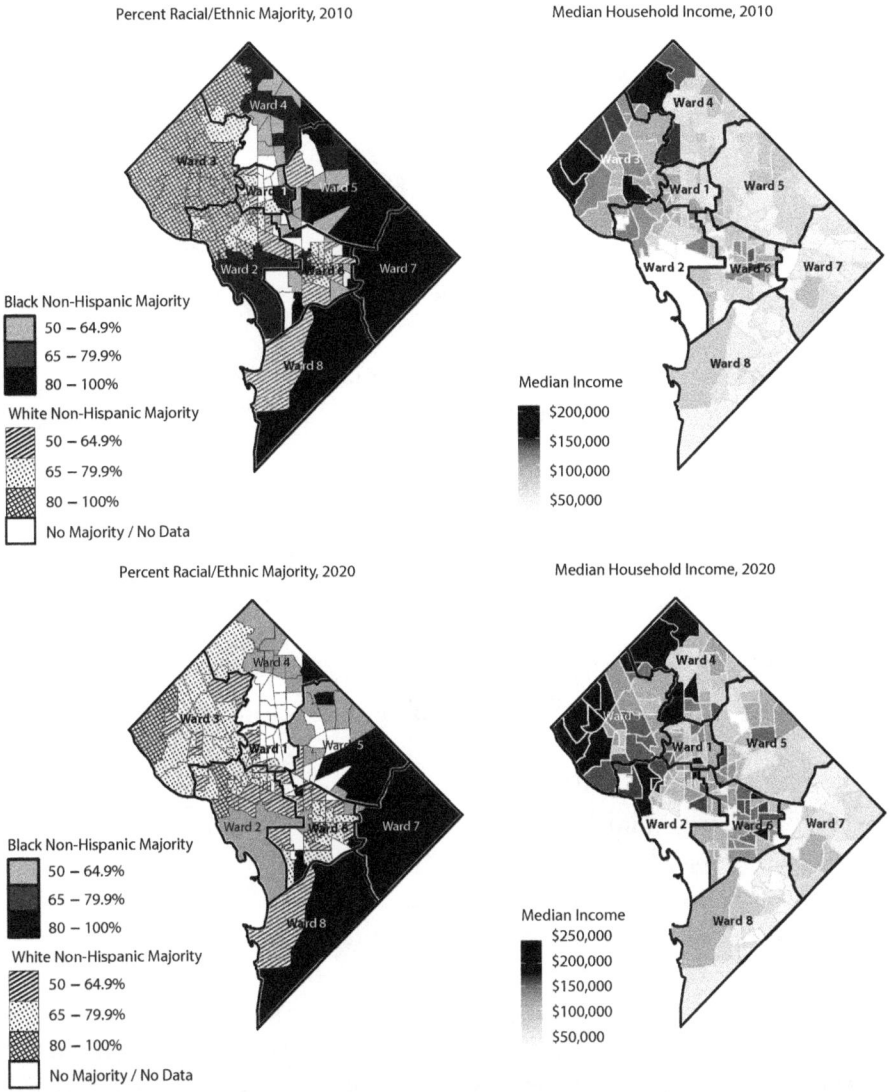

Percent Racial/Ethnic Majority, 2010

Black Non-Hispanic Majority
- 50 – 64.9%
- 65 – 79.9%
- 80 – 100%

White Non-Hispanic Majority
- 50 – 64.9%
- 65 – 79.9%
- 80 – 100%
- No Majority / No Data

Median Household Income, 2010

Median Income
- $200,000
- $150,000
- $100,000
- $50,000

Percent Racial/Ethnic Majority, 2020

Black Non-Hispanic Majority
- 50 – 64.9%
- 65 – 79.9%
- 80 – 100%

White Non-Hispanic Majority
- 50 – 64.9%
- 65 – 79.9%
- 80 – 100%
- No Majority / No Data

Median Household Income, 2020

Median Income
- $250,000
- $200,000
- $150,000
- $100,000
- $50,000

FIGURE 7. Racial residential distribution and median household income, DC, 2010–20. Data sources: American Community Survey; US Census (accessed from IPUMS).

the city. (I use shorthand for the city's quadrants: SE, NW, NE, SW). The maps on the left illustrate the city's racial residential distribution by ward, drawing from the 2010 and 2020 censuses, while the maps on the right illustrate the city's median household-income distribution, drawing from the 2010 and 2020 American Community Surveys. The maps clearly illustrate that Black people

Infant Mortality Rate by Ward, 2010

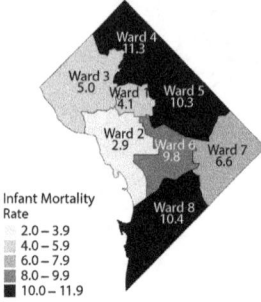

Homicide/Assault Crude Death Rate by Ward, 2010

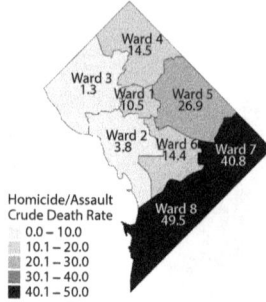

HIV/AIDS Crude Death Rate by Ward, 2010

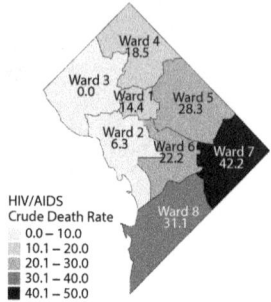

FIGURE 8. Infant mortality, homicide/assault, and HIV/AIDS death rates by ward, DC, 2010. Data source: Reproduced from District of Columbia Department of Health 2014.

are both more likely to live in the east and south of the city and more likely to have lower incomes compared to White people. Inequality across wards is also striking. Between 2010 and 2014, Ward 3 in the NW, the richest ward, was 82% White and 6% Black, with a median household income of $109,909 and a 3.9% unemployment rate.[11] By contrast, Ward 8 in the SE, the city's poorest, was 93.7% Black and 4.3% White. It had a median household income of $31,642 and a 14.1% unemployment rate.[12] Stark inequality continued into the next decade, even with gentrification. Between 2017 and 2021, Ward 3 was 75.6% White and 8.7% Black and had a median income of $133,750 and a 4.2% unemployment rate. By contrast, Ward 8 was 84.1% Black and 9.3% White. It had a median household income of $42,697 and a 15.8% unemployment rate.[13]

The spatialized racial distribution of SES translates into health outcomes, as illustrated in the maps in Figure 8, which were reproduced using data from a 2014 DC government report.[14] The maps show striking health inequalities across the city in infant mortality rates, homicide and assault rates, as well as AIDS deaths, with the darker areas showing disproportionate death in the poorest and Blackest wards in the NE and SE of the city. Overall life expectancy follows the same patterns, as illustrated in Figure 9, reproduced from a 2019 DC government health report, which shows strikingly high life expectancy in the NW, in Woodley Park (51) in particular (89.4 years), and strikingly low life expectancy in the SE, in St. Elizabeth's (47) in particular (68.4 years). This is a 21-year life-expectancy gap between neighborhoods located about 8.5 miles apart.[15]

So on the face of it, the story appears to be simple. Contemporary health vulnerabilities in the city are fixed in particular spaces, spaces that are pre-

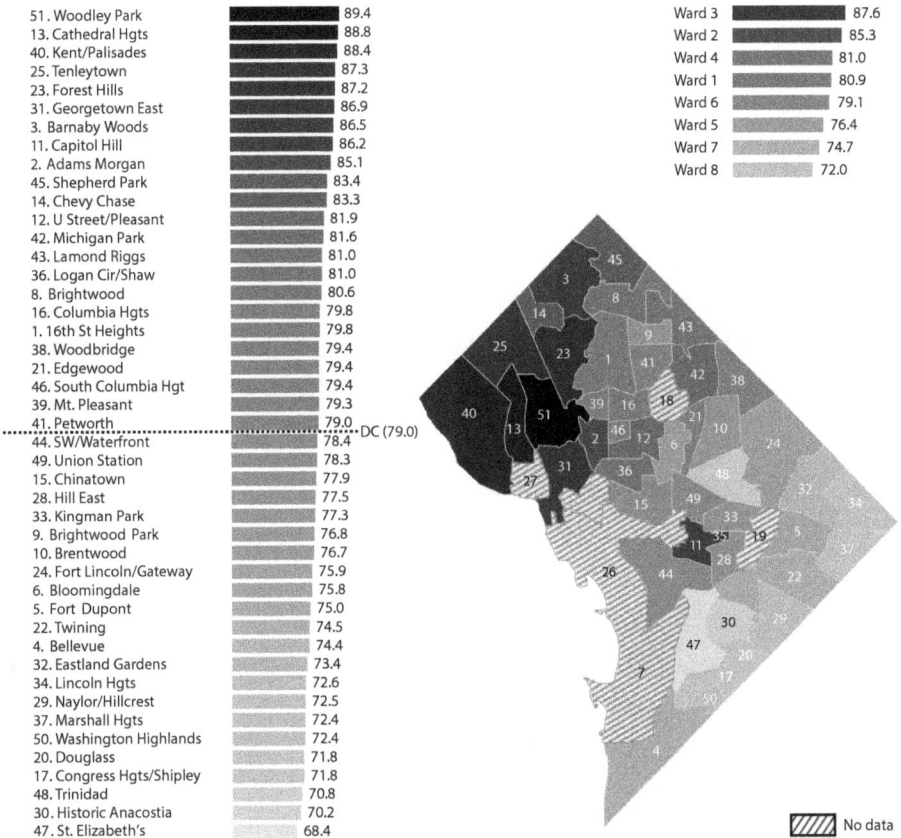

51. Woodley Park	89.4
13. Cathedral Hgts	88.8
40. Kent/Palisades	88.4
25. Tenleytown	87.3
23. Forest Hills	87.2
31. Georgetown East	86.9
3. Barnaby Woods	86.5
11. Capitol Hill	86.2
2. Adams Morgan	85.1
45. Shepherd Park	83.4
14. Chevy Chase	83.3
12. U Street/Pleasant	81.9
42. Michigan Park	81.6
43. Lamond Riggs	81.0
36. Logan Cir/Shaw	81.0
8. Brightwood	80.6
16. Columbia Hgts	79.8
1. 16th St Heights	79.8
38. Woodbridge	79.4
21. Edgewood	79.4
46. South Columbia Hgt	79.4
39. Mt. Pleasant	79.3
41. Petworth	79.0 · DC (79.0)
44. SW/Waterfront	78.4
49. Union Station	78.3
15. Chinatown	77.9
28. Hill East	77.5
33. Kingman Park	77.3
9. Brightwood Park	76.8
10. Brentwood	76.7
24. Fort Lincoln/Gateway	75.9
6. Bloomingdale	75.8
5. Fort Dupont	75.0
22. Twining	74.5
4. Bellevue	74.4
32. Eastland Gardens	73.4
34. Lincoln Hgts	72.6
29. Naylor/Hillcrest	72.5
37. Marshall Hgts	72.4
50. Washington Highlands	72.4
20. Douglass	71.8
17. Congress Hgts/Shipley	71.8
48. Trinidad	70.8
30. Historic Anacostia	70.2
47. St. Elizabeth's	68.4

Ward 3	87.6
Ward 2	85.3
Ward 4	81.0
Ward 1	80.9
Ward 6	79.1
Ward 5	76.4
Ward 7	74.7
Ward 8	72.0

No data

FIGURE 9. Life expectancy at birth by DC neighborhood, 2011–15. Data source: Reproduced from District of Columbia Department of Health 2019.

dominantly Black. And Black people have worse health and premature death compared to White people because they are poorer and live in poor neighborhoods. However, as I will illustrate in this Part, the connection between Black residential spaces, poverty, and poor health outcomes is neither merely contemporary nor accidental. It is by design. Indeed, placing this connection in historical context[16] suggests not only why the city continues to combat racialized health crises decade after decade but also why they are so intransigent and hard to improve without significant political will.

• • •

PART I PLAYLIST

Odetta	No More Auction Block for Me (1960)
Charles Mingus	Original Faubus Fables (1960)
John Coltrane	Alabama (1964)
2Pac	Changes (1992)
Nina Simone	Mississippi Goddam (1964)
Tracy Chapman	Across the Lines (1988)
Michael Jackson	They Don't Care About Us (1996)
The Freedom Singers	We Shall Not Be Moved (1963)
Mahalia Jackson	How I Got Over (1963)
The Staples Singers	Freedom Highway (1965)
Sweet Honey in the Rock	Keep Your Eyes on the Prize/ Hold On (2000)
Junkyard Band	The Word (1986)
Duke Ellington	It Don't Mean a Thing (1931)
Chuck Brown & The Soul Searchers	It Don't Mean a Thing (If it Don't Have the Go-Go Swing) (1986)
Trouble Funk	Pump Me Up (1982)
Parliament	Chocolate City (1975)

ONE

The First Era

1790–1890

MIGRATION AND THE GROWTH OF THE BLACK POPULATION IN DC

From the city's beginnings in 1790, race had a distinctive place in Washington, DC. As historian Howard Gilette Jr. described, the city was "a central battleground for the future of race relations in America," repopulating land originally owned by Native Americans, and created from and located between two of the largest slave-holding states in the country, Virginia and Maryland.[1] According to the US census, in 1800, the year the US capital moved to Washington, DC, a third of the DC population (30.4%) was Black, and 84% was enslaved (Figure 10). However, over the ensuing decades, while Black people remained about a third of the DC population, an increasing proportion were free (by 1830, 50.5% were free, and by 1850, 73.2% were free).

Enslaved and free Black people engaged in a wide variety of occupations in the city, as Letitia Woods Brown, writing on DC between 1790 and 1846, described:

> The Navy Yard and its accompanying shops and businesses operated as an economic center for much of the Negro population. Free Negroes and slaves could find a variety of work in the area ... The payrates for work at the Yard were apparently rather attractive in terms of contemporary pay scales ... If a man worked a 240-day work-year at the Navy Yard at $1.25 a day, he earned, at $300, a higher annual income than any public servant employed by the Corporation of Georgetown for the year 1828 except the Mayor who received $600 and the Clerk of the Corporation who was paid $1000. The Clerk of the Market was paid $225 per annum, the Captain of the Watch was paid $200, and the Clerk

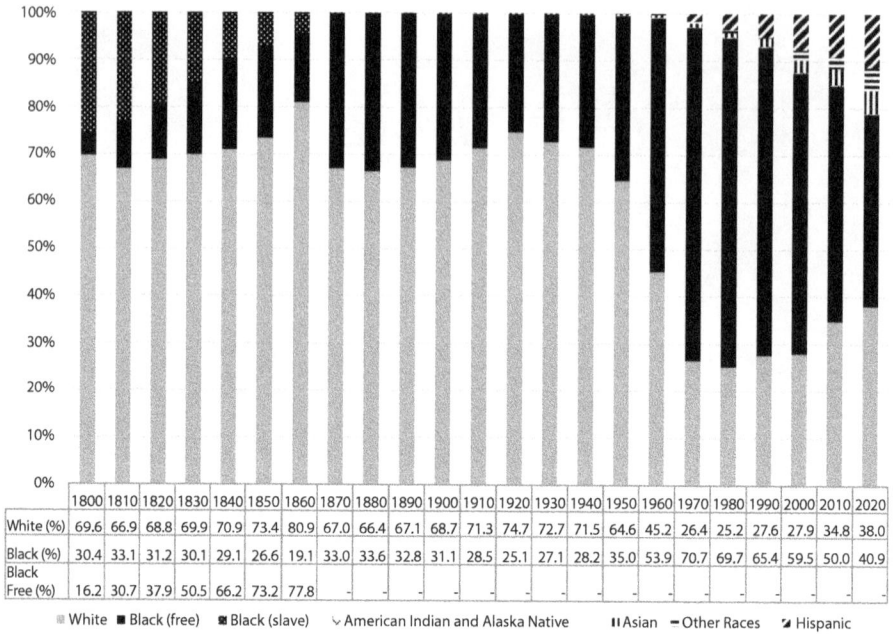

	1800	1810	1820	1830	1840	1850	1860	1870	1880	1890	1900	1910	1920	1930	1940	1950	1960	1970	1980	1990	2000	2010	2020
White (%)	69.6	66.9	68.8	69.9	70.9	73.4	80.9	67.0	66.4	67.1	68.7	71.3	74.7	72.7	71.5	64.6	45.2	26.4	25.2	27.6	27.9	34.8	38.0
Black (%)	30.4	33.1	31.2	30.1	29.1	26.6	19.1	33.0	33.6	32.8	31.1	28.5	25.1	27.1	28.2	35.0	53.9	70.7	69.7	65.4	59.5	50.0	40.9
Black Free (%)	16.2	30.7	37.9	50.5	66.2	73.2	77.8	-															

White   Black (free)   Black (slave)   American Indian and Alaska Native   Asian   Other Races   Hispanic

FIGURE 10. Racial/ethnic distribution of DC, 1800–2020. Data source: US Census Bureau (IPUMS).

of the Board of Common Council earned $150. Police officers were paid $150 ... and the two Superintendents of Fire Engines were paid $25.[2]

In addition, Black people were running their own businesses, working in hotels and boarding houses, doing retail and service work and domestic service in homes, as well as engaging in jobs as carpenters, laborers, blacksmiths, painters, plumbers, teachers, ministers, and physicians. Others worked for the federal and city governments in a variety of capacities.[3]

However, as the free Black population expanded and prospered, officials started to place restrictions on Black mobility around the city through Black codes, which included introducing nighttime curfews and adding requirements that "free Black [people] carry certificates of freedom at all times ... register ... with the mayor, post ... bond[s] for good behavior" ($20 in 1820, rising to $1,000 by 1836), and secure White character witnesses (rising from one in 1820 to five witnesses by 1836).[4] There were also increasing restrictions on Black economic opportunity and mobility. Black people began to be excluded from federal employment, and from 1831, restrictions were passed by the Washington Corporation Council to limit Black businesses by restricting access to and taxing licenses for businesses run by Black people, including lucrative restaurants and bars.[5]

The national battle over slavery took a particular form in DC, "a center of slavery and the slave trade."[6] The "Radical Republicans pressed for the end of slavery in the District" while "local residents [worried about being] overrun with Black refugees from the South."[7] Up to that point, there had been a delicate balance in Congress between the South (slave holding states) and the North (free states); thus, what happened in the nation's capital was not just a local matter but one of national significance. One of the five "bleeding wounds of the republic" elucidated by Henry Clay, a senator from Kentucky, was slavery and the slave trade in Washington, DC.[8] The Compromise of 1850 partially resolved the issue by proposing the abolition of the slave trade, but not slavery in the District.[9] It took another 12 years before slavery was abolished in the nation's capital. In 1860, just before the abolition of slavery in DC, while Black people had dropped to 19.1% of DC's population, 77.8% of them were free (see Figure 10). On April 16, 1862, President Lincoln signed the DC Compensated Emancipation Act for the city.[10]

The Black population continued to grow rapidly in the post-slavery Reconstruction era—so much so that it had "the largest urban concentration of Blacks in the US until World War I—even more than New York City."[11] By 1880, of the 177,624 people in DC, 33.6% were Black (see Figure 10). Migration into Washington was not just driven by the growth of the federal government and the city's status as a haven for free Black people and slaves escaping from other states, but also by the Civil War, when the city's population dramatically swelled. During Reconstruction, Black rights dramatically expanded—by some accounts, to the point of having more rights than other Black people in the US. As a national report noted:

> The popularly elected Assembly of the District passed a [1872] law giving Negroes equal rights in restaurants, hotels, barber shops, and other places of public accommodation. Stiff penalties were provided for violation ... In Washington the Negro ... has greater advantages than elsewhere in the Union ... the law requires that he shall be permitted if he can afford to do so, to eat in the best restaurants, sleep in the best hotels, and be admitted to the best theaters patronized by Whites.[12]

The implication was that there were Black people who were wealthy enough to fully enjoy the best the city had to offer. Indeed, Black wealth had dramatically increased. As a report from the National Committee on Segregation in the Nation's Capital (hereafter, Segregation Report) noted: "At the time of the Emancipation Act [1862], they ['free Negroes'] outnumbered slaves in the District of Columbia by 3 to 1. They were paying taxes on $650,000 worth of real estate and constituted one-fifth of all the owners of land in the District."[13] (For context, the 2022 DC Black home ownership rate was 34%.)[14]

A distinct part of Washington's Black society was complex lines of inequality based on slave and free status; among those who were free, generational family duration in DC (with longer duration linked to property ownership and early establishment of family wealth); educational achievement; occupational status gradations (often anchored by federal employment); wealth generated from business, investments, and property ownership; distinctions of skin color (one popular test used a brown paper bag) and degree of Black blood ("octoroons" [one Black great grandparent], "quadroons" [one Black grandparent], and "mulattos" [one Black parent]); and finally, social class comprising some combination of these factors, with the highest class having multiple streams of income.[15] Washington, DC, was deemed "the capital of the colored aristocracy"[16] and was presumed by Du Bois to have "probably the wealthiest group [of Black people] in the country."[17] These complex inter- and intraracial inequalities and dynamics were reflected in residential arrangements.

SPATIAL RACIAL AND CLASS CONTAINMENT

Social containment with respect to race and class was institutionalized by the city's taxation system and physical design. This began as early as the 1820s and '30s when, as Constance McLaughlin Green described:

> The method the city early adopted in distributing funds for poor relief, policing, and other public purposes penalized the poorer parts of the city. Each ward collected its own taxes, paid a small part into the city treasury and spent the rest within its own limits; each ward independently solicited contributions for relief of its own poverty-stricken inhabitants. The result was small separate financial kingdoms with unequal opportunity for growth.[18]

In this way, richer areas could afford better improvements, which further attracted wealthy people, while poorer areas "lost progressively the capacity to attract the well-to-do."[19] These class containment dynamics mapped onto the racial classification system and were expressed in fine-tuned residential patterns that unfolded throughout the century.

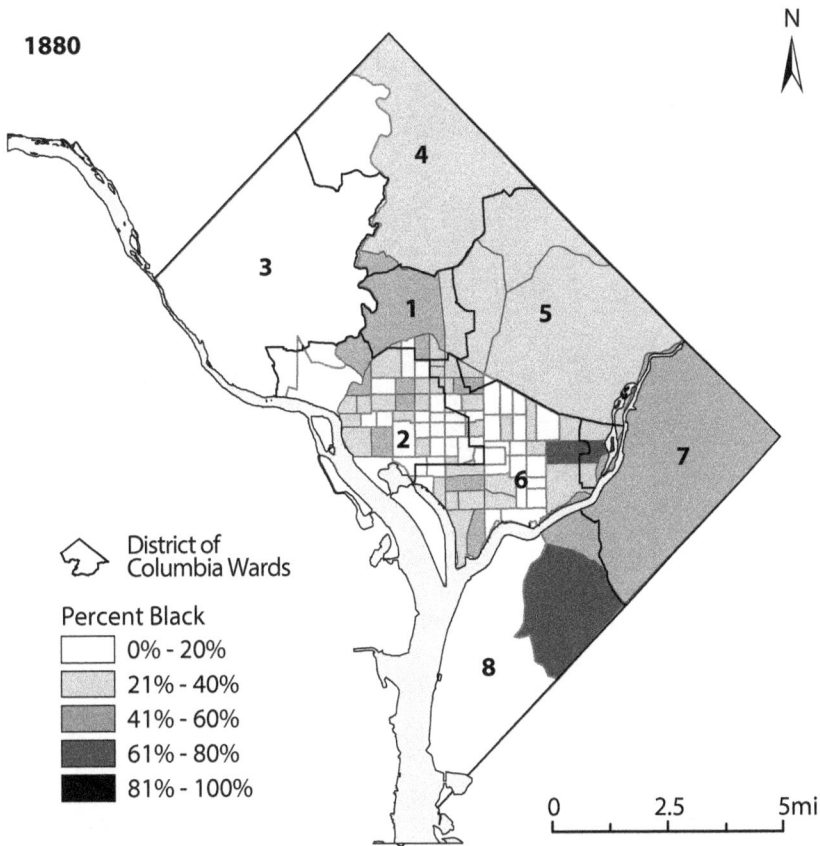

N

District of
Columbia Wards

Percent Black

	0% - 20%
	21% - 40%
	41% - 60%
	61% - 80%
	81% - 100%

0   2.5   5mi

FIGURE 11. Racial settlement patterns in DC, 1880. Data source: US Census Bureau; John R. Logan, Jason Jindrich, Hyoungjin Shin, and Weiwei Zhang, 2011, Mapping America in 1880: The Urban Transition Historical GIS Project, *Historical Methods* 44(1):49–60, https://s4.ad.brown.edu/Projects/UTP/Default.aspx.

Macrolevel Patterns

Figure 11 shows macrolevel racial settlement patterns in Washington, DC, in 1880, drawing on the earliest available geocoded census data. In Figure 11 and in subsequent census-derived figures, modern-day ward lines are superimposed to enable easy location and comparisons. The figure illustrates almost exclusively White enclaves in Ward 3, part of Ward 4, and most of Ward 8, almost exclusively Black enclaves in part of Ward 8 and part of Ward 6, and an otherwise even dispersion of Black people throughout the rest of the city. However, the apparent racial dispersal belies the fact that at

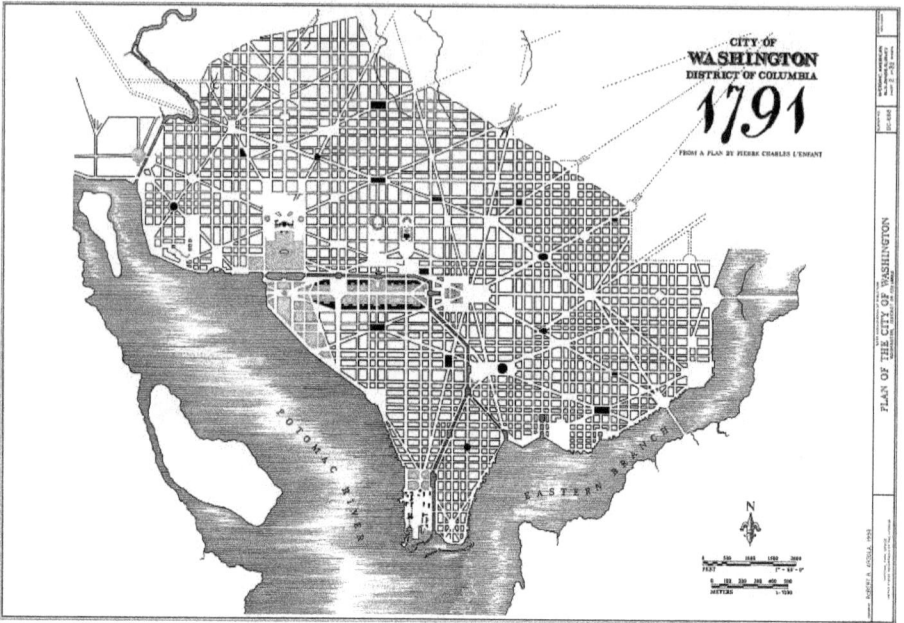

FIGURE 12. Pierre L'Enfant's Plan. Source: Library of Congress, https://tile.loc.gov/storage-services/
service/pnp/habshaer/dc/dc0700/dc0776/sheet/00002v.jpg.

the street level, housing was both racially and economically segregated, creating the complex residential geography described below. This pattern largely
reflected the dominant settlement pattern in the Southern US—that of tertiary segregation, whose aim was to balance racial social distance with work
proximity.[20] A key constraint was the limited ability for people to separate
themselves by race or class while still remaining within easy walking or
horse-carriage riding distance to their workplaces and social lives prior to the
transportation revolution.[21]

Microlevel Patterns

Washington, DC, owes its elegant layout, depicted in Figure 12, to Frenchman
Pierre L'Enfant, who "envision[ed] a grand capital of wide avenues, public
squares, and inspiring buildings in what was then a district of hills, forests,
marshes and plantations."[22] In the initial plan, the physical layout of the city,
with its wide avenues, lent itself to grand houses along the street fronts with
substantial land in the backyards and along alleys.

Sample Area, 1880–88

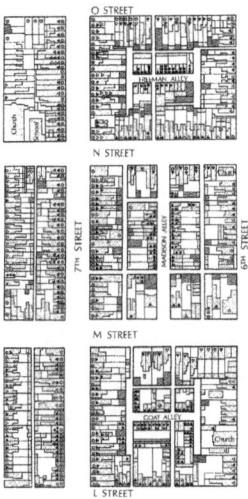

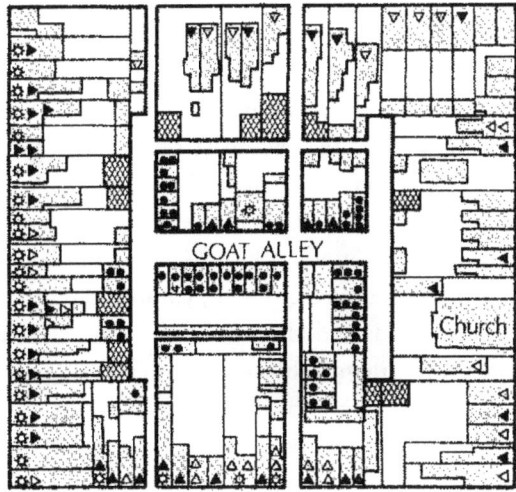

FIGURE 13. Racial/nativity residential arrangements in DC, 1880–88. Source: James Borchert, *Alley Life in Washington: Family, Community, Religion, and Folklife in the City, 1850–1970* (University of Illinois Press, 1980). Copyright © 1980 by the Board of Trustees of the University of Illinois. Used with permission of the University of Illinois Press.

Throughout the century, there were rapid waves of White and Black in-migration, accelerated in the 1860s by thousands of former slaves following the Civil War. Migrants faced the challenge of finding housing in close proximity to work. Sensing a lucrative business opportunity, landowners rapidly constructed housing of widely varying—and often substandard—quality in their rear lots facing the alleys. This was a mix of shacks, shanties, tenements, and wooden and brick row houses.[23] As Paul Groves described, "Alley properties were handsome investments, commonly realizing from 10–20 percent per annum on initial capital, and rent even for the more affluent alley dweller could take as much as 40 percent of his income."[24] Indeed, James Borchert found that "nearly every survey reported that return on investment for alley property was at least twice that for street property."[25]

Street-front, backyard, and alley residential arrangements were organized by race and nativity, as illustrated by the maps in Figure 13 constructed by historian James Borchert[26] using a combination of 1880–88 census data and city directories. The figure illustrates rows of White circles representing native-born White people on the street fronts, rows of Black triangles representing foreign-born White people in their backyards, and rows of Black circles representing Black people in the internal or blind and hidden alleys—Freeman Alley, Madison Alley, and Goat Alley, in this case. Overall, wealthier White and some wealthy Black families found housing predominantly on street fronts, the latter most often within Black enclaves but sometimes near White people. Borchert found that Black people comprised about 9% of the street-front population in the area he sampled.[27] Poor immigrant White (German and Irish) and poor Black families found housing in overcrowded, confined, and predominantly racially segregated backyards and alleys behind the main houses.[28] This pattern also held in predominantly Black enclaves, where poorer Black people lived in alleys while wealthier Black people lived on street fronts. (Some Black people lived where they worked, e.g., live-in domestic servants).[29] In general, darker-skinned, poorer, and more recent Black migrants were more likely to live in alleys, while those who were lighter skinned, able to move to higher income jobs, and/or those who were more established in the city experienced alleys as "holding stations" on their way to better alleys/slums or street-front homes in Black enclaves.[30]

Two particular Black enclaves warrant special attention. The first were those created by the Bureau of Refugees, Freedmen, and Abandoned Lands (or the Freedmen's Bureau) to accommodate former slaves who surged into the city during and following the Civil War (1861–65) and were "congregated in squalid camps and festering slums."[31] The Bureau "sensitive to White criticism ... looked to create 'Negro colonies' in areas that were either already Black or were inhabited and thus far from White neighbors."[32] The result was the creation of Barry Farm in 1867 (in current Anacostia, Ward 8).[33] The second type of enclave, at the other end of the economic spectrum, was comprised of Black "aristocrats."[34] However, even they struggled to secure housing and had to pay a premium. As Willard Gatewood described:

> In no areas, perhaps, did aristocrats of color in Washington confront the color line so persistently as in their efforts to secure adequate housing. As early as 1881, the *People's Advocate* complained about the shortage of "houses for our people", noting that the crisis was especially acute for those of "the official class" because respectable homes were simply out of reach for anyone classified as a Negro.[35]

Many elite Black people eventually settled in LeDroit Park (current Ward 1) in NW DC, near Howard University.[36] It was a predominantly White neigh-

TABLE 1
CITY OF WASHINGTON: ALLEY POPULATION, 1858–1913

	Total Alley Population	Number of Inhabited Alleys	Percent of Alley Inhabitants White	Black
1858	715	53	65.1	34.9
1871	1,345	170	17.9	81.1
1880	8,551	187	11.4	88.6
1897	18,233	246	11.7	88.3
1913	10,689	228	8.7	91.3

Sources: For 1858 and 1871 rough estimates of alley population were derived by using the 1880 ratio of *occupied* alley inhabitants to *total* alley inhabitants (1:2.33). Occupied alley inhabitants and alley count from Boyd's *Directory of Washington and Georgetown* (Washington, D.C.: 1858) and *Directory of Washington, Georgetown and Alexandria, 1871* (Washington, D.C.: 1871).
For 1880, 1880 Census of Population Manuscript Schedules for Washington, D.C.
For 1897, *Report of Commissioners of the District of Columbia, 1897* (Washington, D.C.: 1898).
For 1913, District of Columbia, *Board of Commissioners Annual Report* (Washington, D.C.: 1914).

FIGURE 14. Alley population of Washington City, 1853–1913. Source: Paul A. Groves, The "Hidden" Population: Washington Alley Dwellers in the Late Nineteenth Century, *The Professional Geographer* 26(3):270–76. Copyright © 1974 American Association of Geographers. Reprinted by permission of Taylor & Francis Ltd, https://www.tandfonline .com, on behalf of 1974 American Association of Geographers.

borhood that gradually transformed into a Black elite neighborhood following lawsuits by white homeowners.[37]

Most Black people did not live in alleys. Many lived in slums and tenements as well as in wood and brick homes and on small-hold farms further out.[38] However, within alleys, as Figure 14 from Groves[39] illustrates, there was a clear difference between racial residential trends before and after the end of slavery in 1862. As the figure illustrates, while in the late 1850s, two-thirds of alley dwellers were White, by 1871, after the end of slavery, the racial composition of alleys was reversed, with 81.1% of households being Black while 17.9% were White.[40]

A primary reason for the racial changeover was persistent racial discrimination not just in housing by landlords but also in occupations by employers, during and after Reconstruction.[41] In the case of the latter, Black people were excluded from unions, which controlled construction work, encountered promotion ceilings, and were paid half as much as White laborers for the same job, contributing to higher rates and longer periods of unemployment, as well as lower pay.[42] Restricting Black income and employment also restricted the financial means to secure better housing relative to poor and/or immigrant White people. Housing patterns thus reflected the social containment of Black people through the expansion and contraction of their economic life chances as the century progressed.

Living in alleys and slums was consequential for Black health outcomes, and they were universally acknowledged as hazardous for health in Board of Health (BOH) reports (1872–90) to the District commissioners (who were presidentially appointed to run the city and who submitted annual reports to Congress). Street-front residents would typically throw their garbage into the alleys for removal by the city; this included decomposing animal and vegetable matter, as well as dead household pests like rats, which were killed with arsenic and tossed into the backyard. Privies (pit latrines) were also located in the backyard, were limited in number, and alleys often did not have running water or sewers. The city could not or did not keep up with cleaning the alleys, which was an expensive endeavor.

While BOH reports vacillated in attributing the ensuing ill health of alley inhabitants to their personal "habits," they were often accompanied by frank acknowledgements that the environment in which alley residents lived was a direct cause of their health outcomes. As an 1872 BOH report clearly described at a time when about 81% of the alley population was Black:

> No portions of a city contribute more to generate disease than its ill-regu-lated, neglected alleys; these, unless closely watched and constantly cleaned contain more or less animal and vegetable matter in and near them constantly undergoing decomposition, and giving rise to gaseous emanations highly offensive and pernicious because [of] the receptacles of filthy accumulations from the houses and backyards with which they connect.[43]

In a supplemental report presented on July 22, 1872, titled "Filthy Alleys," health officer T. S. Verdi went on to describe what was "permanently existing at all hours in every part of the city, behind the palatial mansion as well as in front of the poor man's hut," elaborating:

> I allude to the one hundred miles or more of alleys which run through our squares, and which receive the filth that flows from almost every house in our city. They are generally illy paved and undrained, yet are used as the repository of all disgusting and foul refuse of our dwellings, there hidden from public gaze … A general inspection of said alleys would bring dismay to the stoutest heart and make one doubt the intelligence of the community that has planted in the rear of its dwellings the fatal poison that is to cast it into its grave.[44]

He went on to recommend sewer installation and more frequent alley cleaning. The sheer expense of these ventures, in the context of a Congress who were "relatively unconcerned with the city's routine health problems,"[45] meant the most amenable means at the disposal of the health department was condemning buildings as "unfit for human habitation."[46] However, this would leave poor tenants with an even more limited supply of housing.

It was not only the condition of the alley streets that caused health problems but of the alley dwellings themselves, along with dwellings in tenements and slums where increasing numbers lived as the century progressed. While there was clear variation in housing quality,[47] many were in very poor condition. As a health officer noted in the 1877 BOH report:

> A shanty is defined by Worcester to be "a mean cabin" and that is evidently what they mean by the term in Washington and Georgetown, for no meaner cabins for temporary or permanent shelter can be found than some of our wretched poor are born and exist and die in, here at the capital of the United States. And strange, as it may seem, none so mean that they have not an owner mean enough to charge rent for them. Down in the alleys, below grade, with combination roof of felt, tar, shingles; rags, tin, gravel, boards and holes; floors damp and broken; walls begrimed by smoke and age—so domiciled are families, with all the dignity of tenants having rent to pay; perhaps four, five or, maybe, eight, dollars a month, and proud of the distinction, though often greatly exercised to meet their obligations.[48]

Landlords, while collecting substantial sums in rent, were in turn reluctant to improve housing for their tenants. As described in an 1875 BOH report:

> That a house with [a] leaky roof, damp walls, below grade, having decayed floor, in general filthy condition, is a nuisance injurious to health is not difficult to demonstrate, except your listener be the owner of several such, from which he realizes a comfortable income, equal to the full value of the houses each year. When such interested party receives a notice, detailing in exact terms wherein the unsanitary condition of his source of revenue must be corrected, involving more or less expenditure, he immediately feels himself aggrieved, believes himself to be the victim of persecution, condemns the Board of Health itself as a nuisance which he promises to abate at the earliest opportunity, and wants to know what business it is to us, since it is *his* property, and his tenants do not complain . . . the very poor we have with us always, and they must find some place to lay their head. They must seek those shanties or tenement houses where rents are lowest. The most dilapidated and the worst located are

cheapest, and the tenants are the last to complain; are frequently even found testifying on the side of the landlord against a Board seeking to improve the conditions which hazard their own and the public health.[49]

The tenant's defense of the landowner reflected both a shortage of affordable or available housing and fear of losing access to their tight-knit community if their home were to be condemned.[50]

Death in a Syndemic Zone

The health consequence of these living conditions was a syndemic. Board of Health reports described multiple overlapping epidemics and listed the main causes of death as "zymotic" (infectious) diseases such as consumption (tuberculosis), influenza, cholera, measles, scarlet fever, diphtheria, dysentery, croup, whooping cough, typhoid fever, syphilis, and diarrheal diseases, as well as "local diseases" such as asthma, bronchitis, colic, jaundice, and pneumonia. While these epidemics affected the city as a whole, they had their greatest impact on the Black population and were seen by health officers to be clearly exacerbated by the overcrowded and substandard housing conditions in which the Black population predominantly lived. Figure 15 shows estimated mortality rates by race between 1876 and 1890 from the 1890 BOH report (see endnote for comment on estimates).[51]

Overall, Black people died at nearly twice the rate of White people (18.4/1,000 White, 33.6/1,000 "Colored"), and over 60% of Black deaths were among infants and children under the age of five.[52] The reasons for these deaths were obvious to medical inspectors, who repeated their explanations in report after report with what Betty Plummer characterized as "a mixture of genuine concern, racism and paternalism,"[53] even as they acknowledged their own inability to help. Writing in the 1876 BOH report, for example, W. D. Stewart, MD, wrote:

> I cannot better explain this extraordinary waste of human life so largely represented by one class (the colored) than by quoting my remarks on this same subject (from the Annual Report of the Board of Health for 1874, page 232) which are as follows:
>
>> This explanation is readily found in the unsanitary condition of a large majority of their homes, the faulty construction of tenement-houses and shanties, and the overcrowding of these filthy, unventilated abodes where poverty throngs so many of the alleys of Washington and Georgetown ... The hard,

Years.	Population.			Deaths.			Death rate.		
	White.	Colored.	Total.	White.	Colored.	Total.	White.	Colored.	Total.
1876	106,741	50,859	157,600	2,086	2,074	4,160	19.54	40.78	26.40
1877	109,505	52,870	162,375	2,187	2,021	4,208	19.97	38.22	25.91
1878	112,340	54,960	167,300	2,166	2,065	4,231	19.28	37.57	25.29
1879	115,217	57,130	172,377	2,196	2,113	4,309	19.05	36.90	24.99
1880	118,236	59,402	177,638	2,085	2,121	4,206	17.63	35.71	23.68
1881	121,300	61,760	183,060	2,205	1,931	4,136	18.18	31.27	22.59
1882	124,441	64,212	188,653	2,353	2,218	4,571	18.91	34.54	24.23
1883	126,300	65,680	191,980	2,270	2,016	4,286	17.97	30.69	22.33
1884	130,700	69,300	200,000	2,576	2,238	4,814	19.71	32.29	24.07
1885	130,700	69,300	200,000	2,610	2,388	4,998	19.97	34.45	24.99
1886	136,000	69,300	205,300	2,442	2,232	4,674	17.96	32.35	22.80
1887	140,000	70,000	210,000	2,484	2,181	4,665	17.74	31.15	22.21
1888	150,000	75,000	225,000	2,778	2,262	5,040	18.52	30.16	22.40
1889	170,000	80,000	250,000	2,713	2,439	5,152	15.96	30.49	20.60
1890	170,000	80,000	250,000	2,934	2,630	5,564	17.25	32.87	22.25
Mean death rate...							18.40	33.60	23.47

FIGURE 15. District of Columbia mortality rates, 1876–90. Source: DC Board of Health, *Annual Report of the Commissioners of the District of Columbia*, 1890.

exhausting labor, principally washing and scrubbing, that constitutes the only employment available to the mothers of this poor class of the population, directly induces the mortality of their offspring. In many cases, they are driven from the wash-tub or scrubbing brush to the pains of childbed, from which they are compelled, in many instances even a few days or hours, to arise and resume their exhaustive labor for the support of their children.[54]

In an 1875 report, Dr. Parke G. Young, writing on the sixth sanitary division, described continued challenges after birth:

The mother, as soon as delivered, seeks work, neglects to nurse her child, loses her milk, and abandons it almost entirely to the care of others, who, already overburdened by the duties of their own households, invariably abuse the trust. It is improperly fed, dosed with opiates to keep it quiet, badly clothed, kept in the closest of rooms during the hottest summer days, with the fires of winter, and when at last the wretched little one yields to these accumulated abuses, the physician is called to the hopeless task of curing a disease whose causes he cannot remove. For this there is and can be but one remedy—an institution where these infants can be cared for; a place where the mother can place her child while she goes to her daily work. There are many of them who would not only be willing but too happy to pay what they can for this care, could they but obtain it.[55]

Harsh working conditions and lack of paid maternity leave and high-quality childcare were thus acknowledged as key factors in high infant mortality.

An important underlying implication was the necessity for Black women to work outside the home to support themselves and their families. Within alleys, Groves found significant racial differences in women's labor force participation, with 24.2 White women employed per 100 White working men, compared to 90.3 Black women employed per 100 Black working men.[56] He noted that "this would suggest a differing role for the female within the White alley social structure, namely fewer working wives, fewer female heads of households, and more young White females at school."[57] The higher rate of employment for Black women was necessitated by the relative precarity of Black men's work. Women worked in safer and more dependable occupations, such as domestic work within White homes.[58] Black men had higher unemployment and lower pay compared to White men due to discrimination as well as high rates of on-the-job injury, disability, and death.[59]

Ward doctors, a short-term city innovation, thus submitted frustrated reports about their inability to help in the face of structural and environmental constraints. For example, Dr. J. E. Brackett of the fifth sanitary division wrote in the 1875 BOH report:

> There is probably no class of practice that causes so much annoyance to the physician, so difficult to manage, so unsatisfactory, and attended with such unfavorable results as that devolving upon the medical attendant to the poor of our cities and towns. The reasons are obvious; at least to those who are at all familiar with the sanitary and hygienic condition of this class of people inhabiting alleys and filthy streets, crowded together as they are in close and ill-ventilated apartments; inhaling noisome and noxious gases impregnated with the germs of disease; wretchedly protected from the cold, and subsisting upon such nourishment as their slender means will obtain . . . Can it be wondered at that our efforts are sometimes fruitless; our medicines frequently inadequate, and that our time and attention often seem wholly lost? So long as the exciting causes exist, how can we ever hope to combat disease successfully?[60]

Overspending to the tune of $5.2 million ($136 million today) by the Board of Public Works (led by Alexander Shepherd, who worked at a furious pace to improve the city's infrastructure[61]) resulted in significant budget cuts to the Health Department, reducing the number of health inspectors from ten to three and reducing the budget for the city's poor.[62] The significance of these cuts was not lost on health registrar of vital statistics D. W. Bliss, who noted that they were "an enforced retrenchment which trifles with human life"[63]—and in particular, given the unequal mortality rates, Black life.

In sum, in the first era, racial and class containment of poor people, Black people, and especially poor Black people in syndemic zones, led to their disproportionate death rates. This occurred through tertiary residential segregation, which included poorly regulated and overcrowded housing, exploitative and neglectful landlords, and unsanitary neighborhoods and dwellings used as the city's garbage dumps, which the city government was then derelict in cleaning. It also occurred through economic immobility due to racial occupational discrimination and employer exploitation, which combined to limit Black people's economic means to move out of these neighborhoods, leading to regular and elongated exposure to noxious and toxic places. Government cuts to the health department then limited poor people's health care once ill. Thus, multiple institutions—including the government, the real estate industry, and employers—worked together in ways that led directly to higher Black mortality in the city. In the next half century, while the style of social containment took on a new form and acquired a new rationale, the connection between space, race, and health persisted.

TWO

———

The Second Era

1890–1950

BETWEEN 1890 AND 1950, a new strategy of racial containment was pursued in Washington, DC. This reflected, in part, a Jim Crow–era backlash that reversed many post-slavery Reconstruction-era gains, including a return of the color bar restricting Black people from jobs as well as social spaces in the city, such as hotels and restaurants.[1] These processes stood in stark contrast to earlier decades characterized by expanding liberation and equality and expanding freedom of mobility. Robert Manning observed, "The most striking aspect of the White backlash [was] the spatial displacement and concentration of the widely dispersed African American population, within and outside the District, into racially confined neighborhoods . . . [in effect, a] social construction of urban apartheid."[2] A number of federal, District, and private institutions and policy instruments, along with local residents, worked in concert to redesign the racial geography of the city, mirroring a pattern described by Arnold Hirsch in *Making the Second Ghetto*.[3] As I will illustrate, in the case of DC, this occurred, ironically, in the name of health. A public health rationale was also utilized in cities such as Baltimore, Atlanta, and New York, as documented by Samuel Roberts Jr. in *Infectious Fear*.[4] And the overall effect was to reconstitute the relationship between space, race, and health and thus reproduce racial health inequality for the next generation.

ALLEY HOUSING DESTRUCTION AND URBAN RENEWAL

Over several years at the end of the 19th and early 20th centuries, District physicians were joined by social activists in campaigning for the removal of alley and slum housing due to their condition and health consequences, alongside advocating for the construction of good-quality, low-cost housing to accommodate displaced residents.[5] As Mary Clare de Graffenried, a field expert in the Department of Labor and a member of the Women's Anthropological Society, argued in a paper she prepared in spring 1896 following "an investigation of the alleys of Washington . . . inaugurated by the Committee on 'Housing of the People of the Washington Civic Centre'":

> It is unwise policy for a great and growing municipality, on which the eyes of the nation are turned, to permit or to multiply these wretched habitations in the heart of populous blocks . . . the poor can be housed cheaply without being housed meanly and in a way that induces vice and mortality.[6]

By 1903, the drumbeat had reached Congress and the White House. A visit by President Theodore Roosevelt's friend Jacob Riis to Washington's alleys was followed by a report to Congress.[7] Danish-born Riis was a journalist who had famously documented New York City tenements in his book *How the Other Half Lives*. As James Ring, an administrative officer of the National Capital Housing Authority (NCHA) described:

> Riis toured the slums of Washington and a few days later, having been invited to address a joint meeting of the Senate and House Committees on the District of Columbia, he related the results of his trip. In writing of this meeting later, Riis said: "When I argued the case against Washington slums . . . one smooth-shaven Senator was quite indifferent even to the unheard-of contagious disease record in Willow Tree Alley till I said that the clothes lines full of towels hung across the alley. They were from the Senate barber shop which had its washing done there. At that, my Senator sat up straight and wiped his chin thoughtfully, and after that he took an interest."[8]

The senator's reaction underscored the separate but nonetheless physically close and intertwined nature of front street/back alley racial residential arrangements. In a 1904 speech, Roosevelt made clear to the nation the connection between poor housing and poor health outcomes, noting:

> The death-rate statistics show a terrible increase in mortality, and especially in infant mortality, in overcrowded tenements . . . The slum exacts a heavy total of death from those who dwell therein; and this is the case not merely in the great crowded slums of high buildings in New York and Chicago, but in the alley slums of Washington. In Washington people cannot afford to ignore the harm that this causes.[9]

He went on to note that "the local death rates, especially from preventable diseases, are so unduly high as to suggest that the exceptional wholesomeness of Washington's better sections is offset by bad conditions in her poorer neighborhoods." He called for "a systematic investigation" as well as "an appropriate building code" and hoped for "the reformation of existing evils." He felt this endeavor was important because "the Nation's Capital should be made a model for other municipalities [which was] an ideal which appeals to all patriotic citizens everywhere." Thus, the endeavor to fix the "housing problem" in Washington was to set the tone for national efforts in the coming decades, and the theme of housing improvement in the name of health[10] became a key rationale for the subsequent urban renewal program.

THE GOVERNMENT ACTS:
HOUSING POLICY FOR THE POOR

Activist efforts reached a sad crescendo when a deathbed wish by First Lady Ellen Wilson, wife of President Woodrow Wilson, calling for the removal of alley housing provided the final impetus to the congressional passage of an act "banning the use of alley dwellings after July 1, 1918."[11] Passed on September 25, 1914, it was "an Act to provide, in the interest of public health, comfort, morals, and safety, for the discontinuance of the use as dwellings of buildings situated in the alleys in the District of Columbia." The act made it "unlawful in the District of Columbia to erect, place, or construct any dwelling" without "sewer, water mains and gas or electric light," or in alleys narrower than 30 feet, or in hidden alleys, among other regulations. A fine of $10-$100 (about $300-$3,000 in 2024 dollars) was to be applied to each violation day.[12] However, World War I stymied efforts to enforce the act. Continued activist efforts finally led to President Franklin D. Roosevelt (the fifth cousin of Theodore Roosevelt) signing the District of Columbia Alley Dwelling Act in 1934.[13] The acts were significant as hundreds of property owners and landlords[14] stood to lose their lucrative rentals, especially given how large the profit margins were (see Chapter 1). The Alley Dwelling Act set up the Alley Dwelling Authority, which was tasked with implementation.[15]

Overall, a series of national acts and authorities focused on housing were set up during Franklin D. Roosevelt's term, including several directed at prospective or current home-owning Americans, such as the Home Owners'

Loan Corporation in 1933, which provided mortgage relief, the National Housing Act in 1934, and the Federal Housing Administration (FHA) in 1934. These acts were designed, in part, to shore up home ownership in the middle of the Great Depression. More controversially, however, the Alley Dwelling Act was joined by other acts and presidential orders focused on low-income and very poor Americans, including the Wagner–Steagull Housing Act in 1937, which focused on public housing and led to the creation of the United States Housing Authority to provide loans for the construction of public housing, and specifically for DC, the National Capital Housing Authority (NCHA), responsible for public housing in the District.[16]

John Bradner Smith, counsel for the FHA, commented in 1936 that "it has been asserted on good authority that one-third of the wage earners in this country do not earn enough money to afford what we could call decent housing."[17] Thus, the country's "entering the housing field," and in particular constructing public housing, was seen as an attempt to solve the widespread unemployment problem and the "housing problem" at the same time through a public works program.[18] Since low-rent homes could not go to high-income people, and these federal loans were only going to public housing agencies, he perceived that the government would not be interfering or competing with private enterprise, a key part of the controversy around public housing.[19]

The planned road from alley and slum housing to newly constructed public housing was paved with ostensibly good intentions. As a report of the NCHA covering its first ten years (1934–44) noted of its overall aim, "The objective remains constant, a city rid of all its slums, a city with *good* dwellings for *all* its people"[20] (my emphasis). John Ihdler, the executive officer and secretary of the authority, was the driving force behind its work and attempts to fulfil this objective. Throughout the report, there was an emphasis on the authority's aim to provide "good" housing. They frequently referred to "good low-rent housing" and providing "good dwellings for families of low income," and in particular they felt "the need for increasing the supply of good dwellings for Negro families of low income."[21] However, these aims were undermined by historical contingencies such as the Great Depression and World War II, the imposition of racialized institutional logics on the implementation of new housing policies, as well as a range of intersecting racialized policies. As I will illustrate, all these worked together to recreate disproportionate Black death.

A key constraint for the NCHA was an increase in demand for low-rent housing that far outstripped initial estimates. In addition to a burgeoning in-migrating Black population, the Great Depression (1929–41), with its attendant job losses, contributed to an increase in White and Black demand for low-cost housing.[22] Further, in the first 40 years of the 1900s, Black opportunities for employment and occupational mobility shrank due to new racialized employment policies. Previously, there had been robust Black participation and mobility in the federal government. However, the T. Roosevelt and Taft administrations began to racially segregate workers, and during President Wilson's administration, segregation and limited hiring and promotion of Black people became the de facto government policy.[23] The National Segregation Report, released in 1948 and researched by some of the nation's top sociologists, including the University of Chicago's Louis Wirth (who chaired the committee), Joseph Lohman, and E. Franklin Frazier, a Howard University sociologist and the first Black president of the American Sociological Association, among others,[24] noted:

> As late as 1938, 90% of all the government's Negro employees were confined to the lowest custodial labor status . . . Until 1940, the State department refused to hire colored people in Washington except as chauffeurs, messengers or janitors. (Between 1924 and 1940 no Negro was employed in the Department above the custodial level. The number of Negroes in the professional Foreign Service is less than half as large as it was forty years ago.)[25]

The loss of federal government jobs would have especially impacted the most educated Black people, leading to underemployment. This might explain why on Malcolm X's first visit to the city in 1941, he noted in his autobiography, "The old 'Colonial' railroaders had told me about Washington having a lot of 'middle class' Negroes with Howard University degrees, who were working as laborers, janitors, porters, guards, taxi-drivers, and the like. For the Negro in Washington, mail carrying was a prestige job."[26]

The Segregation Report, describing the Black job ceiling, noted that "three-fourths of all Negro job holders were employed as laborers, domestics, or service workers, while only one-eighth of White employees were in these categories."[27] It observed that Black people were often the "last to be promoted . . . first to be demoted . . . last to be hired . . . first to be fired."[28] Official and unofficial government and local racial policies limiting economic opportunity and occupational mobility in the second era meant that there would be greater demand for low-cost housing among Black people relative to their White counterparts.

Adding to the overall demand for housing were the many construction workers engaged in Depression-era public works projects to improve the city's infrastructure. In addition, World War II (1939–45) contributed to a rapid expansion of the federal government as large numbers of war workers and their families moved to the city and needed housing.[29] The NCHA was newly tasked with providing temporary housing for the war workers. Their new mandate made it clear that war workers were to be prioritized over low-income tenants and upgrades to existing poor Black housing.[30] There were also complex intraracial class implications. As the NCHA documented, because of a racial segregation policy, housing incoming Black war workers and their families was accomplished by deprioritizing the rehousing of low-income Black people displaced from demolished alley housing, and by displacing older Black homeowners and small-hold farmers. The latter's lands were initially seized under eminent domain to create new public housing for displaced Black tenants; war needs led to its use for temporary housing for Black war workers instead.[31] The racial and class containment principle thus led first to low-income Black tenants displacing Black home owners and then to higher-income Black people displacing their lower-income counterparts, inadvertently compounding their housing problems.

URBAN RENEWAL

Before alley housing could be demolished and cleared to make way for new housing, areas for improvement needed to be identified. Officials used the metaphors of "rotten fruit" and "infection" in their description of initial targets for alley-house removal.[32] Initial authority projects in 1935 involved replacing alley houses with garages to deal with a rising demand for city parking. As the NCHA report put it:

> These garage projects were an expression of the Authority's desire to test the theory of removing rot spots in otherwise good neighborhoods. i.e. to check the process under which slums had spread from inhabited alleys to the street properties and then across the streets. So in these instances it merely cut out the rotten core, hoping that the sounder areas would care for themselves.[33]

Around the same time, the American Public Health Association introduced a more "objective" way of identifying houses for removal, with a shift to the language of "blight." As Carolyn Swope describes, the housing appraisal method they developed in the 1930s

> identified key aspects of housing that influenced health and developed guidelines and an appraisal method for users to evaluate local housing. This method included inspection forms with a set of detailed housing and neighborhood conditions that were individually assigned scores and scaled; it was intended to be a "simple and objective" way to create "a concise and quantitative picture" of housing problems ... Planners and other urban officials used the collected data to create supposedly objective justification for which neighborhoods were deemed blighted and targeted for renewal.[34]

Swope went on to note that "the APHA found that Black people paid the same amount as White people for substantially worse housing conditions across every housing cost bracket."[35] There was thus a clear rationale for improving housing for Black families and thus a greater need to target Black housing for renewal. The method thus provided a seemingly objective way of identifying inferior housing that was detrimental to health, while also meaning that Black families were more likely, *a priori,* to suffer from displacement due to prior housing discrimination.

The NCHA acknowledged in 1938 that "for Negroes, very little new housing has been built, even for those who can afford to pay good rents";[36] this limited them to older housing stock. They went on to rather passively describe landlords' thinking and subsequent actions: "When a dwelling has deteriorated beyond a certain point or when the neighborhood has deteriorated, there is relaxation of attempts to keep it in good condition and repair. Then the rent goes down."[37]

Dwelling deterioration "beyond a certain point" was surely due to the lack of maintenance, and Black neighborhood deterioration similarly reflected collective neglect by area landlords and dereliction by the city in enforcing housing regulations. (Presumably if landlords were displeased with tenants, they would not lack for new tenants given the very high demand for low-rent housing and the ability of some Black people to "pay good rents.") Thus the Segregation Report observed that "the physical ghettoes ... give racism a base by the Lincoln Memorial,"[38] and Malcolm X described how he "was astounded to find in the nation's capital, just a few blocks from Capitol Hill, thousands of Negroes living worse than any I'd ever seen in the poorest sections of Roxbury; in dirt-floor shacks along unspeakably filthy lanes with names like Pig Alley and Goat Alley."[39] But he also "saw other Negroes better off, they lived in blocks of rundown red brick houses."[40]

The NCHA gradually shifted from a "rot removal" approach to clearing alley houses and slums altogether, while retaining street-front housing. (In the case of Baltimore, Samuel Roberts documents how "infected house theory" was used to justify slum clearance of segregated Black neighborhoods where tuberculosis cases were high).[41] Following the racial containment principle, slums were first replaced with low-rent public housing for either White families or Black families.[42] (I describe public housing in more detail later.) This was then followed by the targeting of entire Black neighborhoods for destruction. The latter approach was accelerated by World War II, with new needs for land for war-related buildings, such as the Navy Yard, housing for war workers, and new military highways, especially in SE and SW DC where there had been more predominantly Black neighborhoods (as opposed to neighborhoods with tertiary street-front/backyard segregation). As the Segregation Report described:

> Large areas formerly occupied by Negroes have been condemned for government buildings, parks, schools and highway systems. In recent years, many Negro families have been dislodged by the new Federal buildings on Constitution Avenue, by war housing projects for Whites in the Garfield section of the southeast, by the expansion of the Navy yard, and the super highway network built to service the Pentagon Building and the National Airport... Colored people are displaced by public improvements more often than Whites because they are concentrated in blighted downtown areas that are suitable for public construction. And once unhoused, they are worse off than Whites because they cannot move freely in the District.[43]

Many simply moved into yet-to-be demolished slums, exacerbating the situation there. As reporter Agnes E. Meyer, writing in *The Washington Post* in 1944 under the headline "Negro Housing—Capital Sets Record for U.S. in Unalleviated Wretchedness of Slums," described:

> In my journey through the war centers I have visited the worst possible housing. But not in the Negro slums of Detroit, not even in the Southern cities, have I seen human beings subjected to such unalleviated wretchedness as in the alleys of our own city of Washington. ... The crowding in the slums of the District has also been intensified by the fact that not only housing but the areas formerly occupied by Negroes have decreased. Various developments such as public buildings, war housing projects for Whites and new roads have swept away many acres of ground heretofore open to Negro occupancy.[44]

Neighborhoods were not just cleared for federal and war needs or because the areas had alley and slum dwellings, however. Large swaths of Black non-alley/slum dwellings across the city were subject to demolition, ostensibly because they were labeled as blight and thus condemned in the name of urban renewal, public health, and the City Beautiful movement.[45] However, land was also cleared for private development to create housing to compete with the suburbs, where increasing numbers of middle class and affluent White people were moving.

The Case of Southwest DC

Alley and slum housing, precisely because it was in some of the oldest parts of the city and in walking distance to central locations, was often located on prime land. As such, part of the early debate was about the best use of cleared land, and in particular, whether, as a news article put it, DC should be "ceding in perpetuum the best city land to the lowest income families and in all probability creating new slums for the future"[46] or whether the land should instead be sold to private developers. Then, either the private market could meet the low-income housing demand, especially for displaced people, or public housing could be constructed for them elsewhere. This latter argument eventually made its way into law in 1945 when Congress passed the District of Columbia Redevelopment Act (including creating the Redevelopment Land Agency [RLA] in DC) and the National Housing Act in 1949. These acts together enabled private developers to have priority in redeveloping newly cleared slum areas with non–low rent housing, and it also allowed the RLA to legally acquire land through eminent domain and convey it to private developers at subsidized rates.[47] This process became formally known as "urban renewal" in the Housing Act of 1954.[48] The case of SW DC is instructive.

After the 1945 and 1949 laws, a new city planning process in 1950 identified SW DC, home to over 20,000 Black and immigrant Jewish residents and business owners, as a priority "problem area" of the city, and it was prioritized for renewal. As Amy Lavine described, the planning report found that "out of the entire 550 acre area, 43% of the residences had only outhouses, 44% did not have showers or baths, 70% had no central heating, and 21% did not have electricity." Some parts were overcrowded, with "death rates from tuberculosis [that] were 136% higher and mortality from syphilis . . . a staggering 489% above the city average."[49] Thus, quality of housing along with health were jointly used to justify its problem-area designation. However, as Asch and Musgrove noted, "[The] Southwest also featured fine row houses of brick or wood with carefully tended front and back lawns. Indeed the Homebuilders' Association of Metropolitan Washington found that many homes were 'as sound and in many cases as large as fashionable homes in Georgetown.'"[50]

The alternative, of course, was to retain existing quality housing, rehabilitate and upgrade the worst parts of the neighborhood, and improve health care access (curative medication for syphilis and TB had been in use since at least 1943[51]). Instead, the renewal plan called for building condemnation, eminent domain to acquire the land, demolition of the entire area, and land conveyance to private developers (who were required to set aside some affordable housing units) and to the government to build a new highway. A lawsuit fighting the government's use of eminent domain to obtain privately owned land was lodged by businessmen and eventually made its way to the Supreme Court in the 1954 *Berman v. Parker*. In deciding for the city, the court stated, "If those who govern the District of Columbia decide that the Nation's Capital should be beautiful as well as sanitary, there is nothing in the [Constitution] that stands in the way."[52] In addition to devastating losses for Jewish business people, a reporter in the *Pittsburgh-Washington Courier* wrote in 1949:

> The plea that "thousands of Negroes will lose their life savings and become renters or objects of charity; hundreds of Negro business enterprises will be wiped out; hundreds of Negro churches will be destroyed and their membership scattered; Negro professional men will lose their clientele" is seen as a poor excuse for not making Washington the most beautiful city in the world.[53]

The area was subsequently demolished and new award-winning units for 3,600 people were built and priced to attract wealthy residents.[54] New tenants were predominantly White, and affordable housing was abandoned. As Francesca Russello Ammon described:

> By 1960, only 2 percent of all occupied units had black residents ... [and it was] determined that it would not be feasible to offer one-third of the units at an affordable rent, arguing that cost increases had made the rent limit impractical and that affordable housing was available in other parts of the city. The RLA responded in 1959 by removing this provision from the entire Southwest project.[55]

Thus, thousands of former Black residents were permanently displaced from SW DC.

CONSTRUCTION OF PUBLIC HOUSING:
FROM TENANTS TO STATE DEPENDENTS

As the ranks of displaced people climbed, public housing became not just a mandate but an imperative. District housing authorities (variously the Alley Dwelling Authority, NCHA, and RLA) were painfully aware of the costs of congressional and city policies as the reality of Black people's inability to find alternative housing on the private market became immediately apparent, a problem that was compounded with each subsequent demolition. Their own efforts to relocate displaced residents were frustrating, and private developers preferred to build to sell, as opposed to building rentals, especially for low-income tenants.[56]

Congressional actions also added significant constraints on the construction of public housing, as the housing authority was no longer able to build on newly cleared land and had to find land elsewhere. The containment principle provided further limitations, as they could only build public housing for a racial group in areas where that racial group already lived. Often land on which slums were located was prohibitively expensive or prioritized for private developers, leading the authority to seek locations far from the city center, where Black tenants did not necessarily want to move.[57] The National Association of Home Builders as well as the National Association of Real Estate Boards[58] also put negative pressure on public housing in Washington, DC, seeing victory in the District as helping to secure national victory in halting public housing altogether. As the National Association of Home Builders put it, "We are fearful that if subsidized housing is accepted in this country, that subsidized medicine, subsidized food production, and eventually completely subsidized industry will follow, destroying our unique American system of private enterprise, and gradually changing us into a socialistic state."[59]

It was also clear, however, that the battle was not just about public housing for low-income people but also about race. There was fierce resistance from White citizen's associations to the siting of public housing in or near their neighborhoods, especially Black public housing projects, with some upzoning their properties to prevent construction of public housing units.[60] In the case of Parkside Dwellings, for example, the authority, on a limited budget, finally located an inexpensive site in SE DC "near the banks of the Anacostia River and adjoining the abandoned Benning race track." While there were "7 white families living in old houses" in the area, it had been "trending toward complete Negro occupancy for many years."[61] As the NCHA went on to report:

> Soon after these phases of project development were begun, the Authority received protests from associations of white persons in the northeast Anacostia area. These protests were not against the construction of a public housing property but against the proposal, which had been announced by the Authority, that the dwellings to be constructed would be for Negro occupancy.[62]

John Ihdler, the executive officer of the authority met with citizen association representatives and elaborated on the strategy of racial containment the authority had pursued in siting the project to try to appease their concerns, describing

> that the project site was bounded by industrial property on one side, by a broad avenue and trolley tracks on another, by the old race track on a third side and by a public park on a fourth; that the site was not adjacent to any neighborhood with predominantly white occupancy; and that the necessity for additional housing for Negro families was critical.[63]

By 1965, DC's housing agency had constructed 37 public housing projects, more than half of which were located in the SE, with many others located in the NE and SW quadrants of the city. Over 41,000 people lived in the projects,[64] and many of the 20,000 people displaced by the demolitions in the SW were funneled into public housing.[65] In 1940, 83% of public housing residents were Black;[66] by 1965, 98% were Black, and 60% of residents lived at or below the poverty line.[67] While, at least initially, Black housing quality was significantly better than before, the overall effect of the urban renewal effort was to move thousands of Black people from owning their homes, or paying rent to private owners and living in close proximity to White people, to being public housing tenants located in racially contained and distant locations.

CREATING A NEW RACIAL GEOGRAPHY

The new form of racial containment was constructed with many layers of redundancy, involving multiple institutions, which worked to entrench racial economic inequality through housing (with intergenerational implications).[68] Housing, in turn, was a primary mechanism for the reproduction of racial health inequality.

Public resistance to the authority's public housing efforts led on more than one occasion to "vigorous attack on the NCHA" at congressional hearings. The NCHA report describes "Mr Harry S. Wender, President of the Federation of Citizens' Associations . . . testifying [as] an individual citizen [and] speaking of the 'numerous controversies before the Zoning Commission and courts on zoning questions' having to do with low-cost housing, both private and public, and on criticisms of NCHA." The report quoted him saying:

> I think it is only fair for me to say publicly now what has been privately said [on] many occasions in recent months, and which has been said, of course, in citizen association meetings and has been reported in the press, that if we are to have a proper picture at this hearing of this problem, we must understand that the race problem cannot be removed from the public housing picture.[69]

A principal way in which the race problem was expressed was "through the sincere rhetoric of home ownership and property values."[70] In other words, White property owners were genuinely concerned that the siting of Black housing near White housing would bring down the value of their homes. (As noted earlier, there was less objection to White public housing.)

Indeed, the connection between race and land value was an important lynchpin underlying the new racial geography of the second era, and it became a key means through which White supremacist ideology about Black inferiority became institutionalized. Once the idea that the presence of Black people devalued a place took hold, keeping Black people out of one's neighborhood could then become tied to the apparently race-neutral goal of preserving property values. This then led to a self-perpetuating process of White flight from neighborhoods when Black families moved in, racial covenants to prevent Black people from buying homes in a neighborhood, and protests (including violent protests[71]) to keep Black public housing from being constructed in or near a neighborhood. It also meant that once land became designated as a predominantly Black area, it became cheaper to buy, resulting in both depressed home values for Black property owners as well as cheaper land in Black areas for the construction of public housing, thus leading to a concentration of public housing in Black areas. In addition, they were convenient city sacrifice zones; cheap lands that were unattractive to private developers and occupied by marginalized groups were viable sites for municipal dumps, major highways, and other such uses.[72]

This attachment of race to land value was expressed in article 34 of the National Association of Real Estate Board's Code of Ethics in 1924, which stated that "a Realtor should never be instrumental in introducing into a neighborhood a character of property or occupancy, members of any race or nationality, or any individuals whose presence will clearly be detrimental to property values in that neighborhood."[73] Describing the work of Richard Ely, who founded the Institute for Research in Land Economics in 1920, Winling and Michney described how economists in conjunction with the National Association of Real Estate Boards worked together to devise "the nature of [land] value" and how it was to be determined. The goal was to create a more explicit racialized system of land value and to "standardize professional real estate work," with the thinking that this would ultimately reduce racial conflict. As they put it:

> In economists' (and appraisers') way of thinking, racial exclusion was not a moral consideration but rather a legal and practical one, because separating Black from white was deemed fundamental to preserving real estate values ... racial deed restrictions and covenants to manage residential real estate markets ... were intended to preempt African American access to white neighborhoods and stabilize property values of white-owned homes.[74]

These ideas were subsequently codified in various ways in the 1932 Federal Home Loan Bank Act, the 1933 Home Owners' Loan Act and its linked corporation, the Home Owners' Loan Corporation, and the 1934 National Housing Act and linked Federal Housing Administration.[75] Michney and Winling note that "it was the NAACP's discovery in December 1938, of Section 223 in the FHA *Underwriters Manual* requiring racial segregation ... that conclusively confirmed the existence of a systematic policy of discrimination and prompted more assertive demands for reform."[76] In Washington, DC, these land and housing policies played out in a variety of ways, working to turbocharge already ongoing actions of different federal and local governments and private actors who worked in concert, both intentionally and unintentionally, to produce a new racial geography throughout the second era. This process was also overseen and officially sanctioned and pursued by a long series of senators and House representatives sitting on the District committees that controlled city government. In 1946, for example, Senator Theodore G. Bilbo from Mississippi, chairman of the Senate District committee, explicitly said, "I wanted this position so I could keep Washington a segregated city."[77]

Federal and District Government, Developers, Real Estate Agents, and Lending Institutions

As the District government pushed poor tenants out of alley/slum housing and blighted areas into racially segregated public housing, developers and lending institutions moved to dispossess more well-to-do Black people from their historic homes to create exclusively White neighborhoods. A particular focus of these efforts was Georgetown.[78] As the 1948 Segregation Report detailed:

> Since the 1920s, this old part of Washington has been promoted as a quaint, historic, desirable place for White people to live. The dispossession of Negro residents is part of the redevelopment project, and is jointly managed by the city's leading realtors and their allied banks and trust companies. A few Negro home-owners have succumbed to inflated prices and have sold willingly. Others have been compelled to sell after being refused loans for repairs and improvements. As a matter of policy, the lending institutions of Washington deny credit to colored people in regions being prepared for Whites. Many Negro tenants have been evicted so that White owners could remodel or rent or sell to Whites at substantially increased prices. And as the White developers have moved into Georgetown, they have covenanted it block by block with racial restrictions to keep any Negro from returning.[79]

Once designated as a White area, the city's real estate community considered it a matter of ethics to keep it that way. The Washington Real Estate Board Code of Ethics stated as early as 1921 (and later expanded):

> No property in a White section should ever be sold, rented, advertised or offered to colored people. In case of doubt, advice from the Public Affairs Committee should be obtained. (As a general rule, the Board takes the position that any neighborhood is White if 50% or more of its inhabitants are White.)[80]

The federal and District governments supported these racial containment efforts in a variety of ways. Manning described how

> both the Federal and District governments promoted passive segregation policies . . . These include restrictive covenants for preventing property transfers to specified groups (primarily Blacks and Jews), denying construction permits and/or financing for African American housing developments outside the designated Black zones, condemning Black-owned residential property in the "public interest" (highways, public buildings, parks, White housing), permitting suburban communities to reject federal funds for public housing, and administering federal mortgage loan (FHA, VA) programmes so that Blacks would not be able to purchase homes in the suburbs.[81]

> 5. The Negro problem has not improved. In communities where there is any possibility of infiltration, application for insurance should be rejected.

FIGURE 16. "The Negro Problem," excerpt from a Federal Housing Administration report, 1940. Source: Federal Housing Administration, *Interim Report on Conditions in the Washington D.C. Housing Market, as of June 1, 1940*, p. viii. Uncovered by Sarah Shoenfeld, Mapping Segregation in D.C. (Prologue DC, 2019). For the report, see https://www.dcpolicycenter.org/publications/mapping-segregation-fha/.

A confidential FHA report, uncovered by historian Sarah Shoenfeld at Prologue DC, titled *Interim Report on Conditions in the Washington, D.C. Housing Market as of June 1, 1940* offered as one of its conclusions: "The Negro problem has not improved. In communities where there is any possibility of infiltration, application for insurance should be rejected"[82] (shown in print in Figure 16). This guidance brought the full weight of the federal government to bear, adding another layer of redundancy to efforts by homeowners' racial covenants, real estate agents' codes of ethics, and developers' strategies to ensure racial containment. Banks followed their cue in their mortgage approval/denial process, rating Black neighborhoods "hazardous for mortgage lending."[83]

The 1937 government map in Figure 17, uncovered by Sarah Shoenfeld and Mara Cherkasky at Prologue DC as part of the project "Mapping Segregation," shows the FHA's coding of the city and its suburbs.[84] The darker A areas were the best, loan worthy areas, and lighter H areas were the worst. The map illustrates the beginnings of intergenerational wealth creation among White families who were able to buy homes in the northwest of the city. While thousands of Black people eventually bought homes in the city, especially after White migration to the suburbs began in earnest in the second half of the century,[85] thousands of others were consigned to lives as renters and to the vagaries of the rental market in the eastern and southern parts of the city.[86]

NET EFFECT OF RACIAL CONTAINMENT EFFORTS

Figure 18 illustrates the net effects of these efforts. Between 1880 and 1930, residential patterns shifted from Southern-style tertiary segregation to Northern-style primary segregation,[87] with the races geographically separated. This occurred despite large overall population increases recorded in the census (from 177,624 in 1880 to 486,869 in 1930) and Black population

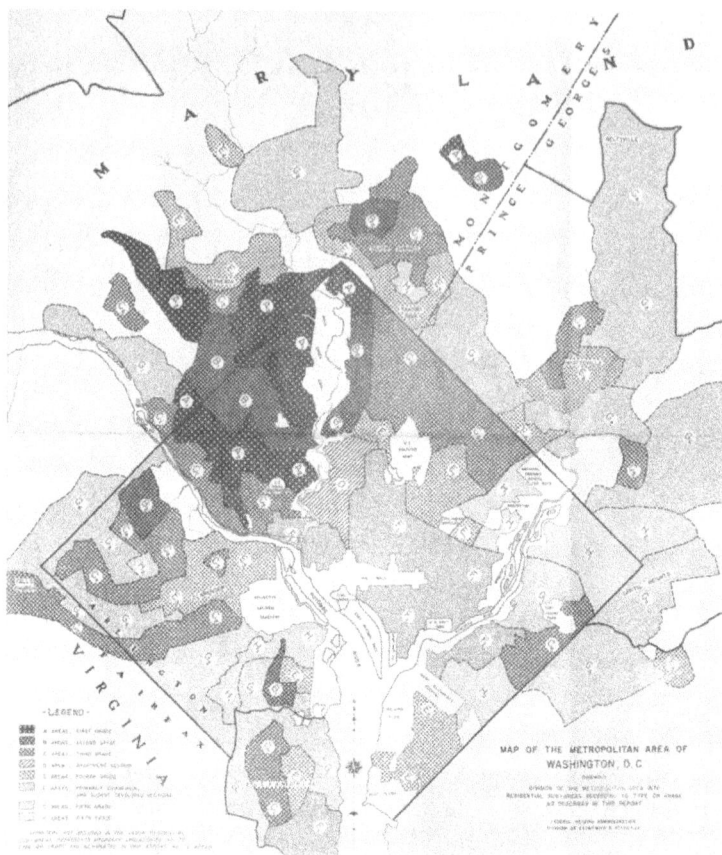

FIGURE 17. Federal Housing Administration rating map, DC, 1937. Sources: Sarah Shoenfeld, Mapping Segregation in D.C., https://mapping segregationdc.org/resident-sub-areas.html; https://mappingsegregationdc.org /assets/fha-commitments-in-metropolitan-dc-12–31–1936.pdf; https:// mappingsegregationdc.org/assets/residential-sub-areas-for-website-rev.pdf. Housing Market Analysis, Washington, DC, July 1937, Federal Housing Administration, Division of Economics and Statistics, August 5, 1937, pp. 19–26. (Research and Statistics Division, Records Relating to Housing Market Analyses, 1935–42, Box 17, RG 31, National Archives.) National Archives and Records Administration.

increases (from 59,596 in 1880 to 132,068 in 1930), showing the sheer impact of early passive and active containment policies and actions by the government, real estate agencies, developers, and landlords *before* the official start of urban renewal. As the population continued to expand between 1930 and 1950 (to an overall 802,178 in 1950, of whom 280,803 were Black), new policies and practices in that period ensured that the approximately 150,000 new

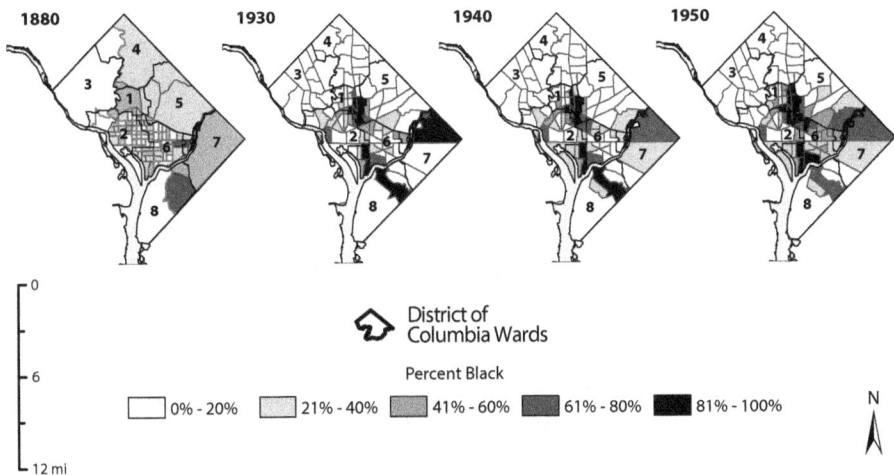

FIGURE 18. Racial containment in Washington, DC, 1880–1950. 1880 data source: US Census Bureau; John R. Logan, Jason Jindrich, Hyoungjin Shin, and Weiwei Zhang, 2011, Mapping America in 1880: The Urban Transition Historical GIS Project, *Historical Methods* 44(1):49–60, https://s4.ad .brown.edu/Projects/UTP/Default.aspx. 1930–1950 data source: US Census Bureau (NHGIS, IPUMS).

Black additions were carefully funneled and absorbed into the new racial geography. The maps make clear what observers noted: "Looked at it in one way, the colored people are being contained."[88]

These citywide dynamics contributed to a severe housing crisis for many Black people, reeling from the destruction of their homes, churches, businesses, communities, and livelihoods, and from a kind of trauma Mindy Fullilove has called "root shock."[89] Shut out of White-only suburbs, they also confronted employment and housing racial discrimination in the city, reducing the stock of housing they could access. As a result of the limited supply for Black people, the Segregation Report documented Black people renting and buying homes at rates as high as 30% more than White people.[90] Many poorer families simply doubled up, resulting in severe overcrowding. The report described:

> A sample census survey made in 1947 indicates that a Negro family is two and a half times as likely as a White family to live in a dwelling containing six or more persons. A Negro family is also:
>
> 9 times as likely to live in a house needing structural repair
> 4 times as likely to lack a private flush toilet
> 10 times as likely to lack central heating
> 11 times as likely to lack running water
> 8 times as likely to lack electric lights[91]

Comparison of death rates of street and alley residents with respect to race and age.

Age.	Death rate.					
	White.		Colored.		Total.	
	Alley.	Street.	Alley.	Street.	Alley.	Street.
Under 1 year........................	170.73	114.85	402.06	286.59	373.49	158.66
1 to 4 years........................	23.26	11.71	31.65	31.34	30.82	16.75
5 to 20 years.......................	....	3.61	8.77	9.96	7.84	5.25
21 years and over..................	12.57	10.10	28.75	23.94	27.05	18.08
All ages...........................	14.30	14.73	31.94	25.84	30.09	17.56

FIGURE 19. Mortality rates of DC residents by race and place, 1910. Source: DC Board of Health, *Annual Report of the Commissioners of the District of Columbia*, 1910.

HEALTH CONSEQUENCES

Overall, these dynamics contributed to the reproduction of racial inequality in mortality between 1890 and 1950.[92] In 1900, Black residents died at almost twice (1.75) the rate of White people (death rates were 30.31/1,000 for Black people and 17.36/1,000 for White people).[93] And residents died young. The Board of Health (BOH) report noted that 31% of deaths occurred among children aged 5 and younger, and "the average age of all decedents was 32 years, 2 months and 24 days; of the whites alone, 39 yrs, 2 months, and 11 days and of the colored, 25 years, 3 months and 6 days."[94] By 1910, though death rates had declined, in a continuation of previous trends, Black people died at almost twice (1.81) the rate of White people (the White death rate was 14.73/1,000 while the Black death rate was 26.7/1,000).[95] The 1910 BOH report also examined mortality differences by age, race, and location, uncovering stark inequality.[96] As Figure 19 illustrates, overall, regardless of race, almost 40% of infants in alley dwellings died before the age of 1, and they had 2.4 times higher death rates (373.49/1,000) than infants in street-front dwellings (158.66/1,000). Further highlighting the significance of class containment, within-race differences were stark; infants in alley dwellings had approximately 1.5 times higher death rates compared to same-race infants in street-front dwellings. However, between-race differences were even more stark; Black infants in both alley and street-front dwellings had approximately 2.5 times higher death rates compared to their respective White counterparts. Disproportionate Black death was thus a combination of both race and class, mediated through the location of their housing.

Overall, most deaths in 1910 were attributed to pulmonary tuberculosis and pneumonia (caused by viruses, bacteria, and fungi). Diarrhea was particularly hazardous for Black children under the age of two compared to White infants.[97] These diseases can be rife in overcrowded, unsanitary, and polluted settings. The 1920 BOH report recorded clear declines in mortality since 1900. While the average age at death in 1919 was 42 years, 11 months,[98] when disaggregated by race, the average White age at death was 46 years, 6 months while the average Black age at death was 36 years, 5 months—a 10-year difference in the average age of death. There was a 9-year difference between Black and White men and an 11-year difference between women.[99] In addition to the influenza epidemic, the major causes of death in 1920 continued to be TB and pneumonia.[100] By mid-century, the 1948 Segregation Report observed: "The life expectancy of a Colored resident of Washington is ten to twelve years less than that of a White resident. In 1944, his chances of dying were 37% greater. Elsewhere in the nation, the Colored death rate was only 19% higher than the White death rate."[101] Further, "Colored babies born in the District were almost twice as likely to die as White babies, and Negro mothers were six times as likely to die as White mothers."[102] The Segregation Report also noted that compared to White residents, Black residents were "more than four times as likely to die from [TB] . . . because they are segregated by race in the worst jobs and dwellings."[103] It pointed out that "Colored people who had moderate incomes and lived in adequate houses" had lower death rates than White people living in slum areas, highlighting the role of poverty and low quality housing in shaping death outcomes.

The Board of Health's 1950 report documented worsening racial inequality five years after the statistics reported in the Segregation Report. In 1949, non-White people (the new racial label for Black people in the BOH report[104]) were 43% more likely to die than White people.[105] The epidemiological transition from infectious to chronic diseases had begun, and heart disease and cancer accounted for a "staggering" 45.9% of deaths in DC.[106] However, TB continued to claim many more Black (123.4/100,000) than White lives (21.5/100,000).[107] The infant mortality rate was 26.4/1,000 live births, a significant improvement from 10 years earlier (48/1,000). However, non-White infants were 36% more likely to die than White infants.[108] Notably, the city was especially proud of the "new all-time record low maternal death rate"[109] and noted a slow but steady decrease in the racial gap, with non-White mothers now having only 2.3 times higher death rates than White mothers.

The Segregation Report also highlighted racial inequalities in health care access. Only two public hospitals accepted people of color. Ironically, while, the "District health department spen[t] two thirds of its funds on the care of colored people and they occupy a third of the hospital beds . . . the facilities available to them are inferior and far short of their greater need."[110] Black people primarily used public hospitals because even though some private hospitals were funded with public money, "private hospitals allot only 14.5% of beds to Negro wards; so 78% of public hospital beds are occupied by Negros."[111] What is striking is that the report discusses this as being significantly worse than 60 years before, noting:

> In 1889, the United States Senate asked for a report on the racial policies of Washington's hospitals, and all of the eleven which then served the city replied that no person was denied admission on account of 'race, color or previous condition of servitude.' Now, a fourth of the 12 private hospitals exclude Negroes altogether, and the remainder allot them a limited number of beds in segregated wards.[112]

The report noted that Howard University (established in 1868) had "one of the country's two medical schools for Negroes." The report documented that it had at one point a third (26/72) of the nation's "certified Negro specialists and 200 licensed Negro practitioners," but they were

> barred by the District Medical Society, and from the American Medical Association [AMA]. They are barred from all the twelve private hospitals of the city, and from federally supported St Elizabeth's Hospital for mental diseases. There is only one hospital (348 bed Freedmen's) in the city to which a Negro physician can take a private patient.[113]

In other words, the city had numerous Black doctors and specialists, but they were barred from treating patients in most of the city's hospitals. (Full AMA access with fortified non-discrimination policies occurred in 1968 after decades of protest).[114] The Segregation Report concluded the section, noting:

> As long as Colored people are segregated in the worst slums and the worst jobs, their health will be inferior to that of unsegregated White people . . . those who need hospital attention the most will get the least.[115]

In sum, considerable efforts by health activists, a succession of presidents, a first lady, and one arm of the government, the NCHA, to improve housing and health conditions for the poorest, especially Black, residents of

Washington, DC, were undermined by the actions of a variety of other government and private actors and institutions, such as other presidents, the congressional District committees, the FHA, real estate developers, banks, White citizen associations, the American Public Health Association, the AMA, and the District Medical Society, among others. Collectively, they worked to modernize and beautify the city, extract maximal profit from prime land, and create and institutionalize a new form of racial containment. The result was severely reduced availability of housing and overcrowded environments for Black people in racially contained parts of the city. And this reproduced new syndemic zones of economic disadvantage and multiple overlapping epidemics, the latter of which were poorly controlled due to racialized neglect—such as condemning homes as opposed to treating people—and denial of adequate health care access to hospitals. In the process, these actors also contributed to a reproduction of the relationship between space, race, health, and disproportionate Black death.

THREE

The Third Era

1950–PRESENT

AFTER 1950, NEW FORMS of racial containment emerged and solidified: the "chocolate city/vanilla suburbs," a term popularized by the band Parliament, and the "cappuccino city," coined by Derek Hyra to describe the late 20th and early 21st century influx of White migrants who began gentrifying low-income Black neighborhoods.[1] Alongside residential shifts, there was a changing governance structure as residents gained partial independence from Congress and Black leaders won mayorships for the first time. However, as I will show, the connection between space, race, and health not only persisted but was exacerbated in the third era. Once DC became a chocolate city, a paradoxical question emerged: Why did racial health inequalities not just persist but widen under Black leadership? In this final chapter of Part 1, I describe the common and unique governance challenges that came with these new forms of racial containment for Black mayors and for DC's mayors in particular. I show how when the city gained partial self-governance, power came with impossible strings attached by the predominantly White Congress, giving Black leaders limited options to achieve contradictory ends. Their solutions resulted either in a questioning of Black legitimacy to lead or in a judgment of Black leaders as competent but whose policies generally resulted in class containment activities that benefitted middle class and affluent White and Black people and came at the expense of poor Black people. The latter's disproportionate presence in the city contributed to the overall widening of racial health inequality.

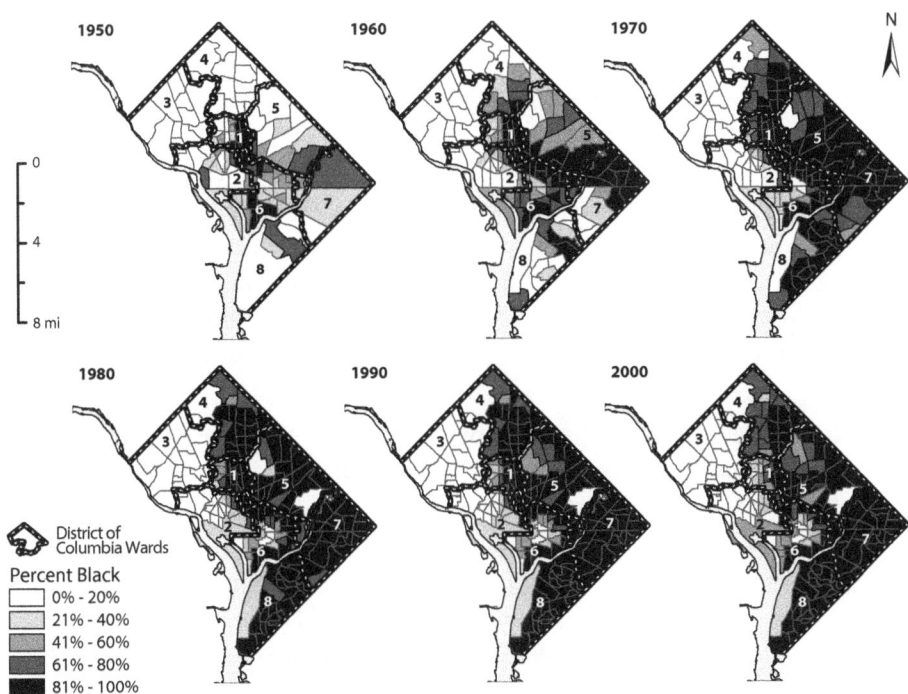

FIGURE 20. "Chocolate City," 1950–2000. Data source: US Census Bureau (NHGIS, IPUMS).

THE NEW RACIAL CONTAINMENT:
FROM CHOCOLATE CITY/VANILLA SUBURBS
TO CAPPUCCINO CITY

Figure 20 illustrates the racial transformation of the city between 1950 and 2000. In 1950, the city was 35% Black, by 1960, it was 53.9% Black, and by 1970, Washington, DC, was a "chocolate city" at 70.7% Black (see Figure 10). Nonetheless, the maps illustrate a clear racial separation, with Black residents to the east and White residents to the west.

The city began to transition to a cappuccino city in the 1990s, as White people returned (25.2% in 1980, 27.6% in 1990, 27.9% in 2000), and Black people began to migrate out (69.7% in 1980, 65.4% in 1990, 59.5% in 2000).[2] By 2010, White and Black people comprised 34.8% and 50% of the city, respectively, and in 2020 DC was no longer a chocolate city, with a 38% White and 40.9% Black population (see Figure 10). (While as discussed in the Introduction, the book narrowly focuses on the non-Hispanic Black/

White gap, it is nonetheless important to note that the city became multicultural over this period. The non-Black/White population—most of whom were Hispanic and Asian—was 2.9% in 1970, 5.1% in 1980, 7% in 1990, 12.5% in 2000, 15.2% in 2010, and 21.1% in 2020 [see Figure 10]).

A number of factors underlay these Black/White settlement patterns. At the beginning of the third era, racial containment now worked to keep Black people in the city through federal-loan or insurance denials for purchasing suburban homes, suburban racial covenants, and discriminatory real estate agent practices before—and even some years after—the 1968 Fair Housing Act.[3] Meanwhile, thousands of renting and homeownership opportunities in the city opened up for Black residents,[4] and over 250,000 Black in-migrants were drawn to the chocolate city between 1950 and 1970.[5] Residential opportunities were created by over 350,000 White people leaving between 1950 and 1980[6] to take advantage of the rapid development of suburban Maryland and Virginia homes, federal employment, as branches of the government moved to the suburbs, and a dramatically expanded highway system to ease commuting.[7] They also left in the aftermath of riots following Martin Luther King Jr.'s assassination in 1968.[8] White out-migration mirrored nationwide trends.[9]

Suburban racial composition changed when developments welcoming Black people in Maryland and Virginia began to be constructed, as Karyn Lacy documented.[10] The period also marked a large expansion of middle class Black people, following the civil rights era ending of legal racial discrimination and a resumption of unrestricted federal employment. The subsequent exodus of many middle class and affluent Black people from the city reflected not just economic mobility but also pent-up demand after decades of denial and a desire for access to more space and, among the affluent, more luxury.[11] They were also taking advantage of new suburban job opportunities and escaping worsening city service delivery and schools.[12] While in 1947, Black people comprised 2.3% of the total Black population in the larger metropolitan statistical area (MSA), this increased over the half century, with most of the Black MSA population living in the suburbs after 1990 (20.7% in 1960, 25% in 1970, 47.5% in 1980, 61.6% in 1990, 82.7% in 2000).[13]

Within the city, racial containment dynamics through cappuccino-style gentrification led to dramatic neighborhood changes. For example, between 1980 and 2000, in Wards 1 (which includes neighborhoods such as Columbia Heights) and 2 (which includes neighborhoods such as Shaw), the Black pro-

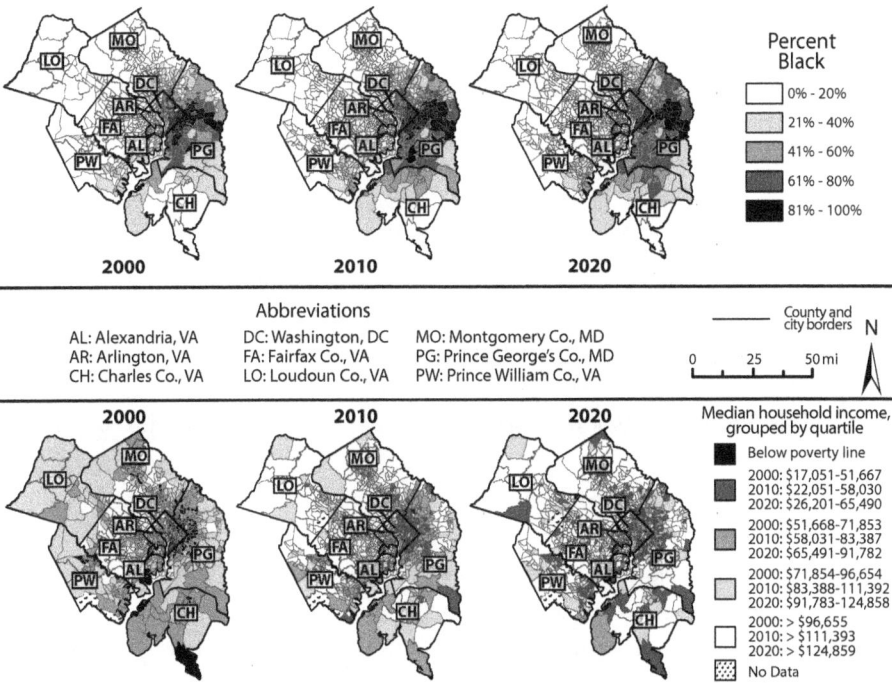

FIGURE 21. Race and income distribution in DC and its suburbs, 2000–2020. Data source: US Census Bureau (NHGIS, IPUMS).

portions of the population reduced from 70% to 46% and from 35% to 23%, respectively.[14] Overall, these dynamics served both to concentrate Black people into particular neighborhoods and to increasingly shift the class composition of out-migraters towards poorer Black people, displaced out of the city and into Prince George's (PG) County in Maryland.[15] The city itself became more unequal. The suburban exodus led to not only population declines but also to job and retail sales losses.[16] Journalists Harry Jaffe and Tom Sherwood noted that "nearly one-third of those remaining [in the city] — 180,000 — were on the public assistance rolls,"[17] and the city's poorest were concentrated in Wards 7 and 8, which were 97% and 98% Black by 2000.[18] By 2010 and 2020, as illustrated in Figure 7, wards with the highest concentrations of Black people also had the highest proportions living in poverty.[19]

Racial containment was also evident in the suburbs.[20] As Figure 21 illustrates, between 2000 and 2020, while there were integrated suburban areas, many suburbanites lived in predominantly same-race neighborhoods.

Predominantly White suburbs were generally wealthier than predominantly Black suburbs; however, there was wide intraracial inequality, including wealthy, predominantly Black suburbs (e.g., in parts of PG County) and poor, predominantly White suburbs (e.g., in parts of Charles County).[21] Overall, the statistical portrait of the 60-year period illustrates dramatic shifts in the city's inter- and intraracial dynamics. The capital became an iconic Black city with striking Black/White inequality alongside intraracial inequality in the city and suburbs, creating distinct social worlds Jaffe and Sherwood described as "the black middle class ... sandwiched between a small class of Black aristocrats and the poor Blacks," in other words, "a segregated city among Blacks."[22]

This complex statistical portrait might partly explain the paradox of some of the nation's most advantaged and disadvantaged Black people living within the same MSA, with each seemingly masking the other's presence. When viewed with a wide lens, incorporating the entire MSA, DC's Black people are among the most privileged in the country, but when viewed with a narrow focus on those living within the District limits, as I mostly do in this book, some of the city's Black residents are among the most disadvantaged in the nation. The dynamics of widening intraracial inequality among Black people, both economically and residentially—a seeming delinking of Black fates[23]—was reflected in the city's governance and in its health outcomes.

THE PARADOXICAL GOVERNANCE OF
A CHOCOLATE CITY

It was not until 1975 that Washington, DC, was able to have a popularly elected mayor, an elected city government, and partial self-governance, 100 years after power was wrested from it by Congress.[24] (In 1967, Walter Washington was appointed as "mayor-commissioner" by President Lyndon Johnson in a transitional role before becoming mayor in 1975.) For the past 50 years, the city has been led by Black mayors, as shown in Table 1. The task of the DC mayor is unique compared to other mayors, combining functions of a state governor, city mayor, and county official. (DC is often compared to states, including in federal statistics; its population has been approximately 600,000–800,000 between 1950 and 2020;[25] the smallest US states—Wyoming and Vermont—have about 600,000 people. Further, the city notes

TABLE 1 Mayors of Washington, DC, 1975–present

Walter Washington	1967–75 (mayor-commissioner)
	1975–79 (mayor)
Marion Barry	1979–91
Sharon Pratt Kelly	1991–95
Marion Barry	1995–99
Anthony A. Williams	1999–2007
Adrian Fenty	2007–11
Vincent C. Gray	2011–15
Muriel Bowser	2015–present

that it is "treated as a state in more than 500 federal laws.")[26] Writing in the mid-1990s, Meyers succinctly summarized the task in this way:

> The District is a unique jurisdiction. No other city in America has the District's *state* functions of welfare and Medicaid responsibility, maintenance of a state court, prison and parole system, a state-level university, a state-level employment service and job training administration, disability compensation, state occupational safety and health enforcement, state licensing and utility and banking regulation, motor vehicle registration, and the like, in addition to such *county* functions as a county hospital, nursing homes, community mental health facilities, alcohol and drug abuse services and public libraries along with the usual *city* services such as police, fire, public works, traffic control and recreation. *[my italics]*[27]

(As I explain in Part 5, in 1997, the federal government took over some of these costly functions, including "a $2 billion unfunded pension liability, which had been accumulated entirely by the Federal Government," which the city inherited when it gained home rule; it "had grown to $5 billion, almost entirely as a function of interest" by 1997.)[28] Marion Barry, DC's longest-serving mayor, describing his job in 1997, said:

> I have the responsibilities of a governor . . . no other mayor in America has to worry and manage a state prison or a Medicaid program . . . or a welfare program, food stamp program, state [mental] health program . . . Seventy percent of all the income earned in Washington is earned by people outside of the District of Columbia. We cannot tax that income. We could get $700 million, if we could.[29]

Indeed, the city was unable to pay for all these functions the usual way—congressional law did not permit the city to tax the income of city workers who did not live in DC. Further, the city could not tax the federal government for property, a significant reduction in potential revenue. This challenge was clear early on. After the first decade of home rule, David Goldfield put it this way:

> The federal government accounts for more than one-third of the city's property. Over the past 40 years, taxable property in the District has shrunk by 24%. Not only the federal government, but the expansion of local government, embassies and chanceries for foreign governments, the increased number of streets, and the development of the subway system have served to reduce taxable property.[30]

The context of out-migration to the suburbs becomes especially relevant here. DC mayors were having to not only accomplish state/city/county governance tasks for a population at least the size of a state, but they also needed large revenue generation to run the city, even while their tax base declined by thousands of people year by year, as the middle class and wealthy migrated out to the suburbs, enriching Maryland and Virginia.

In addition, when the city won partial self-governance, it inherited a budget deficit and had a congressional mandate to balance the budget.[31] If they did not, Congress had the right to take over city finances. Further, Congress retained the ability to veto city legislation, impose its own legislation, and to scrutinize, approve, or reject city budgets, even when revenue was generated from DC residents' own taxes.[32] Despite this level of congressional oversight and authority, DC was not allowed to have a congressional representative, only a nonvoting delegate. Civil rights activist and founding member of the Congressional Black Caucus Walter Fauntroy served as the city's delegate from 1971 to 1991, followed by Eleanor Holmes Norton (1991–present). This arrangement—a city larger than some states, paying taxes but with no ability to raise revenue through a commuter tax, controlled by Congress but with no voting or legislative representatives—was controversially described by city son Stokely Carmichael and Charles Hamilton as a Black colony under White "indirect rule."[33] The city's displeasure with congressional oversight has been evident since at least 1800,[34] and city residents have been unsuccessfully agitating for statehood since the 1890s.[35]

Finally, there was the question of legitimacy and a politics of respectability.[36] DC was part of a wave of cities that ushered in the first cohort of Black mayors in the late '60s and '70s.[37] The nation was watching whether Black people could run cities, and DC's mayors were not unique in having something to prove. Expectations were not just external but also came from fellow Black people, with their own finally in power. And the challenge was acute as mayors oversaw growing intraracial inequality between poor and "truly disadvantaged" and wealthier Black people.[38] In the eyes of some observers, such as H. Paul Friesema, "black mayors' arrival in city halls brought them only a 'hollow prize,'"[39] as they were ultimately set up to fail with respect to significantly improving Black life chances. Roger Biles quoted C. Eric Lincoln as saying: "Anyone who expected the election of a black mayor to end the problems of crime, poverty, housing, unemployment and the countless other frustrations of the cities is both politically and intellectually naïve. There is no magic in being black."[40]

Biles pessimistically concluded in his historical assessment of Black mayors that "vying against a century of neglect, racism and malfeasance, black mayors could only hope to hold the line against further degeneration."[41] Indeed, as early as 1969, Friesema noted, "There are serious reasons to question expectations that [black electoral success] can significantly improve Negro life" given the loss of resources to the suburbs, "rising indifference to city problems by white dominated state and national legislative bodies," "pressures for tangible increases in public services," the limited ability of cities to affect individual income, and the problems that occur when "municipal boundaries become racial boundaries."[42] Neil Kraus and Todd Swanstrom further observed that "whites and minorities have sorted themselves into separate political systems,"[43] cementing very large racial economic disparities between the city and the suburbs, even while there were disproportionately more needs in the city. This reflected the ultimate goal of the new version of racial containment—combining physical racial segregation with the clustering of privilege and resources in White (and to a lesser extent Black) suburbia. In this sense, DC was similar to other Black-led cities; however, the key difference was that its equivalent "state" government was Congress, whose representatives, including Maryland's and Virginia's, institutionalized the hoarding of billions of DC's potential commuter tax dollars over the ensuing decades.

In sum, right from the start, Washington, DC, began its partial self-governance with a gargantuan set of governance responsibilities, alongside a financial crisis, a limited ability to generate revenue, a population crisis as the tax base declined, limited legislative independence, and the constant threat of losing newly gained control to Congress if it failed.

CONTINUED DISPLACEMENT OF POOR BLACK
PEOPLE TO GENERATE REVENUE

Since the 1970s, DC's Black mayors pursued two main solutions to the financial conundrum they were presented with. The first, followed by several mayors, was pursuing a new form of "urban renewal" through business and real estate development incentives in order to increase property tax income. The second, kicked off by Mayor Anthony Williams, added the goal of increasing the tax base by increasing DC's population by 100,000.[44]

Describing gentrification in the 1970s but reflecting a pattern repeated over and over in the subsequent decades,[45] Goldfield described that

> private neighborhood redevelopment in Washington has generated a vicious side effect: the displacement of hundreds, perhaps thousands of poor, Black households by middle-income Black and White newcomers ... Between Oct 1972 and Sept 1974 for example, one of out every five sales of homes in the District involved two or more sales of the same property, 80% within 10 months of each other. For those homeowners or tenants who manage to escape the initial wave of sales, inflated property taxes and higher rents brought on by the rapid increase in property values eventually force displacement ... The process is very rapid. It amounts to reverse blockbusting. When an area becomes a "hot" market, all properties are sold, within two years or less. During that time, one socioeconomic class has totally replaced another—gentrification has occurred.[46]

Real estate speculation was not just driven by domestic investors but also foreign ones,[47] and most of those displaced were low-income renters. The local government was not just passively observing displacement but actively participating in it. As Goldfield noted, "Between 1974 and 1977, the District's own renewal policies in the downtown areas displaced over 4,000 households, 95% of which were renters. In 1977, 90% of all displaced households were low income."[48] Displaced individuals and families struggled to find new housing given a 2% rental vacancy rate and increasingly limited housing stock for the poor. Repeating dynamics from the prior two racial containment eras, this "forced the poor to double and triple-up in shoddy rooming houses and deteriorating private dwellings."[49] Anacostia (Ward 8) and Maryland's PG County were "the last refuge of the displaced poor."[50] Twenty-three years after these observations, in 2003, Gillette noted that "the County Executive of Prince George's County took the unusual step of accusing Washington's mayor of actively exporting its poorer residents to his jurisdiction."[51] Indeed, parts of PG County are now colloquially called Ward 9.[52]

City officials were aware of the predominantly Black poor's plight but, caught in a double bind, did not take steps to redress it, not wanting to "tamper with the tax windfall that private redevelopment has become."[53] Additionally, there were barriers to poorer Black people's relocation, as Sabihya Prince discovered among residents whose property was earmarked for upgrading: "Hindrances to taking up residence in the new mixed income community included limits connected to poor credit or the arrest records of children, grandchildren and other family members."[54] Given the city's nation-leading mass incarceration rates (see Part 4), screening residents for the opportunity to return to upgraded housing could lead to permanent displacement. Seen in historical context, there is an eerie similarity to the second-era pattern of poor Black displacement, overcrowding, and struggling to find alternative affordable housing, even while the responsible actors had changed.

Federal incentives introduced in the late 1990s, such as President Clinton's well-intentioned "Good Neighbor Policy," arguably exacerbated these trends. The policy was "a plan to make the U.S. government a helpful participant in Washington's livelihood" by contributing to a new city initiative, business improvement districts (BIDs).[55] As geographer Nathaniel Lewis described,

> [The Policy] prompted the U.S. General Services Administration, which manages most federal buildings, to join and subsequently fund the Downtown D.C. BID in 1997 ... Since 2000, [it] has helped facilitate over 100 new construction projects—close to 15 new projects each year ... Over 50,000 more people work in Downtown D.C. today than in 1996, an increase of about 42%, compared with only 2% in non-BID areas of Downtown and 3% in the entire District of Columbia.[56]

New housing stock for affluent buyers was constructed at federal expense and introduced to the market at prices that low-income families could not afford, contributing to their clustering in the poorest wards or out of the city altogether. Indeed, Lewis observed a racial patterning in the placement of BIDs:

> The poorest, mostly Black neighborhoods (e.g. Anacostia, Congress Heights) in southeast and northeast Washington do not have BIDs despite the presence of commercial areas that support large residential populations. Instead, BIDs are centered in areas that are heavily touristed (e.g. Capitol Hill),

sites of federal government buildings (e.g. Downtown D.C.), traditionally wealthy areas (e.g. Adams Morgan, Georgetown), or areas that are being rapidly developed for a growing wealthy professional class (e.g. NoMa, Capitol Riverfront).[57]

A BID was placed in Anacostia in 2012, and the business community response was limited.[58] The Matthew effect[59] was thus at work: As White people returned to the city, the wealthiest predominantly White and gentrifying White areas were further enriched and revitalized by the federal government and private business, while the poorest predominantly Black areas continued to be ignored. Tanya Golash-Boza described this recurrent racial capitalist pattern as Black "dispossession, displacement and disinvestment, followed by . . . [White] racialized reinvestment."[60]

A NEW WRINKLE: PUBLIC HOUSING DETERIORATION

Even while the city's poor struggled to find affordable housing, those who had secured a public housing unit were also troubled in the third era. Within a sort of separate-but-equal logic, the promise of public housing was that despite racially segregated projects, residents would at least be in modern buildings with a full set of amenities, such as running water, central heating, electricity, and indoor toilets, which significantly improved on alley and slum dwellings, hopefully quelling racial resentment and conflict.[61] However, the problematic reality of this logic materialized within a few years of construction; public housing buildings began to deteriorate, with residents experiencing flooding, shifting foundations, fires, peeling walls and ceilings, high air pollution, and drifting garbage among other problems.[62] These experiences were the consequence of a series of decisions made by housing officials during the construction process, as well as racialized transportation and land use policies, which mapped onto racialized housing policies. Racial containment ensured that the full effect of these overlapping decisions and policies by different institutional actors was disproportionately concentrated on low-income Black residents, reproducing and exacerbating their disproportionately poor health in the third era.

Racial dynamics underlay the city's transportation policies, with health consequences. For example, the Suitland Parkway, opened in 1944 to connect military installations, was designed to run directly through the Barry Farm playground—a large recreation park in Anacostia (Ward 8)—splitting up the neighborhood, curtailing its children's recreation area,[63] and exposing them to highway pollution. After World War II, the government increased its investment in expanding the city's transportation infrastructure on newly cleared land in the form of a mass transit expansion into the suburbs. This included "a 33-mile rail system" as well as "329 miles of new interstate highways," mostly funded by the Federal-Aid Highway Act of 1956, which provided 90% of the funding.[64] As with other innovations, DC was to be a "national model of urban revitalization,"[65] and as President John F. Kennedy later put it, "a national model for coordinated metropolitan development."[66] An initial neighborhood-neutral "radial" highway design would have affected every quadrant of the city; however, as documented by Howard Gillette, during implementation, despite Black resident protests, Democratic and Republican congressmen and influential lawyers living in the city, among other actors, used their power and influence to force through freeway plans that preserved affluent White neighborhoods and disproportionately ran through Black neighborhoods.[67] Land cleared for highways was made available for use in the construction of public housing, such as Sheridan Terrace and Kenilworth Courts, placing predominantly Black residents in close proximity to suburban commuters' car pollution. As Janet Currie and others have demonstrated, air pollution exposure contributes to a wide range of poor health outcomes for children, including infant mortality.[68]

Housing officials were constrained by limited land options for the construction of public housing, a limited budget, which could be co-opted for other government needs (such as temporary housing for war workers as described earlier), and pressure to rapidly relocate displaced tenants struggling to find alternative housing.[69] However, as Justin Shapiro documented, this contributed to the selection of cheaper but environmentally problematic sites. For example, the Barry Farm public housing complex in Anacostia was sited on uneven land. Shapiro described the end result of construction:

> In the end, the entire complex sloped towards the Anacostia River. Water naturally moved from the highest point towards the northeast of the complex towards the lower southwest portion. This would prove to be a problem later on, as it provided opportunities for flooding and pooling towards the low-lying sections of the complex.[70]

Eventually, flooding began to compromise the complex's integrity, leading to "gaping holes in walls and ceilings, flaky plaster, and rusting gutters."[71] To add insult to injury, tenants were charged for repairs. Shapiro also described the case of Kenilworth Courts.[72] The complex was sited near the six-lane Kenilworth Avenue Freeway and next to the city's municipal dump, which was "operated as an open-burn landfill"[73] which generated "toxic incinerator ash."[74] As Shapiro describes:

> Area 'E' was directly across from the Kenilworth Courts public housing complex. [It] was to receive six hundred cubic yards of ash residue per day, six days per week for several weeks. The residue was to be delivered while still smoldering. Once deposited it would be quenched and compacted to six inches each day ... Dumping would not cease until the early 1970s, which meant that Kenilworth Courts tenants faced months during which trucks carrying incinerator ash and refuse from other parts of the city ran down Kenilworth Avenue Freeway to deposit their loads on the site near their homes. When the dumping finally did end, the Kenilworth Park contained about four million tons of "raw refuse, incinerator ash, and other burned residue ... [it had] an average depth of 25 feet, and covered an area of about 145 acres."[75]

In sum, within a decade of finalizing public housing construction, DC's solution to the housing problem had indeed "simply shifted elsewhere,"[76] but this time, it was neatly contained, away and out of sight of White society. And the first era alley and slum conditions that second era public housing had been designed to eliminate had simply been reproduced in the third era—in the case of Kenilworth Courts, almost exactly, as the city literally dumped its garbage at its doorstep.

OVERWHELMING SERVICE PROVISION NEEDS

With limited revenue and large public assistance needs, Black mayors were faced with the challenging task of maintaining or even improving city services with a limited budget. Exacerbating this situation was their inheritance of decades of poor decisions, neglect, and indifference. Shapiro describes a congressional allocation in 1952 of $38,000 to work on 7,707 units, noting, "This means that the Congressional allocation for maintenance and operations was $4.93 per unit ... equivalent to $47.70 in 2020."[77] Walter Washington, during his tenure leading the NCHA in the early '60s, had been willing to meet with tenants but had a limited budget to help. By the early '70s, when he was mayor-commissioner, DC's deteriorating public housing complexes were in crisis. The housing authority was insolvent and owed $2 million in unpaid rent because tenants were protesting the lack of maintenance. A request submitted to HUD for $19.6 million resulted in a $10 million allocation, and a request for $900,000 from HUD to the city's criminal justice office for a tenant security program resulted in a $190,000 allocation.[78] Sterling Tucker, DC City Council vice-chair, highlighted the needs, including,

> increased trash collection and police protection at public housing projects, the temporary loan of departments of environmental services and general services crews to repair public housing units, and the loan of city housing inspectors to survey defective housing units."

He lamented that "without [federal] funds . . . between 300 and 400 of the authority's 700 employees will have to be fired and efforts to upgrade the quality of public housing in the city will die."[79] By then, the NCHA had lost federal support and "in a political twist . . . was left without increases in federal funding necessary to offset costs of repairs . . . [HUD] refused to increase its subsidies to the District of Columbia because the city had been found in violation of several federal regulations."[80] During construction, the NCHA had used its federal status to flout the city's building regulations for site locations, permits, and inspections, but now that the consequences of those violations was manifesting in deteriorating buildings, federal maintenance money was withheld or limited.[81]

Various efforts were made in the ensuing years to deal with immediate problems, even as other major problems worsened. For example, in 1974, HUD granted $2 million for "patchwork maintenance." However, patchwork maintenance had limited utility when the major issues were structural.[82] Even when Black mayors began to allocate significant money to public housing, their efforts were futile, inadequate, or entirely absent. In 1981, at Barry Farm in Anacostia, for example, the building manager told reporter Edward Sargent that "there's a lot of flooding, water bangs up against the buildings and the structures begin to sink and rot . . . we just don't have enough manpower, money or supplies to take care of all the problems."[83] Barry Farm had entirely missed out on a $9.9 million allocation from the Barry administration to improve public housing.[84] At Sheridan Terrace, also located in Anacostia, a "federal audit noted that between 1988 and 1992 nearly half of all ordered repairs went unmade." Years of neglect meant that units that had only needed minor repairs now required, "comprehensive modernization."[85] Several units were empty, boarded up awaiting repair and serving as host to a thriving drug trade unfolding in city-owned infrastructure.[86] (See Part 3). Mayor Barry set up a commission to repair public housing units, but more units needed major repair by the end of the project. Mayor Sharon Kelly, his successor, set up a strike force to deal with repairs, but almost 75% of the units lay vacant by the end of the two-year project due to requirements for major repair.[87] Efforts by the city department responsible for public housing were also undermined by rapid leadership turnover—there had been 13 directors between 1979 and 1995.[88] Millions of federal dollars went unspent, and many units sat vacant, in need of repair, while thousands of poor families awaited a public housing unit.[89] Frustrated tenants protested both through withholding rent and through filing individual and class action lawsuits.[90] The public housing agency went into court-ordered receivership in 1995, and David Gilmore was put in charge of the receivership. William Knox, his new director of operations, told reporter Vernon Loeb:

> The last time the agency inspected all of its 11,500 units for code violations was three years ago . . . that exercise produced 58,000 work orders that swamped the system. Many of the repairs were never made . . . we have 11,500 units . . . and two licensed plumbers . . . Simply put, you're looking at neglect—neglect that results from human failure, bureaucratic failure, a condescending attitude toward poor people. There are instances, as I walk through this place, of conditions that no human being should have to live in.[91]

With a dedicated team and drawing on millions of unspent federal money, public housing in the city was eventually turned around.[92] However, by then, the SAVA syndemic of the third era had already wreaked havoc on its tenants. As I will illustrate in Part 3, public housing often served as ground zero and a "sacrifice zone" for the city syndemic.

DID BLACK PEOPLE BENEFIT? EXPANDING BLACK PROSPERITY, DEEPENING RACIAL INEQUALITY

While many journalists and scholars were scathing in their critique of Marion Barry, the city's longest-serving mayor, they give him credit for his many attempts to help Black people living in the city's poorest wards, such as Anacostia, albeit often unsuccessfully, as illustrated above. They also note his significant efforts to enable Black prosperity. For example, in what Jaffe and

Sherwood characterized as "an honest attempt to bring Blacks and women to the table in what had been a Whites-only affair," in a "heavy-handed" manner that was "doing openly what Irish, Italian and Jewish politicians had done behind closed doors," Barry "raise[d] the percentage of the city's business with minority contractors from just over 10 percent to 35 percent. He demanded that developers who wanted to build on city property bring Blacks into joint ventures."[93] As such, many Black business people benefited richly from the city's construction and gentrification boom that had generated over $700 million in property tax revenue annually at its height.[94] Another strategy was increasing the size of city government—to the point of excess. At its height in 1988, almost a decade into Barry's term, Jaffe and Sherwood observed that 1 in 13 DC residents were city employees.[95] They went on to note that this was "more government workers per capita than any other city or state government, including New York, Chicago, Houston, Philadelphia and Detroit. Barry's work force soaked up half the city's budget, which had grown from $1.2bn to $3.2bn under Barry's regime."[96] This strategy was successful in enabling many Black people to get stable, salaried, middle-class jobs. However, the cost, along with widespread corruption in his administration leading to criminal indictments and grossly inefficient city services overseen by him and a number of subsequent mayors, contributed to lawsuits, many agencies being put into receiverships, and a major budget crisis.[97] (Part 5 also examines contributions of the city syndemic to this crisis). Congress took over the city's finances in 1995, put in place a financial control board, assumed some major city costs, and worked to bring DC back to a balanced budget.[98] Anthony Williams, who had served on the successful financial control board, won election for mayor and demonstrated that Black people could run an efficient government—an image boost needed after the controversial Barry years.[99] He did this by cutting local government jobs, introducing BIDs, cutting programs, and engaging in a range of strategies to increase the tax base, including attracting more affluent residents to the city.[100]

Starting from Williams's term in 1999, and maintained in the following years through continued use of technocratic expertise under Mayors Fenty, Gray, and Bowser, DC's budget was balanced, its tax base was increasing as affluent residents streamed into the city and lived in gentrified residences and neighborhoods, business was booming, and all was well with Congress. However, over the past five decades of Black mayoral leadership as described in the Part overview, its infant and maternal mortality rates, its homicide and

HIV rates, which all disproportionately affected Black people, along with its racial life expectancy gap, have been or are the worst in the nation.[101]

HEALTH CONSEQUENCES

"A Brief Moment in the Sun," 1960

Reflecting an initial "brief moment in the sun,"[102] an improvement in the Black standard of living at the beginning of the era, racial health inequality had narrowed by 1960, though wide racial gaps remained. This narrowing reflected the positive effects of moving out of overcrowded and deteriorating alley and slum housing to brand new public housing with modern amenities, as well as increased rates of home ownership among Black people moving into previously White neighborhoods, as residents departed for the sub-urbs.[103] It also occurred despite the fact that "more than one-fourth of the District residents are medically indigent and must rely on this Department for medical care and rehabilitation."[104] While overall life expectancy at birth was 66.6 years, the racial gap had narrowed. There was a 4.41-year gap between White (65.4 years) and Black (60.99 years) men and a 6.76-year gap between White (73.34 years) and Black (66.58 years) women.[105] Maternal mortality remained high. The overall rate was 60.4/100,000 live births, higher among Black (67.2/100,000) compared to White (46.2/100,000) mothers.[106] The city's infant mortality rate was 36.4/1,000 live births and was also unequal (White 29.4/1,000, Black 39.6/1,000).[107] Notably, both the White and Black infant mortality rates were equivalent to those found in the third poorest and poorest poverty ventiles of the nation's counties, respectively.[108] While heart disease, cardiovascular disease, and cancer remained the top causes of death,[109] the 1960 Board of Health report noted that "the District of Columbia had the highest rates of veneral [sic] disease infection (syphilis and gonorrhea) in the nation."[110] Thus, while earlier infectious diseases such as TB and influenza had declined, sexually transmitted epidemics became prominent, exacerbated by HIV as the era progressed.

Widening Inequality, 1970–2020

Over the next 50 years, the overall racial life-expectancy gap widened. In the 1969–71 decennial life tables, DC's life expectancy was 65.7 years, and the gap between White (66.08 years) and Black (58.96 years) men had widened by almost 3 years, to 7.12 years. Among women, however, the life-expectancy gap narrowed by a quarter year to 6.5 years (White 74.8 years, Black 68.3 years).[111] The leading causes of death continued to be heart disease, cardiovascular disease, and cancer.[112] In 1970, the infant mortality rate had declined to 28.9/1,000 live births, with a smaller racial gap (White 23/1,000; Black 29.7/1,000).[113] Maternal mortality rates remained wide (55.7/100,000 live births overall; 15/100,000 White women; 52.8/100,000 Black women).[114]

In the 1979–81 decennial life tables, overall life expectancy increased to 69.2 years; however, the gap between White (71.24 years) and Black (61.88 years) men had widened by a further 3 years to an almost 10-year difference in life expectancy (9.4 years).[115] Homicide was the leading cause of death for Black men, followed by heart disease and cancer, while heart disease was the leading cause of death for White men, followed by suicide and cancer.[116] Among women, the gap continued to narrow, with a 5.9 year difference (White 77.9 years, Black 72 years).[117] For both Black and White women, cancer was the leading cause of death; however, for Black women, heart and liver disease and cirrhosis were the second and third leading causes of death respectively, while for White women, it was suicide and heart disease, respectively.[118] Overall infant mortality had declined in 1980 (24.6/1,000 live births), but racial inequality had widened; Black infants were twice as likely to die (26.6/1,000 live births) as White infants (13.1/1,000 live births).[119] By 1988, the city's infant mortality rate, at 23.2/1,000 live births, was "higher than that of any [US] city with a population of 500,000 or more."[120] Ahmed and colleagues conducted a review of certificates of infant death and found that 86% of deaths were among Black children and 9.8% among White children, and 67% of the deaths were preventable.

In the 1989–91 decennial life tables, DC's life expectancy had decreased by 1.2 years to 68 years. The gap between White (76.1 years) and Black (64.4 years) people had further widened to 11.7 years. There was a 9.5-year gap for women (White 81.1 years, Black 71.6 years), representing an end to the multidecade narrowing trends. White and Black men could expect to live 71.4 years and 57.5 years, respectively (a 13.9-year gap).[121] Men's life tables reveal that health inequality began in the first year of life and dramatically widened over time. Exposed to 1989–91 mortality rates, Black male infants would die twice as much as White infants, 13- to 14-year-olds would die almost five times more, and 20- to 21-year-olds, nine times more.[122]

In the 1999–2001 decennial life tables, DC life expectancy had increased by 5 years to 73.1 years, reflecting a recovery from the mortality shock of the

White, 2000

LO
79.5

MO
79.6

AR
FA 80.5 DC 80.4
80.8
AL
79.7
PW
77.5

DC

PG
79.6

CH
76.1

85 – 87.9
82 – 84.9
79 – 81.9
76 – 78.9

White, 2010

LO
82.9

MO
82.3

AR
FA 83.3 DC 84.6
83.5
AL
82.9
PW
80.5

PG
82.3

CH
78.6

White, 2019

LO
84.0

MO
83.2

AR
FA 85.7 DC 87.1
84.9
AL
85.0
PW
81.4

PG
83.2

CH
78.8

Black, 2000

LO
76.0

MO
74.6

AR
FA 73.6 DC 67.6
77.6
AL
73.4
PW
74.8

PG
74.6

CH
74.0

79.5 – 83.4
75.5 – 79.4
71.5 – 75.4
67.5 – 71.4

Black, 2010

LO
80.7

MO
78.3

AR
FA 77.9 DC 72.8
81.3
AL
77.7
PW
79.3

PG
78.3

CH
77.9

Black, 2019

LO
82.3

MO
79.4

AR
FA 80.1 DC 71.6
83.2
AL
79.8
PW
80.6

PG
79.4

CH
78.2

AL: Alexandria, VA
LO: Loudoun Co., VA

AR: Arlington, VA
MO: Montgomery Co., MD

CH: Charles Co., VA
PG: Prince George's Co., MD

DC: Washington, DC
PW: Prince William Co., VA

FA: Fairfax Co., VA

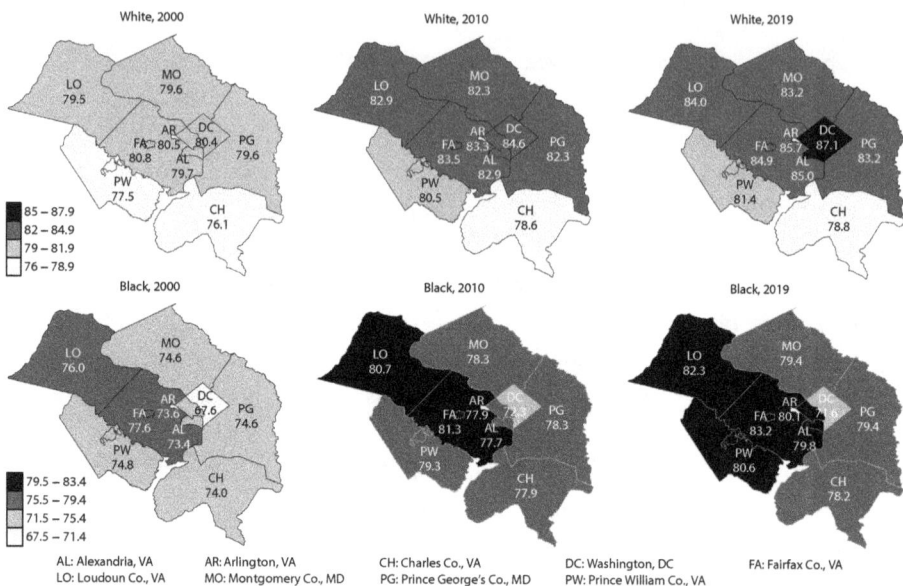

FIGURE 22. Life expectancy in DC and its suburbs, 2000–2019. Data source: Global Health Data Exchange.

1990s.[123] The gap between White (81.5 years) and Black people (69.6 years) was 11.9 years. However, while men gained over 7 years in life expectancy, the gap between White (78.9 years) and Black (64.6 years) men had further widened to 14.3 years. Among women, both White (84.3 years) and Black (74.5 years) women gained about 3 years in life expectancy over the decade; however, the racial gap had widened to 9.8 years. Infant mortality continued to disproportionately affect Black families; over 90% of infant deaths were of Black infants.[124] These statistics thus illustrate that the tale of two cities in 2010 and 2020 described in the Part overview is merely a continuation of 50 years of incrementally widening racial life expectancy gaps between Black and White people.

It is important to place DC's life expectancy in the context of its surrounding suburbs. In Figure 22, for each racial group, lighter colors reflect lower life expectancy and darker colors higher life expectancy. In 2000, among White MSA residents, those living in Fairfax County had the highest life expectancy (80.8 years) while those living in Charles County had the lowest life expectancy (76.1 yrs), a 4.7-year gap. Among Black MSA residents, Fairfax County residents also had the highest life expectancy (77.6 years) while DC residents had the lowest (67.6 years), a 10-year gap. The highest suburban Black life expectancy (Fairfax) was equivalent to the second lowest suburban White life expectancy (Prince William). In 2010, among White MSA residents, DC residents had the highest life expectancy (84.6 years) while Charles County residents had the lowest (78.6 years), a 6-year gap. Among Black MSA residents, Fairfax County residents had the highest life expectancy (81.3 years) while DC residents had the lowest (72.3 years), a 9-year gap. The highest Black MSA life expectancy was now higher than the two lowest White counties (Prince William and Charles Counties) but lower than all the rest. In 2019, among White MSA residents, DC residents still had the highest life expectancy (87.1 years), and Charles County residents had the lowest (78.8 years). The 8.3-year gap is almost double the gap in 2000, reflecting widening inequality among White people. Among Black MSA residents, Fairfax County residents still had the highest life expectancy (83.2 years), while DC residents had the lowest (71.6 years), a 11.6-year gap, and one that remained relatively stable over the 19-year period. The highest Black MSA life expectancy was now equivalent to that of residents in the sixth and seventh (out of nine) highest White MSA counties (PG and Montgomery Counties).

Overall, these findings illustrate inter- and intraracial health inequality for both White and Black MSA residents and underscore the stark racial health inequality among DC residents in particular compared to their suburban counterparts. While racial health inequality followed Black people into the suburbs, it was significantly blunted, and Black suburbanites derived a decade's worth of life-expectancy advantage relative to their city counterparts.

CONCLUSIONS

In sum, this Part illustrates how the design and reconstitution of DC's racialized geography created, institutionalized, and reproduced racialized vulnerability to illness and premature death across generations of African Americans. A key mechanism for this process was racial containment, which shifted forms throughout the city's history—from tertiary segregation (front street/back yard/alley) in the first era to primary segregation (containment to specific neighborhoods within the city) in the second era. In the third era, the city shifted to a chocolate city/vanilla suburbs formation (when DC was predominantly Black), and then to a cappuccino city (with White people moving in and poorer Black people being gentrified out). Racial containment was orchestrated by a range of government and private actors and institutions, and it worked to contain poor Black people in spaces—from alleys and slums to deteriorating projects to neglected and poorly serviced neighborhoods—that were, variously, overcrowded, near garbage dumps, subject to flooding, and air polluted, among other factors contributing to detrimental health outcomes. In this way, racial containment created syndemic zones—spaces where multiple overlapping infectious and chronic disease epidemics flourished, contributing to persistent and widening racial health inequality.

The Part also shows how while the first 180 years (1790–1970) of the city's history reflected a clearer story of racism driving the shifting residential distribution of Black and White people in the city and subsequent racial health inequalities, these dynamics continued even after the city was led by Black mayors. The predominantly White Congress retained legal and budgetary authority over the city, and it did not permit the city to benefit from hundreds of millions of potential commuter tax dollars. This forced Black mayors to turn to residential gentrification and large commercial developments as major revenue sources to maintain a balanced budget and thus retain home rule, even though they displaced poor Black people. Congressional strings thus connected the racialized institutional logics of the prior two eras to the third one, resulting in the continued enactment of racial containment by Black actors. This was undergirded by class containment. DC's Black mayors facilitated the growth of the Black middle class and Black wealth in the city and its suburbs but did little to improve the life chances of Black people—especially poor Black people—within DC's borders. While it is certainly arguable whether they were able to, what is clear is that Black mayors essentially participated in and presided over the reproduction and even exacerbation of racial health inequality in Washington, DC, in the third era.

In Parts 2–5, I examine how racial containment structured the social dynamics underlying the SAVA syndemic, as well as individual experiences of life within syndemic zones. I also explore how and why efforts to control the city's health crises were so often frustrated and why, even when interventions were extraordinarily successful, they had so little effect on racial health inequality.

PART TWO

Sex, Love, and HIV in a
Syndemic Zone

HIV/AIDS RATE IN D.C. HITS 3%. CONSIDERED A 'SEVERE' EPIDEMIC, EVERY MODE OF TRANSMISSION IS INCREASING, CITY STUDY FINDS ... At least 3 percent of District residents have HIV or AIDS, a total that far surpasses the 1 percent threshold that constitutes a "generalized and severe" epidemic.... "Our rates are higher than West Africa," said Shannon L. Hader, director of the District's HIV/AIDS Administration, who once led the Federal Centers for Disease Control and Prevention's work in Zimbabwe. "They're on par with Uganda and some parts of Kenya."

JOSE ANTONIO VARGAS AND
DARRYL FEARS (*POST*—MAR 14, 2009)

Primary [HIV] risk may simply be engaging in normative heterosexual sexual behavior within a network with a high prevalence of HIV.

MANYA MAGNUS ET AL (2009:1282)

WHY HAVE AFRICAN AMERICANS been disproportionately affected by the HIV epidemic in Washington, DC? In this Part, I examine how racial containment structured sexual life in the city in ways that amplified the spread of HIV among Black people. I draw on historical and contemporary literature reviews, census data (1880–2020), and longitudinal HIV surveillance data (1983–2022), as well as 10 key informant interviews conducted between 2011 and 2023 and 37 life history interviews with African Americans living with HIV who were gay, bisexual, or heterosexual men, women, or transgender women,[1] conducted in 2011, a few years after the city's HIV/AIDS epidemic had acquired a "worst in the nation" status.[2] My aims are threefold: to locate the lives of my respondents within the city's history; to examine how individual choices combined with community relational norms and practices and structural constraints to shape disproportionate Black HIV acquisition and transmission; and to shed light on the dynamics of intimate life in a racially contained syndemic zone. In the introduction to this Part, I discuss my guiding conceptual framework, the puzzle of disproportionate Black HIV vulnerability, and the city's HIV epidemic. I then discuss the epidemic among gay and bisexual men (Chapter 4), followed by the epidemic among heterosexual men and women as well as transgender women (Chapter 5).

CONCEPTUAL FRAMEWORK

The Low Likelihood of HIV Acquisition

HIV (human immunodeficiency virus) is a virus that attacks the immune system, causing such severe damage that after about 6–10 years, a person who acquires it typically develops AIDS (Acquired Immune Deficiency Syndrome) and can die of an infection they might otherwise easily fight off, in the absence of medication.[3] While the per-exposure probability of getting HIV is particularly high through blood transfusions (9,250/10,000), sexual acquisition is especially hard. For unprotected sex, there is an estimated 138/10,000 probability in receptive anal sex, a 11/10,000 probability in insertive anal sex, an 8/10,000 probability in receptive penile-vaginal sex, and a 4/10,000 probability in insertive penile-vaginal sex.[4] Vaginal-vaginal and oral sexual transmission appear to be extremely rare.[5] However, these low HIV transmission probabilities increase if a participant is newly infected (26 times more infectious) or has AIDS (7 times more infectious), because they have a high HIV viral load.[6] Having another sexually transmitted infection (STI) also amplifies the probability of HIV acquisition.[7] The low likelihood of acquiring HIV makes clear that it is not just about sexual practice—number of partners, frequency of partner turnover, or type of sex one has—but also about bad sexual luck—that is, the probability of encountering a partner who is (newly) infected with HIV. However, these encounters are not random; sexual luck is sociostructurally created and maintained. In other words, the structure of sexual life in America, above and beyond individual decision-making, doesn't just shape who has sex with whom, but it also ultimately shapes HIV exposure.

Racial Homogamy and the Structure of Sexual Life

At an individual level, romantic relationships are experienced and often portrayed as based on spontaneity and seeming randomness. However, the distribution of STIs, such as HIV, make visible the structure of sexual life in America and its master organizing principle—racial homogamy. That is, whether by preference, convenience, racism or ethnocentrism, the law, or lack of alternative options, White and Black Americans have been and still are more likely to have relationships with people of the same race.[8] Indeed, a phylogenetic study conducted by Alexandra Oster and colleagues tracking HIV transmission pathways found 81% same-race transmission links among African Americans, with 9% and 8% linked to White and Hispanic people, respectively. They found 62% same-race links among White people, with 20% and 12% linked to Hispanic and Black people, respectively.[9] Racial homogamy extends beyond sexual relationships to many aspects of everyday life in America, such as where and with whom people live, work, go to school, worship, socialize and date, though there has been slow but significant diversification in the most recent two decades.[10] The widespread nature of racial homogamy across many social institutions reflects the overlapping and redundant racial containment processes described in the Introduction and Part 1. As such, same-race partnering is not so much "natural" as it is a conscious product of sociostructural engineering of the kinds of potential partners people are most likely to meet in their everyday lives. Racial containment and its byproduct, homogamy, have also been observed in virtual algorithm-created environments, which both reproduce and even more keenly reinforce them through what Ruha Benjamin calls "the new Jim Code."[11]

Sexual life is also organized through racially homogamous sexual economies and sexual networks, both of which are consequential for HIV transmission. In sexual economies, sexual partnerships are governed by factors like supply, demand, and meeting places, as well as "prevailing community norms, expectations and sanctions determining 'appropriate' sexual behavior for people in a given setting."[12] The key status characteristics systematically stratifying sexual economies are gender, sexual orientation, race/ethnicity, and to a lesser degree, social class.[13] For example, a Black heterosexual economy with a greater supply of men relative to women may result in different sexual norms and expectations (e.g., around relationship leverage) than one with a greater supply of women. Sexual networks characterize the structure of people's sexual linkages with each other. Some partnership configurations are more efficient at transmitting infections than others, such as tight-knit social groups with high partner turnover (core groups), having overlapping partnerships (concurrency), or having a partner who is currently or was previously concurrent or part of a core group (bridging ties).[14] These arrangements increase HIV risk if someone in the sexual network is newly infected and thus has a high viral load. Further, because these partnerships are often trusting, with participants who know each other well, regular condom use and frequent HIV testing may be less likely.

THE PUZZLE OF DISPROPORTIONATE
BLACK HIV VULNERABILITY

Many Americans regularly roll the dice and have unprotected sex. This is evident from the fact that almost half of all pregnancies are unintended.[15]

STIs are also unintended. In a 2021 study, Kreisel and colleagues estimated that 1 in 5 Americans have an STI; of the estimated 67.6 million infections, 26.2 million were new STI cases.[16] Chesson and colleagues estimated that this would elicit an estimated lifetime direct treatment cost of $15.9 billion.[17] (STIs in both studies included chlamydia, genital herpes, gonorrhea, hepatitis B, HPV, syphilis, trichomoniasis, as well as HIV). HIV is thus just one of many STIs circulating in the US; however, it is distinctive in being one of the few STIs that is incurable and often fatal without medication. It is also the most expensive STI to treat. Chesson and colleagues calculated that the estimated 32,600 people with newly acquired sexually transmitted HIV would account for an estimated $13.7 billion in lifetime direct treatment costs, about $420,285 per person.[18] In a 2024 report, the CDC estimated that in 2022 there were 1.24 million Americans living with HIV and 31,800 new infections.[19] Over 700,000 have died of HIV/AIDS-related illness,[20] with an estimated 19,310 deaths of people with diagnosed HIV in 2022.[21] African Americans experience disproportionate risk for contracting HIV and dying from AIDS.[22] Hess and colleagues estimated a lifetime HIV risk of 1 in 22 for Black men, 1 in 54 for Black women, 1 in 140 for White men, and 1 in 941 for White women.[23] While they comprise 12% of the US population, Black people account for 40% of Americans living with HIV, just over a third of new HIV infections (37%), and 42% of AIDS deaths.[24] So far, more than 290,000 Black people have died of AIDS.[25]

There is no cure for HIV/AIDS; however, highly active antiretroviral therapy (HAART/ART) became widely available in the US in the mid-1990s. It prolongs the lives of people with HIV, reduces the virus to undetectable levels, thus restoring immune function, and dramatically reduces infectivity when strictly adhered to. Further, medication combined with condom use almost eliminates HIV transmission (by 99.2%).[26] This has transformed HIV into a medication-managed chronic disease, and widespread ART use is a major tool in community HIV prevention. However, continued new HIV diagnoses and AIDS deaths highlight the insufficiency of ART availability and effectiveness. Taking ART assumes HIV awareness; however, in 2022, only 36% of Americans had ever had an HIV test.[27] Further, the high prevalence of unintended pregnancies and STIs in the US indicates that many couples do not use condoms; indeed, among those aged 15–44, only a quarter of women (23.8%) and a third of men (33.7%) used a condom during their last sexual encounter.[28] Thus, most Americans do not use condoms, do not know their HIV status, and likely do not know their partner's HIV status. In this sense, people who get HIV are not especially different from other Americans.

Indeed, at an individual level, African Americans' disproportionate HIV vulnerability is a puzzle. Overall, many quantitative studies that directly compare individual HIV risk factors, such as number of partners or condom and drug injection use among Black and White people, find few or no significant differences between groups, and where differences exist, Black people have fewer sexual partners, higher rates of condom use, are more likely to have had an HIV test, and are less likely to inject drugs. They nonetheless have higher rates of STIs and HIV compared to other racial/ethnic groups.[29] Hallfors and colleagues, based on their nationally representative study, concluded that "White young adults in the United States are at elevated STD and HIV risk when they engage in high-risk behaviors. Black young adults, however, are at high risk even when their behaviors are normative. Factors other than individual risk behaviors and covariates appear to account for racial disparities, indicating the need for population-level interventions."[30] Magnus and colleagues came to the same conclusion in their DC epidemic research, as highlighted in the epigraph that opened this Part.[31] Overall, these studies suggest that while HIV prevention efforts solely targeted at individual behavior change might be highly effective for White people, they are insufficient for Black people. The scientific recognition of the limitations of solely individual-level approaches to understanding and reducing racial HIV inequality led scholars such as Sevgi Aral, Adaora Adimora, Judy Auerbach, Sam Friedman, and Kim Blankenship, among many others, to call for further examination of the role of racialized and intersecting social structures in uniquely shaping and exacerbating Black HIV vulnerability.[32]

Racial containment processes racialize institutions in ways that differentially structure HIV risk. For example, the racialization of the health care system[33] is evident in racially unequal awareness and availability of and access to ART and pre-exposure prophylaxis medication, which reduce HIV acquisition and transmission as well as AIDS death.[34] It can thus become complicit in higher Black HIV/AIDS rates. Another key institution is the same-race neighborhood, which contributes to racial homogamy. When racial homogamy is a dominant norm in a sexual economy, there are dramatic consequences for the spread of disease. It creates a distinct sexual geography[35] of vulnerability, especially among minority groups in racially contained neighborhoods, by concentrating and locking in disease and overlapping with other potentially amplifying epidemics to create a syndemic zone (see the Introduction). This results in generalized risk for residents regardless of whether they engage in high- or low-risk sexual activity. In addition, Ed Laumann and Yoosik Youm found that African Americans are more likely to partner disassortatively on risk (i.e., form high risk–low risk partnerships), thus making low risk people more vulnerable than they otherwise would be.[36] Partnerships between older and younger men, monogamous and concurrent heterosexuals, homosexual and bisexual men, and bisexual men and heterosexual women have been especially consequential for HIV acquisition and transmission.[37] In these cases, a monogamous HIV-negative person is not protected. Long-term partners are locked into arrangements where trust is likely high, leading to lack of HIV testing, regular unprotected sex, and thus a higher risk of HIV transmission if one of the participants has HIV. These national dynamics played out in DC in a particularly acute way.

THE DC HIV EPIDEMIC

In March 2009, *The Washington Post* reported that 3% of the city's population was living with HIV.[38] Manya Magnus and colleagues at George Washington University and the DC government's HIV/AIDS agency (the HIV/AIDS Administration [HAA], which later became the HIV/AIDS, Hepatitis, STD, and TB Administration [HAHSTA]) noted in a study that "with an HIV/AIDS case rate nearly 10 times the United States rate, its [Washington, DC's] AIDS case rate is higher than that of Baltimore, Philadelphia, New York City, Detroit and Chicago; one in 20 to one in 50 . . . is living with HIV/AIDS."[39] It was startling that one of the nation's worst HIV/AIDS epidemics was unfolding at the nation's lawmakers' own doorsteps.

The 2010 DC HAHSTA report documented the disproportionate impact of the epidemic on African Americans: At least 4.7% of the city's Black population was living with HIV, more than three times the rate of White people (1.5%). Trends by race and gender were even starker: 7.1% of Black men had HIV, compared to 2.9% of White men, and African American women (2.8%)

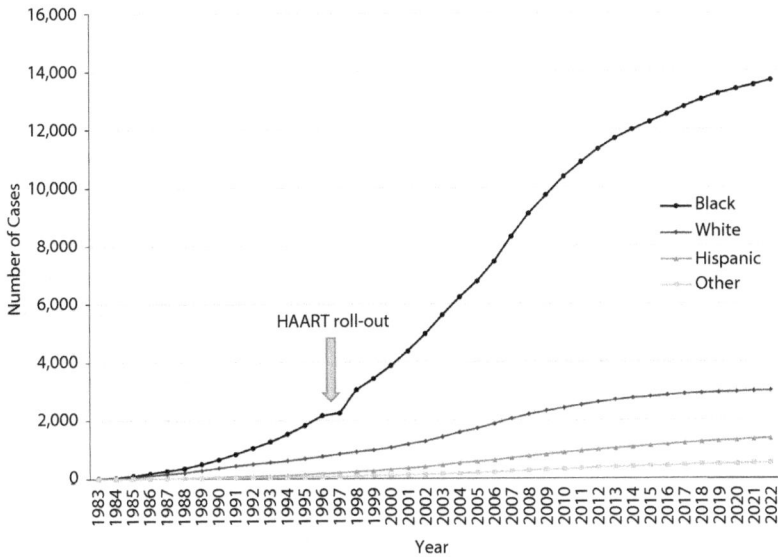

FIGURE 23. Cumulative number of people living with HIV in Washington, DC, by race/ethnicity, 1983–2022. Data sources: DC HAHSTA HIV Surveillance Unit data (1983–2016); DC HAHSTA *Annual Epidemiology and Surveillance Reports* (2017–22).

had 14 times the rate of White women (0.2%); they comprised half (54.6%) of the city's women but 91.1% of women's cases.[40] Overall, this translated into an approximately 1 in 20 chance of encountering a Black partner living with HIV, compared to an approximately 1 in 67 chance of encountering a White partner living with HIV.

Belying the assumption that the epidemic was predominantly a challenge for White gay men, in DC, since the beginning, while significant *proportions* of people with HIV in the early years were White, significant *numbers* of people with HIV have been Black, as illustrated in Figure 23, constructed utilizing data drawn from the city's HIV Surveillance Unit from 1983 through 2022.[41] It is especially notable from Figure 23 that the number of Black people living with HIV skyrocketed from about 1997 onwards, *after* medication capable of reducing HIV infectiousness became widely available. This also occurred while the proportion of Black people declined (from 65.4% in 1990 to 40.9% in 2020) and that of White people increased (from 27.6% to 38%). In other words, the figure is illustrating widening racial HIV inequality over time. The figure illustrates racial homogamy at work, as the HIV epidemic unfolded in racially distinct ways throughout its history. This section (and Part 5) will illustrate how, as with other diseases, this outcome is not accidental.

The DC epidemic was also not limited to a subgroup but was generalized across the population. This was evident both from the fact that more than 1% of the city's population had HIV, as well as from examining modes of HIV acquisition. Across the HAHSTA surveillance data sample from 1983 to 2011, the year of my interviews, 42.6% reported acquiring HIV from sex between men, 27.9% from heterosexual sex, 13.6% from injecting drug use, and the remainder did not know (11%), reported both sexual transmission and injecting drug use (3.6%) or reported other causes (1.3%), such as blood transfusion or perinatal or occupational exposure. Among transgender people in particular, 69.7% reported acquiring HIV through sexual contact, 4.3% through injecting drug use, 6.5% through a combination of sex and drug use, and the remainder did not know (19.5%).[42] (In the 2023 HAHSTA report, among cisgender men and women, 48.9% reported acquisition through sex between men, 27.3% through heterosexual sex, and 8.6% through injecting drug use. The remainder reported acquiring HIV through a combination of sex and drug use [3.9%], did not know [10.1%], or reported other causes [1.2%]. Among transgender people, 74.1% reported sexual acquisition of HIV and 2.6% reported injecting drug use. The remainder reported acquiring HIV through a combination of sex and drug use [8%], did not know [13.5%] or reported other causes [1.8%].)[43] The next two chapters examine the epidemic among Black gay and bisexual men (Chapter 4), and heterosexual men and women, and transgender women (Chapter 5). I examine how historical factors combined with contemporary community norms and relationship dynamics to produce racial HIV inequality as people navigated sex and love in racially contained syndemic zones.

. . .

Ella Fitzgerald and Louis Armstrong	Cheek to Cheek (1956)
Whitney Houston	Saving All My Love For You (1985)
Gwen Guthrie	Can't Love You Tonight (1988)
Queen Latifah	U.N.I.T.Y. (1993)
Coolio	Too Hot (1995)
Lil Nas X	Old Town Road (2018)
Frank Ocean	Ocean in My Room (2019)
Destiny's Child	Survivor (2001)
Mary J. Blige	Real Love (1992)
Lauryn Hill	Doo Wop (That Thing) (1998)
Boyz II Men	End of the Road (1991)
Jill Scott	A Long Walk (2000)
Usher	Confessions Part II (2004)
John Legend	All of Me (2013)
Etta James	At Last (1960)
Wale	The Matrimony feat. Usher (2015)
Rare Essence	Overnight Scenario (1998)

FOUR

The HIV Epidemic Among Gay and Bisexual Men

IN THIS CHAPTER, I INVESTIGATE why Black sexual minority men were disproportionately affected by HIV. I briefly examine both White and Black histories, starting in the late 1800s, to explore how and why they deviated from each other in ways that were consequential for the epidemic, but I primarily focus on the lives and experiences of Black gay and bisexual men.[1] While White and Black men engaged in similar sexual practices, racial containment resulted in their lives unfolding in different institutional and spatial contexts, which structured sexual life differently, leading to differential vulnerability when the HIV/AIDS epidemic arrived.

THE DC CLOSET: SEXUAL CONTAINMENT IN THE LATE 1800S–1970S

Despite desegregation ordinances in 1872 and 1873 in DC, the post-Reconstruction Jim Crow backlash meant that for many, de facto racial containment continued to characterize social life in the ensuing decades.[2] This was the case not just in housing, as described in Part 1, but also in public gathering venues, such as restaurants, theaters, and bars.[3] This resulted in a racially stratified sexual economy with largely homogamous sexual markets.[4] In addition to the racial containment principle, homosexuality was considered a vice that violated the moral code and was thus criminalized. Both the police and the federal government, the city's chief employer, worked together to contain sexual minority life by pushing it into the metaphoric closet. Partner finding thus had to happen discreetly. Between the 1880s and 1950s, Genny Beemyn described both Black and White gay and bisexual men finding partners through cruising in city parks, such as Lafayette and Lincoln Squares, and Franklin and Potomac Parks, as well as in public restrooms ("tearooms"). Longer-term partners would live together as "roommates" in racially segregated rooming houses and apartments, as well as in segregated White and "Colored" YMCAs.[5] Sexual minorities also gathered in mainstream neighborhood bars in Shaw and Columbia Heights, some of which featured drag shows. Beemyn documents Black drag events occurring as early as 1885. By the 1930s, there were apparently enough drag show competitions to elicit a city ban, leading participants to travel to New York or Maryland to perform.[6] Sexual minorities also gathered in private houses and "rent parties" (with an entry charge), which allowed participants to escape police surveillance, harassment, beating, and arrest.[7] The gay/bisexual sexual economy opened up and expanded with the burgeoning of DC's population during World War II, which brought many new patrons, including military personnel, to the city's sexual minority bars. This was part of a national pattern, as documented by Allan Bérubé and John D'Emilio.[8] In DC, the population increase, coupled with liquor laws mandating that alcohol-serving venues must also serve food, led to a proliferation of new spaces to accommodate the growing clientele. These spaces continued to be racially segregated[9] even after the Supreme Court reaffirmed the illegality of restaurant segregation in DC in 1953 following protests and lawsuits led by Mary Church Terrell, a leading African American activist.[10]

The 1950s saw a backlash; in the era of McCarthyism (the "Red Scare" with policing of suspected Communists), there was an ostensible fear that federal employees might be blackmailed because of their sexuality— the so-called Lavender Scare.[11] As a result, thousands were preemptively fired from government jobs if identified as gay.[12] Firing was sometimes accompanied by public naming and shaming in newspapers, making it hard to find another job.[13] Resistance to state surveillance and forced closeting led to the political fight for gay rights both nationally and in Washington, DC.[14] Prominent White DC gay activist Frank Kameny, a World War II veteran and Harvard-trained astronomer in the US Army Map Service, began his activism as a result of being fired by the federal government for being gay.[15] In 1961, a few years later, Kameny cofounded the DC branch of the Mattachine Society, a mostly White gay activist organization, and subsequently led legal and political battles to prohibit federal civil-service and military discrimination against gay people, as well as to fight anti-sodomy laws.[16]

White Sexual Containment

Nationally, among White men, as documented by George Chauncey and others, resistance to discrimination was also accompanied by hardening lines "between the heterosexual and homosexual [now drawn] so sharply and publicly that men were no longer able to participate in a homosexual encounter without suspecting it meant (to the outside world, and to themselves), that they were gay."[17] Previously, homosexuality was based on gender presentation (gender bending versus standard gender presenting men); now, however, it was to be based on sexual identity (gay) and/or practice (having male partners).[18] This ideological shift, combined with resistance to state surveillance, contributed to the creation of "gay ghettos"[19] or gayborhoods, where gay men could be open with their sexuality. As richly described by scholars such as Amin Ghaziani, these were parts of cities, such as LA (West Hollywood), New York (Greenwich Village/Chelsea), Chicago (Boystown), and San Francisco (Castro), where predominantly White gay men constituted significant proportions of the neighborhood.[20] It also made it increasingly difficult for White men to live as straight men who had sex with both men and women, as this was a lifestyle choice that was no longer normalized and tolerated. These gayborhood enclaves—"sexual communities"[21] to which gay men from around the country migrated—became their own spatially distinct sexual economies. Gayborhoods facilitated the (re)emergence and flourishing of institutions specifically catering to men who have sex with men, such as clubs, bars, discos, bathhouses, medical clinics, and community organizations. In short, they (self-)contained and concentrated White gay social life, creating a tight-knit, densely networked community. Gayborhoods offered both social protection and freedom as well as a base for political activism in the fight for gay rights.[22]

In Washington, DC, while there were different gay enclaves in the city, White gay men developed Dupont Circle as a major residential gayborhood in the 1960s and '70s. This development occurred as DC was becoming a chocolate city, and as Kwame Holmes illustrated, the neighborhood positioned itself as being at the leading edge of urban renewal in the city.[23] He noted, "They worked to attach [White] gay commercial development and residency to one of the city's few remaining White middle class neighborhoods, DuPont Circle."[24] The neighborhood was "visibly 'gay' by the mid-1970s,"[25] with an entire social ecosystem including gay restaurants, bookstores, art galleries, bars, and cafes.[26] The *Washington Blade*, the nation's oldest LGBT newspaper, launched in 1969, opened its first office there in 1974.[27] The Whitman-Walker clinic (previously the Gay Men's Venereal Disease Clinic) moved from Georgetown to set up shop near Dupont Circle in 1978.[28]

White gay men also ventured out and created an enclave for partying in the predominantly Black SE, near the Anacostia River. Commercial gay establishments took advantage of abandoned riverfront infrastructure, such as large supply warehouses near the then closed-down Navy Yard, to develop mega club discos, such as Lost and Found (opened in 1971), Grand Central (opened in 1974), and Club Washington, a gay bathhouse, as well as strip clubs, Follies movie theater, Ziegfeld's, and smaller bars and restaurants.[29] Speaking about the rationale for gay commercial development of the area to a reporter, "Frank Kameny, 79, a longtime gay activist, said a perception existed [in the 1970s] that police would ignore gay-oriented businesses if they opened in areas removed from downtown. 'It became an out-of-sight, out-of-mind kind of thing,' he said."[30] This comment, from one of the city's leading gay activists, is striking in capturing the taken-for-granted reality that racial containment had created, the cynical calculation that White gay businessmen were making, and the racial privilege they assumed. While the clubs were out of [White] sight and mind, there were in the backyard of Black residents who had been forcibly displaced out of downtown and relocated there due to urban renewal. Businessmen not only assumed that Black residents would tolerate the clubs (or lacked political power to protest their presence) but also that White sexual minorities would no longer be subject to police criminalization if they located their then-criminalized activity in the Black SE. (Sodomy laws were struck down by the US Supreme Court in 2003). However, as I describe in Parts 3 and 4, Black criminalized activities in the SE were severely punished and residents were overpoliced.

White Sexual Containment Meets Racial Containment

Despite the end of legal segregation, noted earlier, the city's Black sexual minorities continued to be excluded from or discriminated against in White gay residential and social spaces in the city. As historians Kwame Holmes, Genny Beemyn, and Rebecca Dolinsky document, many were excluded from Dupont Circle, and attempts at establishing interracial gay clubs there were short lived.[31] Exclusion or discrimination also occurred in the Navy Yard clubs, located in their own part of the city. Many (though not all) prospective

Black partiers were denied entry to clubs, requested to show more than one form of ID, charged a higher cover price to enter than White patrons, or in some cases, physically thrown out.[32] It was not until 1984, after much protest, activism, and successful filing of human rights complaints, that a bill was passed in the DC City Council to end racist carding practices at White gay clubs,[33] contributing to more diversification.

These racial containment dynamics were part of a national pattern, but they were not inevitable. The nationwide creation of gayborhoods crystallized after the civil rights movement and the end of legal racial segregation in the country. There was thus an opening to create more fully integrated and diverse gayborhoods as communities who had the same sexual orientation and shared histories of oppression. However, this was often not the path taken, as the containment principle was embedded not just in residential aspects of gayborhoods but also in their vibrant social life and institutions. As late as the mid-2000s, for example, Charles Nero, in a piece titled "Why Are All the Gay Ghettoes White?" describes how Black people were excluded from a gayborhood in New Orleans as a result of real estate agents preferentially selling homes to other White gay men, even when poor. In this way, racial solidarity trumped class differences.[34] In Chicago, Ellingson and Schroeder described Black people's overt and covert exclusion from gay enclaves through practices such as triple carding (asking for three different forms of ID) and dress codes.[35] They noted restrictions were lifted during larger public events. In sum, in both historical and contemporary times, and certainly over the past century, while there have likely always been interracial sexual minority coresidence, socializing, and coupling,[36] they have been weighed down by persistent racialized sociostructural, spatial, and normative negative pressure.

Thus, while White gay men created and then escaped to their own neighborhoods and socio-scapes where they could be fully open with their identity and lifestyle, for many Black gay and bisexual men, their sexual and residential lives were spatially integrated with heterosexual people and unfolded within Black neighborhoods.[37] It also meant that while White sexual fluidity had become spatially and structurally limited as strict heterosexual/homosexual dichotomies hardened—at least on the surface[38]—among Black people, queer life, which included sexual fluidity (as sexual practice was less linked to sexual identity and more about the person than their gender) and multioriented identities, unfolded alongside straight life, discreetly or as open secrets.[39]

Postwar DC saw a flourishing of commercial Black gay establishments in Shaw, then a predominantly Black neighborhood.[40] These included restaurant/bars (to accommodate the Alcoholic Beverage Control Board regulations) near Howard University, such as "Kenyon Bar & Grill (opened in 1959) ... Nob Hill Restaurant (opened in 1953) ... Cozy Corner Bar and Grill (opened in 1949), and Rosetta's Golden Nugget Restaurant ... (the 'Black Nugget') ... (opened in 1964)."[41] These clubs were stratified by social class, with establishments catering to both working-class as well as middle- and upper-class Black sexual minorities. In the latter case, discretion was at a premium not just because so many were federal government employees, but also because of the social risk of undermining local and national racial uplift efforts, which many were involved in, as well as their own respectability in the community.[42] As such, there were "nightclubs, theaters, restaurants, [and] gender bending drag performances [which were] extremely popular amongst working class Black audiences,"[43] in addition to more discrete Black social clubs that organized dances, galas, and private house parties for the middle and upper classes, who were lawyers, doctors, and federal employees.[44] That discretion was necessary was made apparent when, reflecting intense homophobia within the Black community, several of the Black-owned gay establishments were targeted and destroyed during the riots following the assassination of Martin Luther King Jr. in 1968.[45] A few places survived, such as Nob Hill[46] (1957–2004), and new establishments were set up in the aftermath, such as the Brass Rail (1973–96), which opened in 1967 but transformed into a predominantly African American club in 1973,[47] and the Club-House (1975–90).[48]

The Black San Francisco

For my respondents, DC in the 1970s and '80s was the "Black gay mecca," a city where they felt they could thrive as Black people and sexual minorities, with a vibrant social life as well as community identity and affirmation as Black. Like Harlem in New York City,[49] DC felt like it had a large sexual minority community, but distinct from New York, DC sexual minorities were living in a predominantly Black city—indeed, the quintessential chocolate city. While many grew up in DC, others moved there permanently as adults, and some socialized in DC while living in the suburbs in their early years before moving there permanently. They were drawn by the prospect of living, working, and socializing in a liberated Black gay space. Chris (all interviewee names are pseudonyms), a gay professional who migrated to DC in 1980, described both the pioneer nature of DC as well as his rich social life there:

> When I moved here in 1980 . . . there were so many house parties of gays and lesbians . . . you didn't necessarily have to go to a club to socialize . . . A lot of Black gays and lesbians moved to DC because DC was considered the Black San Francisco. It had more laws on the books protecting gay people than San Francisco did, quietly. We have gay marriage here in DC. They still don't have it in San Francisco [in 2011] . . . and also there was a very tight-knit Black gay and lesbian community . . . I mean, we had the first Black gay magazine, *Black Light*,[50] in the country. In fact, at one point we had two competing Black gay magazines. Where others had nothing, we had two. We had *Black Light* and one was called *Diplomat* . . . We had social clubs . . . Now there are Black Gay Prides in, like, 23 cities, and I forget how many countries. But DC started it all [in 1991].

Sixty-one-year-old bisexual Gordon grew up in DC, graduated from high school, and joined the Air Force. After returning home from overseas military service, he held a variety of jobs including clerical government work, security, and cleaning. He

> used to . . . try to hit every *[laughs]* every nightclub in the Washington, DC, area. *[laughs]* Man, especially on paydays . . . all I could think of was party, party, party . . . having a good time, you know . . . And, sometimes when I would get tired of the clubs in DC, I would hop on the bus *[laughs]* and go to the clubs in Baltimore! *[laughs]* Party over there till I get tired *[laughs]* . . . So I kept going, kept going . . . back and forth from DC to Baltimore.

In addition to nightclubs, house parties, and social clubs within tight-knit social networks, other gay men lived in "houses" or cliques. Forty-nine-year-old Colin described himself as a "top-of-the-line faggy in Washington, DC, you know . . . I was in that elite." He described belonging to one of three such houses, elaborating:

> Back then we was called the *[names the group]*. It was our clique, you know . . . like After Dark Honeys, Fourth Street Honeys . . . like the House of Khan? . . . It was our house. We had a house *[names location]*, and we had all type of jewelry and furs and top-of-the-line shoes and bags and we were goin' . . . to Manhattan and Queens and Brooklyn, you know. Back then, New York was

the sh-ee-it! And so we would take shuttles, airplanes, you know back and forth . . . it was like, 12 to 15 of us, and we just lived in this house and we just turned it out.

As reflected in this and other accounts, some respondents' social lives stretched across the East Coast but especially within the DC-Maryland-Virginia metro area. Growing up in Richmond, Virginia, 58-year-old bisexual Hiram had always thought that "[DC] was so beautiful and so different, and I just dreamed about living here, all that time, right, and I never knew that I would actually end up living here. So I just kept dreaming . . ." In 1975, when he turned 22, he and his cousin

> would come here [DC] to go to parties and clubs and stuff and then go back home . . . every weekend. On Thursday evening I would pack . . . my luggage, and put it in my trunk, go to work Friday . . . My cousin would meet me [after] work, and we would just jump in the car and drive right from work to the highway, and here we are in DC.

As the city's clubs started opening up, he described going to a mix of Black and interracial clubs, such as the Brass Rail, Bachelor's Mill, Lucy's, the Leather Rack, P Street Beach, and Delta Elite. Their clubbing also extended to Maryland and Philadelphia. Overall, while men's social and sexual lives were focused on Washington, DC, extended sexual networks across the East Coast provided potential pathways through which HIV could enter and then spread within the city.

Once HIV arrived, the city's small size and the concentration of White and Black gay and bisexual social and sexual life, along with the higher risk anal sex carried, made men who had sex with men especially vulnerable, even after medication was widely available. In addition to being one of the "gayest cities in the country" (14.3% of the city's population by one estimate),[51] the racial homogamy principle, and the racially differential odds of encountering HIV—by 2010, a year before my interviews, 1 in 14 Black men had HIV compared to 1 in 34 White men[52]—meant a significantly higher likelihood of Black men encountering HIV in the course of their sexual lives.[53] In Part 5, I describe how racial containment contributed to a racially bifurcated epidemic, proactive White and lagged Black HIV/AIDS activism, and a racially bifurcated city response to the epidemic. Here, I focus on how community norms and intimate relationship dynamics combined with life in a syndemic zone to place Black gay and bisexual men at disproportionate risk of HIV acquisition.

The story of 26-year-old Moses highlights the challenges of intimate life in a syndemic zone. For Moses, clubs were a key part of his transition into a gay identity and lifestyle. As he describes, "I started hangin' around SE at the baseball stadium, with the parties, and still havin' sex and you know, all that, with condoms, without condoms." In thinking through how he might have acquired HIV, his narrative describes multiple exposures to HIV during unprotected sex as well as the larger structural factors that played a role in his vulnerability. His first exposure was in a relationship where his partner did not disclose his HIV status initially. He met his partner in SE, where they lived less than a mile apart. His partner lived with his mother in public housing but also had his own place. As Moses described:

> I was tryin' to get out of SE ... and I met this guy [in SE] and he had an apartment in *[names the location in PG County, Maryland]*. Well, it turns out that the same day I met him is the same day we became boyfriends and ... I moved in the next day. I guess a couple of days went by, like a week or two, and he told me he was HIV positive. And, uh, so, uh, *[silence]* I talked to my mom and she was like—she really didn't want me to be there, but she was like, "If you love him—" which, I really didn't at all, I was just tryin' to get a place to stay, you know. 'Cause I didn't want to stay in SE. There was drugs sellin' where I was livin' at ... It was just too crazy. I knew better, you know? And so I had to get out of that ...

He subsequently described unprotected sex with his boyfriend, even after disclosure, before ending the relationship:

> He got me a job workin' with him ... at a ... company. And one day we had sex in there without a condom, and I knew what I was doin'. And you know, after that I really didn't have sex with him no more, 'cause he wasn't my type. He was attractive, and he had it goin' on. He was five years older than me; I was 20 and he was 25.

They eventually broke up "'cause he started to be violent and shit, so we started to fight ... And so, you know, I moved [back] to SE." Moses then described another relationship where his partner also turned out to have HIV:

> So this [is] how the problem is a bitch. So I started to mess with this other guy ... who told me he was HIV positive. And I was like, "Stop messin' with

him," and then I messed with him, without a condom as well *[snaps fingers]*. So I was actually asking for death. It wasn't like I was tryin' to kill myself, I was just on drugs, and I just was young and dumb, and you know, just tryin' to survive, and just tryin' to be loved and tryin' to love and tryin' to—I don't know, thinkin' I was somethin', whatever.

Subsequent relationships with "undercover" men included "one guy [who] was the type of gay guy that messed with guys like me but who really still messed with females," as well as another such guy "who told me he was HIV positive."

Thus, Moses met a partner in a syndemic zone and moved out, trying to escape drugs, but he ended up in a dependent relationship with an older partner living with HIV who wasn't his type but who was nonetheless providing him with a safe place to stay as well as a job. He then moved back to a syndemic zone where he encountered multiple partners living with HIV, including some who also had sex with women. The zone's overlapping drug epidemic complicated his relationship navigation: He was dependent on drugs and seeking love—often expressed through condomless sex. This dangerous combination would have placed him at heightened risk for HIV even if he had not been drug dependent. It would have required a hypervigilance around HIV testing and condom use to avoid HIV acquisition, even though in his case, all his partners eventually disclosed their HIV status to him.[54] His sexual network linkages provide a picture of how HIV might spread among men who have sex with men and bridge across to women.

Fifty-eight-year-old Hiram had relationships with both men and women, including a marriage to a woman, but "like I said, one [partner] at a time." However, his partners were not monogamous. This was a common theme in narratives of gay and bisexual men, who reported greater relationship openness and tolerance (though not necessarily acceptance) of nonmonogamous partners—all well-documented features of relationships challenging heteronormative (i.e., straight culture's) monogamy norms.[55] Hiram preferred "dealing with straight men, or men that don't, um, deal with the gay lifestyle." Unfortunately, "the only thing I didn't do . . . is back then, is I didn't use a condom . . . it was free love, you know." Hiram attributes his HIV acquisition to a relationship with a male partner of one year who had a concurrent partnership. "I knew I got it from him, 'cause I was only with him, you know . . . So I knew." He described a subsequent relationship with a straight man who had concurrent relationships. "He had three girlfriends while he was dealing with me, and one of the girlfriends he had a child by.

And he still did not stop dealing with me." The relationship ended when the mother of his partner's child "came over to my house" and asked him if her partner "was dealing with a man."

Bisexual men's relationships came under fire in popular media and the Black community when Black heterosexual women's rising HIV vulnerability became widely known. On the one hand, these so-called down low men who had secret sex with men while maintaining relationships and families with women were accused of giving HIV to their women partners. But on the other hand, scholars such as C. Riley Snorton argued that these accusations were simply an extension of a long history of framing and stigmatizing Black men's sexuality more broadly, and sexual minority men's in particular, as disproportionately duplicitous and dangerous.[56] After all, bisexuality, extramarital relationships, and sexual fluidity are not unique to Black men,[57] nor is their impact on HIV transmission. Phylogenetic analysis of US HIV transmission networks by Oster and colleagues found that while men who have sex with men (MSM) of all races/ethnicities mostly get HIV from other MSM (88%), among heterosexual men, half (49%) acquired HIV from heterosexual women and a third (34%) from MSM.[58] Heterosexual women had more transmission links to MSM (29%) than to heterosexual men (21%), and White heterosexual women had more transmission links (39%) to MSM than Black women (25%).[59] However, relatively low White HIV prevalence means that overall, White women are less likely to acquire HIV than Black women simply because Black women are more likely to be living in a syndemic zone with higher community HIV prevalence. In other words, racial containment functions to keep especially White women safe at a structural level, even though they are individually more vulnerable than Black women to HIV acquisition from MSM.

The fearlessness of youth played out in a syndemic zone also made many young Black gay men vulnerable. As 46-year-old James described, when he was in his late teens and early twenties, his attitude was, "I wanna do what I want to do. I want to hang out every night. I would go to the clubs every weekend. I'm not a settle down, I don't want to do the things the settle-down people do." He had an eight-year relationship starting when he was 17, had concurrent relationships along the way, and was diagnosed with HIV in 1989, when he was 24 and at the tail end of his long-term relationship. James never took ART as he was a long-term nonprogressor who remained healthy without medication.[60] James also implicated drug use in his non-use of condoms, noting:

I had sex with no condom, you know, and usually when that happens, not all the time, but a lot of times when that happens, it's because people are getting high, ya know, or when I did it, I was high, 'cause once, when you're high, all morals and scruples go out the window, okay. You don't think about condoms and all that.

Indeed, a crucial factor in the racial bifurcation of the HIV epidemic was delayed Black awareness that HIV was not just "a gay White man's disease," leading to insufficient vigilance around condom use. For 34-year-old Jacob who grew up in DC and was nonmonogamous, "condoms weren't really talked about when I was coming up, um. They were but not to the degree that was as serious as it is now, ya know, um dealing with this epidemic so um." He suspected he might have HIV when he was 19 or 20, saying:

I kind of sort of figured something was going on with me but being as though the stigma of everything . . . if you, ya know, you got tested or . . . if you got that stuff, and that's sort of something I didn't want to do for long, so you know, for a long time I just lived, ya know, hoping and praying that . . . I wasn't infected, um.

He was eventually diagnosed when he was 27 years old. While he got onto ART after diagnosis, which significantly lowered his ability to infect others, for many years after, Jacob did not disclose his HIV status to partners:

For a long time I didn't, I didn't express it um. If somebody asked me I would deny it, and it wasn't like I was in denial 'cause I knew what was going on. I just felt like you don't need to know, you know, and that was even with some of the people that I was having relations with, you know, so . . . I lived like that for a while. [But now] I have to let them know because I have to give that person the opportunity to make a decision, you know, um and that's just where I'm at today. I've been going to groups and stuff, and I hear other people share that they wouldn't tell 'em nothing, and I got to understand that at one point I was there, you know.

Nondisclosure could contribute to the perception that HIV was not a Black problem. Indeed, compared to White people with HIV, Black people experienced slower progress along the HIV care continuum;[61] they tested and were diagnosed later, had later ART uptake, and had lower levels of viral suppression.[62] In combination, this meant that due to racialized sexual economies, while White people could enjoy a kind of "herd immunity" offered by higher ART uptake and viral suppression, Black people with HIV were infectious for longer periods of time. Further, Black communities had higher viral loads than White communities, creating heightened Black community HIV risk.[63]

"THE END OF [WHITE] AIDS" AND WHITE SEXUAL CONTAINMENT

As a result of these dynamics, and as Figure 23 illustrated, White HIV incidence began to taper off soon after ART became widely available, in concert with national trends. The subsequent dramatic reductions in AIDS mortality (see Part 5) led to a national discourse around "the End of AIDS" and "Getting to Zero."[64] Alongside this presumed end of the AIDS emergency and the transformation of HIV into a manageable chronic disease for many, there was also a shift in the sexual residential geography of White gay men. Indeed, alongside talk of a "post-HIV" world, there was also talk of a "post-gay" world[65]—as gay clubs began to close, gayborhoods began to be integrated by young straight families, and sexuality appeared to play a less central role in gay men's residential decision-making.[66] This reflected gay rights movement achievements towards ending discrimination in a range of areas, such as employment and same-sex marriage. However, even in a post-gay world, where historic markers began to be placed in neighborhoods, Amin Ghaziani and Jason Orne described racism and harassment in Boystown when queer youth of color began visiting a community youth center.[67] Adam Green described the racialized encounters of Black men who participated in the downtown gay scene in New York City, which ranged from racialized exclusion, to complete invisibility in gay spaces, to patterned or highly circumscribed inclusion as exoticized men.[68] In other words, a post-gay world was not necessarily a post-racial world.

By the 2000s, Dupont Circle shared many features of other gayborhoods around the country. It began to be integrated by young straight families as it became the leading edge of cappuccino-style gentrification and a White return to the city.[69] Alan Hersker recorded similar complaints among Dupont Circle residents as Ghaziani in Boystown.[70] Commenting on the intrusion of straight people, one of Hersker's respondents noted that this would "continue until . . . the baby carriages get so thick the queens can't roller blade down the street."[71] Hersker also described continued racial exclusion and tensions arising from minority presence in the neighborhood.[72] The sexual integration of Dupont Circle was paralleled by other developments in the late 1990s and early 2000s. By that point, as William Leap described, the gay club district was "attracting a diverse clientele—members of the military, blue-collar workers, farm boys from rural Maryland, residents of the city and the suburbs, of older and younger ages and of White, Black, Hispanic and Asian backgrounds."[73] However, Mayor Anthony Williams's administration created redevelopment plans as part of work to increase the city's revenue through gentrification. Businesses were notified in 2005, and the gay club district, public housing projects with hundreds of residents, and other buildings were razed to make way for the city's new urban renewal scheme, which included a new baseball stadium for the Washington Nationals and high-end housing.[74] As 53-year-old Lionel reminisced:

> They don't have as many clubs . . . we would flourish for clubs. Yeah, but um, they had done away with all that, since . . . in the last 10 years . . . yeah, it's been about 10 years . . . the politicians . . . like I'd say were trying to change the stigma from gay to straight . . . building . . . complexes, and stuff like that . . . so they did away with a lot of the clubs.

Writing about the relatively limited or ambivalent protest from White gay men regarding these plans, Leap described the increasing association of the club district with urban decay and crime, with one of his respondents describing how it was "very isolated" and "reminiscent of an older time for the gay experience."[75] Business owners had to plow the snow from their own streets and conduct their own security to prevent vandalism, due to city neglect and ineffective policing.[76] But now, as Leap showed through an innovative study asking DC gay men to draw maps of their movements, White gay communal residential and social life had spatially dispersed. White sexual containment, as it were, was no longer seen as necessary and was becoming, as with other cities, "reminiscent of an older time."

Black gay clubs around the country also began to close in the 1990s and 2000s, not just because of gentrification but also because of the devastating impact of the AIDS epidemic on gay and bisexual Black male clientele.[77] In DC, both the Club House and the famous Brass Rail closed in 1990 and 1996, respectively. There was also an impact on the close-knit DC network of Black gay house parties—where key patrons and funders of social activities, as well as many clientele, were among the many who died of AIDS. As Chris described:

CHRIS: There were so many house parties ... But a lot of that changed, because ... a lot of people who had the resources, that had the homes, that had the jobs to do that, died, you know. And so, so, now you don't have that kind of house party thing. I mean, there would be social clubs, but all they would do is throw these—these are big house parties, like, you know, like, *The Best of Washington*. Um, which is the only one probably left, but there used to be one called *The Family,* uh, there's one called *The Associates* who do something maybe twice a year. But like, like, a lot of things—that so, you didn't necessarily have to go to a club to socialize, but a lot of that is gone now. In fact, all of it is gone now, just about.

SANYU: So that's primarily because a lot of people died?

CHRIS: Yeah.

As I discuss in Part 5, it was not until the late 2000s that the pace of the city's Black AIDS mortality epidemic began to slow down and the "End of AIDS" discourse became relevant for the Black community. With respect to HIV, while the contemporary socio-scape hosts a rich, more racially integrated social life for sexual minority men, which young men like Moses enjoyed, and the internet has transformed and seemingly de-spatialized matchmaking, young Black men nationally and in DC are now the most vulnerable to HIV acquisition,[78] suggesting that racial containment has merely changed form.

CONCLUSION

In sum, racial and sexual containment in DC contributed to both heightened vulnerability for sexual minority men in general and for Black men in particular. Once the HIV epidemic arrived, for both groups, spatialized containment—in gayborhoods and in clubs, house parties, and other small social gatherings—combined with higher-risk sex to produce disproportionate HIV vulnerability relative to the general population. However, racially differential HIV/AIDS awareness and ART uptake led to dramatically different epidemic trajectories (see Figure 23), producing relative community safety for White men but growing community vulnerability for Black men. This was compounded for Black men living in syndemic zones, among whom interviews revealed syndemic amplification—that is, interacting epidemics like the drug epidemic and the HIV epidemic, which worked together to amplify HIV risk for zone residents and connected others. Residents experienced multiple exposures to HIV in sexual networks and the drug economy, which compromised personal and sexual safety. These sociostructural and institutional features of neighborhoods transformed "free love" norms of nonmonogamy and non-use of condoms into dangerous community norms, making even low-risk Black individuals—monogamous and in long-term partnerships—vulnerable.

FIVE

The HIV Epidemic Among Heterosexual Men, Women, and Trans Women

IN THIS CHAPTER, I EXAMINE how and why heterosexual Black women and men came to be disproportionately impacted by the epidemic. I first discuss the DC heterosexual epidemic and then draw on US census and American Community Survey data (1880–2020) to examine historical and contemporary trends in family formation. I show how and why distorted sexual economies shaped Black heterosexual relationship dynamics and heightened HIV risk in syndemic zones. I discuss the roles of unemployment, mass incarceration, and premature death of young Black men (discussed in the Introduction and Part 1) in creating these distortions in sexual economies. This approach enables me to locate respondents' lives, choices, and health outcomes within the city's larger historical trajectory. I then turn to examining the unique HIV vulnerability of transgender Black women and their relationships with men. I show how they shared the structural features of community life experienced by sexual minority men (Chapter 4) as well as the challenges of distorted relationship markets experienced by cisgender[1] heterosexual women.

The DC HIV epidemic was notable nationally because it was a generalized epidemic, with more than 1% of the city affected. Further, unlike many other US cities where the vast majority of people acquiring HIV were men who have sex with men, in DC, as noted in the Part 2 introduction, about a quarter of people acquired HIV through heterosexual sex. Manya Magnus and colleagues conducted a respondent-driven survey on HIV and sexual behavior risk in predominantly Black low-income neighborhoods in Washington, DC, and found a 5.2% HIV prevalence rate. They concluded that "primary [HIV] risk may simply be engaging in normative heterosexual sexual behavior within a network with a high prevalence of HIV."[2] In other words, when there was a 1 in 20 likelihood of encountering a partner with HIV, even one regular long-term partnership might put someone at a higher risk of HIV acquisition compared to the same choice in a neighborhood with less HIV. Further, the disproportionate vulnerability of Black people in the city as a whole—4.7% were living with HIV compared to 1.5% of White people[3]—suggested a sexual economy with racial homogamy (i.e., same-race partnering) as an organizing principle in the formation of individual partnerships and sexual networks (see Part 2 introduction).

Another striking feature of the city's epidemic was its age distribution: HIV was not a young person's epidemic but one driven by middle-aged adults (here defined as aged 30–59). In the 2010 HAHSTA report, a year before my interviews, HIV prevalence was highest among people in their 40s (7.4%) and 50s (6.1%), and more people in their 60s (1.7%) had HIV than those in their 20s (1.2%). Only 0.1% of teenagers aged 13–19 were living with HIV.[4] This was not just aging survivors: three-quarters (75.6%) of new HIV/AIDS diagnoses were among people aged 30 and over, and half (50.5%) were among those 40 and over.[5] Given that most people may only live 6–10 years in the absence of medication[6] (for which HIV diagnosis through testing is required), this suggests that most new acquisition occurred when people were 30 and over.

This is surprising as we might expect most middle-aged adults to have transitioned out of searching for a partner and be settled into long-term monogamous relationships—presumably the safest relationships for HIV prevention. Yet, ironically, long-term partnerships, such as marriage, can be higher risk than short-term casual partnerships because of repeated HIV exposure during unprotected sex; trusting partners and/or those trying to conceive a child are unlikely to use condoms.[7] The presumed safety also assumes that participants enter such partnerships without HIV and thus tested before sex. However, almost half of people in DC with AIDS (44%) tested less than a year before their diagnosis.[8] The rapid progression from HIV to AIDS implies that many lived with HIV for several years, signaling a low rate of proactive HIV testing, a prerequisite for ART. Another assumption of long-term partnerships being protective is that participants are monogamous or are regularly using condoms if not (and not sharing needles if they inject drugs). A final important assumption is that people are finding partners within low-HIV-prevalence sexual networks, keeping in mind the normal way people partner in the US (as noted in the Part 2 introduction, condom use is low and pre-relationship STI/HIV testing are nonnormative). However, both nationally and in DC, many factors worked together in preceding decades to undermine African Americans' ability to be in such relationships when HIV took hold among heterosexuals. That is, being in long-term, stable relationships, with high levels of proactive HIV testing, high levels of monogamy and/or high levels of condom use to protect against HIV, and selecting partners from low-HIV-prevalence sexual networks. I examine these factors next.

HOW HETEROSEXUAL MARRIAGE CHANGES CREATED THE PERFECT STORM FOR HIV SPREAD

The figures that follow give a population-level view of racial and gendered trends in heterosexual family formation in the US over the past 140 years (see note for same-sex marriage trends.)[9] As Figure 24 illustrates, between 1880 and 1960, non-Hispanic Black people were more likely to have married at least once by age 50 compared to non-Hispanic White people. By 1930, about 94% and 96% of Black men and women, respectively, aged 50 years and older had ever married, compared to about 90% and 91% of White men and women of the same age. A wartime marriage boom between 1940 and 1950 was followed by a convergence in Black and White marriage patterns by 1970. However, over the last 40 years, starting around 1980, when the HIV epidemic also began in earnest, a large racialized transformation in relationship formation occurred. While there was a long-term upward trend in rates of people never marrying (or of first marriages after the age of 50) across all groups, rates of Black people never getting married rose higher and faster than White people. By 2020, 20.6% and 20.5% of Black women and men respectively, had not married by age 50, compared to 6.3% and 8.9% of White women and men, respectively.

As illustrated in Figure 25, overall between 1880 and 2000, men were more likely to report current marriage than women. In 1880, 83.5% of Black men and 81.1% of White men were currently married; their rates remained the same until 1940 and then diverged. For White people, women's trends changed little over the 140 year period, with just under 60% currently married; among men, the proportion married increased between 1950 and 1980 and then steadily decreased. Black women's trends changed little between 1880 and 1960, with just under 50% currently married. Proportions of married Black men and women began to steadily drop from 1960. By 1990, 60.3% of men and 34.4% of women were currently married. After 2000, fewer Black

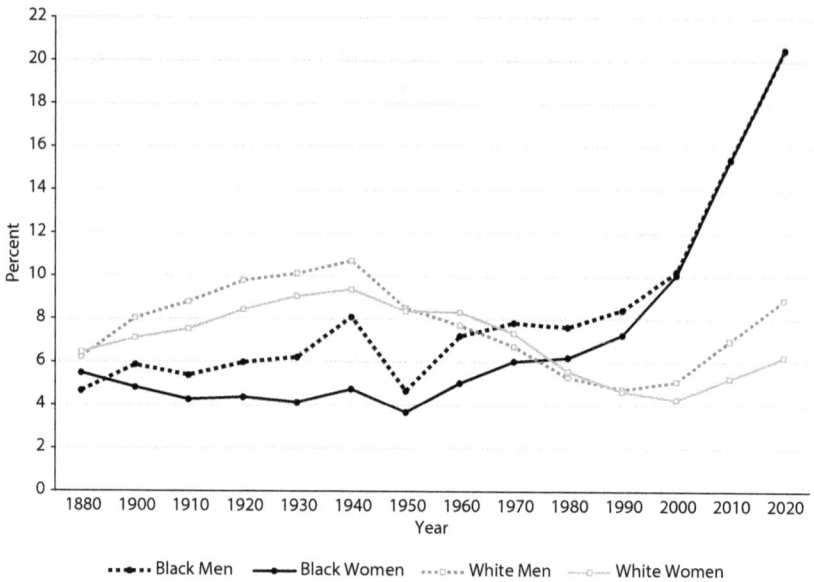

FIGURE 24. Percent never married, US, 50 and older, by race and gender, 1880–2020. Data source: US Census Bureau, American Community Survey (IPUMS).

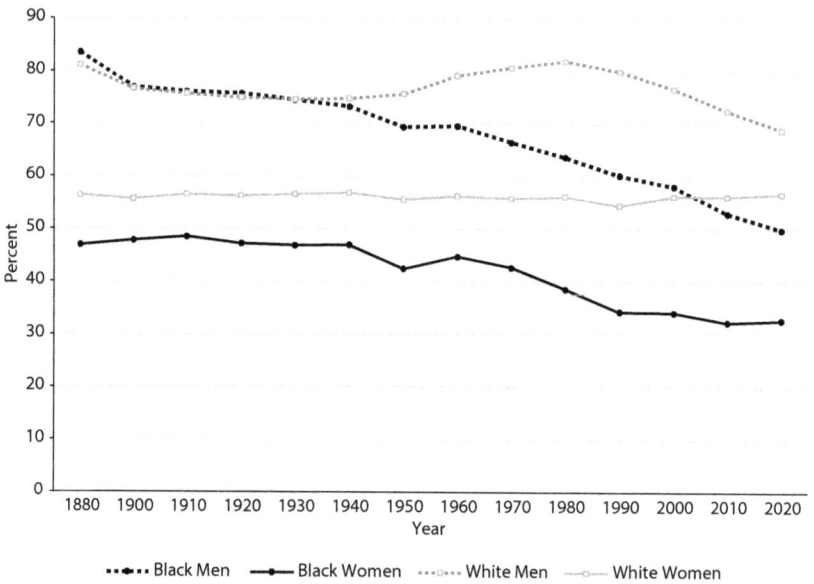

FIGURE 25. Percent currently married, US, 50 and older, by race and gender, 1880–2020. Data source: US Census, American Community Survey (IPUMS).

men were currently married than White women, and by 2020, 49.9% of Black men and 32.8% of Black women were currently married. In terms of other relationship statuses, racial inequality in widowhood significantly declined over time, especially for women (in 1880, 47.1% of Black and 36.7% of White women over 50 were widowed; by 2020, 19.4% of Black and 18.6% of White women were widowed). After 1980, there were significant increases in divorce. Between 1980 and 2020, the Black divorce rate increased from 8.2% to 18.3% for men and from 9% to 22.5% for women, and the White divorce rate increased from 4.7% to 14.8% for men and from 5.7% to 17.2% for women.[10]

Overall, from 1970 onwards, there was a dramatic racial divergence in family formation patterns, with Black people, and Black women in particular, at the leading edge of nationwide trends in declining proportions of married people, through both rising rates of never marrying and divorce. By 2020, among Black women aged 50 and older, only 32.8% were currently married; 20.6% had never married, 22.5% were divorced, 4.7% were separated, and 19.4% were widowed. Even when widening the definition from current marriage to include those who were cohabiting, a Pew study found that 59% of Black and 33% of White people aged 25–54 were unpartnered in 2019, with Black women more likely to be unpartnered (62%) compared to Black men (55%).[11]

Compared to national trends, Washington, DC, is both unique and similar. The city has one of the nation's lowest marriage rates,[12] and as illustrated in Figure 26, the rate of non-Hispanic White people in DC over the age of 50 who never married is higher than their national counterparts (see Figure 24). In 1880, 11.4% of White men and 10% of White women in DC had never married by age 50. This rose to 21.5% of White men and 26% of White women in 1980. By 2020, 21% of White women and 27% of White men were never married. Non-Hispanic Black patterns in DC mirrored those of their national counterparts, though at much higher levels after 1990. In 1880, about 5.5% of Black men and 5.8% of Black women in DC had never married by age 50. By 1970, 9.1% and 11.6% of Black men and women had never married. By 2000, 16.5% and 15.8% of Black men and women never married. By 2020, 38.9% and 34.6% of Black men and women, respectively, had never married by age 50. This suggests historical period and cohort effects[13] among Black people who missed the typical marriage window when they were in their 20s, 30s, and 40s in prior decades.[14]

As Figure 27 illustrates, among people aged 50 and older in DC, many more men than women were currently married. Before 1990, there was relative similarity in the rate of current marriage between Black and White men. In 1880, 78.8% of Black and 74.8% of White men were currently married.

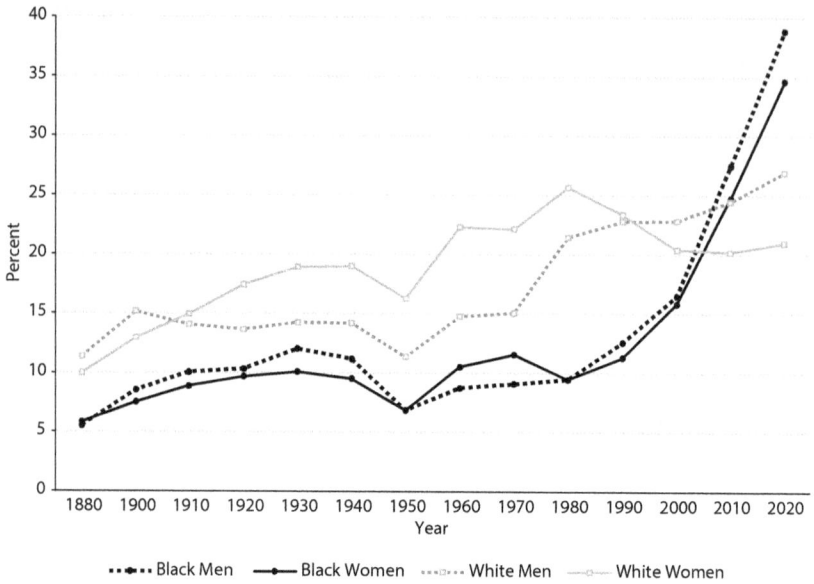

FIGURE 26. Percent never married, DC, 50 and older, by race and gender, 1880–2020. Data source: US Census, American Community Survey (IPUMS).

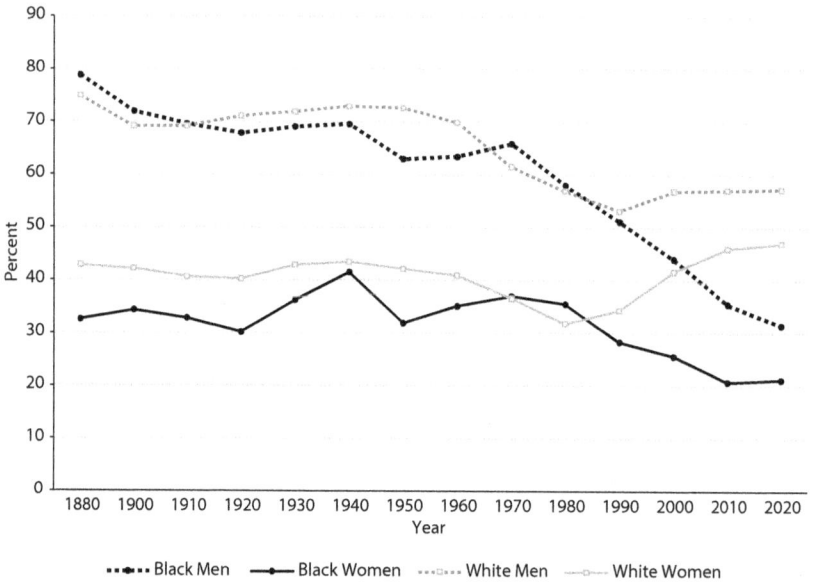

FIGURE 27. Percent currently married, DC, 50 and older, by race and gender, 1880–2020. Data source: US Census, American Community Survey (IPUMS).

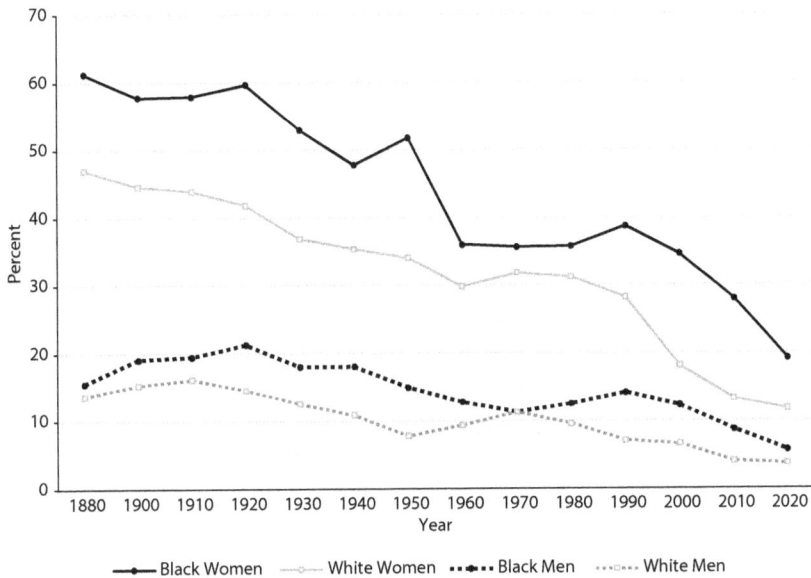

FIGURE 28. Percent widowed, DC, 50 and older, by race and gender, 1880–2020. Data source: US Census, American Community Survey (IPUMS).

Proportions fluctuated between 60% and 70% between 1940 and 1970. However, a racial divergence occurred after 1990, with dramatic declines for Black men, falling to a low of 31.5% married at age 50 or older in 2020 (compared to 57.3% of White men). About 40% of White women were currently married between 1880 and 1960. The proportion declined to 31.8% by 1980 and then steadily rose in ensuing decades. Among Black women, the rate of those currently married fluctuated between 30% and 40% between 1880 and 1980 before declining to 21.2% in 2020 (compared to 47.1% of White women).

The fact that most Black women had married at least once suggests that there was a high level of marriage loss or instability. This is confirmed by examining rates of widowhood/widowerhood, separation, and divorce. As Figure 28 illustrates, in 1880, widowhood rates were exceptionally high: 61.2% of Black and 47% of White women aged 50 or older were widowed. High widowhood rates, especially among Black women, persisted until 1990, before a dramatic decline (38.7% of Black and 28.2% of White women were widowed in 1990; 19.2% of Black and 11.8% of White women were widowed in 2020). Among men aged 50 or older, between 1880 and 1980, widowerhood rates fluctuated between 11%–21% for Black men and 9%–16% for White men. In 2020, about 5.7% of Black and 3.7% of White men were widowers.

This age group also saw significant increases in marital instability between 1980 and 2020. In 1980, divorce rates by race and gender were similar (8.6% of Black men, and 9.9% of Black women, White men, and White women). By 2020, 21% of Black and 19.1% of White women were divorced, and 18.4% of Black and 11.2% of White men were divorced. Black people also had higher rates of separation than White people.

In sum, until 2000, even though about two-thirds of Black people aged 50 or older in DC married at least once, fewer remained married due to higher rates of widowhood, separation, and divorce. After 2000, however, it was apparent that significant proportions of Black cohorts never married during their prime reproductive years. These trends had implications for the city's health more broadly, as marriage is protective of health and life expectancy, especially for men.[15] They were also consequential for the city's HIV epidemic.

Indeed, what these figures illustrate is that by the time the heterosexual HIV epidemic had taken hold, most of the city's Black women were navigating relationships outside of marriage. At an individual level, this meant that those desiring marriage, marrying later, or not at all dealt with elongated periods with casual partners, greater partner turnover, more years of potential HIV exposure, and the need to negotiate condom use multiple times with new partners, compared to married women. At a structural level, a racially contained sexual economy characterized by racial homogamy and life in syndemic zones (with high community-HIV prevalence (or viral load) and other amplifying epidemics, such as drugs) exacerbated HIV risk. Racial homogamy limited many Black women's options and they experienced partner shortages, with consequences for relationship dynamics and subsequent HIV vulnerability.

Partner Shortage

Black women's partner shortage was the result of a number of factors. As described in Part 1, many Black men in DC were missing from the heterosexual economy because they had died. By the 1980s, homicide had become a leading cause of death for young Black men, and by the 1990s, they were 9 times more likely to die by age 20–21 than young White men (Part 1). These were the would-be partners for women born in the '60s and '70s, who were in their 20s and 30s when young men were dying and in their 40s and 50s by the height of the HIV epidemic in the city in the late 2000s and early 2010s. Black men were also absent because of mass incarceration. Eric Lotke estimated that half (49.9%) the city's young Black men (18–35 years) were under criminal

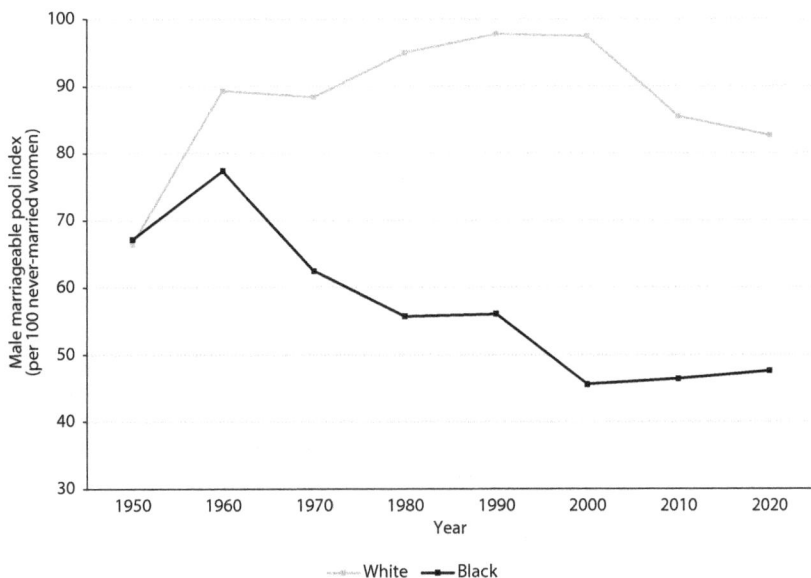

FIGURE 29. DC male marriageable pool index, 1950–2020. Data source: US Census Bureau 1950–2000, American Community Survey 5-year data 2010–2020 (IPUMS), Bureau of Justice Statistics.

justice supervision (imprisoned, on parole, or awaiting trial) by 1997,[16] many for exceptionally long prison terms. Nationally, harsh job market penalties for having a prison record,[17] coupled with high school dropout rates (Part 4), impacted Black men's access to employment and well-paid jobs, and these both contributed to low marriage rates and high divorce rates.[18] Men's un- and underemployment made marriage less attractive for Black women and placed an early strain on Black marriages, especially as Black women were early pioneers of the second shift—combining breadwinning and homemaking.[19]

To encapsulate the state of the heterosexual marriage market, the "male marriageable pool index" was developed by Wilson and Neckerman[20] to estimate the proportion of men in a given community who are not married, dead, unemployed, or incarcerated. Nationally, in 1985, early in the epidemic, Pinderhughes described an index showing 73 Black men per 100 Black women and 43 "marriageable" Black men per 100 Black women. (This was compared to 93 White men per 100 White women and 63 "marriageable" White men per 100 White women).[21] Figure 29 shows estimated trends in the index in DC between 1950 and 2020. The figure depicts dramatically different marriage markets for DC's Black and White women, assuming the racial homogamy principle. After the epidemic began in the early 1980s, while never-married White women (20–49 years) experienced near parity in marriageable partners, similar Black women experienced severe partner shortages, with fewer than 60 marriageable Black men per 100 Black women after 1970 and fewer than 50 marriageable Black men per 100 Black women after 1995.[22]

CONCURRENCY

The shortage of "marriageable" Black men reflects, in sociologist Patricia Hill Collins's words, the "intersecting oppressions of race, gender, class and sexuality [that] provide the backdrop for Black heterosexual love relationships," with consequences for "the micro-politics of intimate love relationships" among Black couples.[23] At the heart of this politics is the inherent gender power imbalance it creates, mapping onto historical legacies to shape contemporary relationship norms and expectations. American Black men experience restrictions to traditional means of performing patriarchally valued heterosexual masculinity, such as owning property, being the breadwinner, and leading a so-called intact family.[24] These limits began during slavery, when many Black men were considered White men's property and were not considered human enough to own property themselves, whose wives were themselves treated as White men's property and were sometimes raped to hasten the production of additional slaves to increase property, and whose children were sold to become other White men's property.[25] Slavery in the US officially ended in 1865; however, since then, a variety of institutional mechanisms have replicated this denial in both explicit and benign ways. The most recent examples are restrictions on the ability to own a home (through job discrimination and mortgage and loan discrimination, aided by government agencies such as FHA and HOLC), mass incarceration (including racially discriminatory arrest, sentencing, and employment on release), restrictions on the ability to be a physically present father (due to mass incarceration, inability to financially provide, rules disincentivizing male partners in public housing), and so on.[26] These limitations have placed a premium on paternity and sexual prowess, regardless of marriage, as a means to establishing valued markers of American masculinity.[27]

As such, partner shortages and their underlying drivers led to several distortions in the Black heterosexual economy, a primary one being concurrency, or overlapping relationships. Concurrency is not only a sexual market response to a surplus of available women relative to men but also a way to perform a more possible, yet valued, masculinity (sexual prowess), as compared to participation in institutions such as marriage, where many financially insecure men are primed to fail.[28] Concurrency, in turn, is hugely consequential for HIV transmission.[29] Studies conducted in the 1990s and 2000s found that concurrency rates were higher among African Americans both within and outside of marriage compared to other groups. In the General Social Survey, about 33% and 15.9% of African American men and women, respectively, reported having ever had extramarital sex, compared to 21.4% and 11.1% of White men and women, respectively.[30] Unmarried African Americans also reported high concurrency.[31] Importantly, both men and women are concurrent, and women sometimes report higher concurrency than men. Thus, both men and women put each other at risk.[32] (As noted earlier, phylogenetic work revealed that about half of US heterosexual men with HIV acquired it from heterosexual women).[33]

Concurrency in a Syndemic Zone

These national dynamics were mirrored in DC, where the rate of concurrency was high,[34] and were reflected in my interviews among heterosexuals living with HIV. When 42-year-old Ida first met her now ex-partner in her teens, he was with a woman with whom he had a daughter. He and Ida eventually got together, but he continued to have concurrent relationships; as she recounted: "He ended up owning his own business. And . . . we moved into a house together . . . he was still seeing his kids' moms. He had a lot of kids, quite a few, later on to find out." She still stayed with him for 20 years, though hurt and ambivalent, because

> he was a good provider in the home. He took care of the home. It was just his, um, cheating, and you know that part, that really kinda, um, made the relationship difficult . . . And I was young. I had fought a lot of his babies' mothers . . . You know . . . I had done went through so much. You know, the cheating, the fighting of womens, the catching him, the taking care of his kids, to go have company come in town and find you the next day in the bed with the baby and the kid's mother. And stuff like that . . . But, I guess, the, the, the fact that he was a provider, a great provider, was enough . . . If my car broke today, tomorrow I had a new car, but the next night he might be out with the car with another girl, you know. So . . .

Ida thus had to weigh his being a "great provider" against his concurrency. In reflecting on why many women tolerated concurrency, 49-year-old Alyssa explained:

> ALYSSA: They'd rather have a man than no man. They'd rather have a man that's gon' cheat on them than to have no man at all . . . Because it's such a shortage of men, of good men that's willing to stay in the home and help them with the children. And then even some women that don't have children just want to have a man in their life. So they'll accept him cheating.
>
> SANYU: Why is there a shortage of men?
>
> ALYSSA: Most of them are locked up first of all, incarcerated. A lot of the straight good men are locked up so you have like, there's only so many of them left on the street. So I'm gonna have either him or nobody, so I'll just deal with him cheating, as long as he comes back to me, he can cheat as much as he wants. And he helps me with my situation, I'll accept him in his situation . . .

Alyssa's own relationship history reflected these dynamics. She described her relationships as "horrible things," recounting how they "lasted like three to four years" with partners who "just wasn't about being with one woman." She went on to note that "each time I was only sleeping with them. But they were always sleeping with other people."

Alyssa was diagnosed with HIV in 1992 when she was 30. She decided to test after two consequential events. She found out that her former boyfriend who injected drugs had died of "the big A." Shortly after, she and her mother were denied additional life insurance, and she "kind of put it together." Among the many emotions she experienced at diagnosis was puzzlement:

> [My physician] told me that "you have contracted the HIV virus." And I was numb. 'Cause I couldn't believe, at first I thought that was a gay White man's disease, first of all, and I didn't, I knew I wasn't gay, I knew I wasn't White. So I couldn't figure out how I could have gotten this.

Thus, despite past relationships with concurrent men, and her most recent boyfriend injecting drugs, the disease was cast in her mind as a sexually and racially contained disease—for gay White men. She did not know she was living in a syndemic zone and had not expected to need to protect herself against HIV. The multiple potential exposures inherent to a syndemic zone were also apparent in an interview with 56-year-old Elijah who was unsure whether he got HIV through injecting drug use or from his wife. As he recounts:

In 1998, um, I found out that I had contracted the HIV virus. And, um, *[silence]* um, uh, it wasn't through sex . . . my cousin was an intravenous drug user, and, uh, that's the only way he had it. And as I look back, that's where— that's the only place I actually got it . . . but, um, uh, my children's mother, um, at the time we had just got married . . . and once I found out I had it, uh, I came back home and I told her that I found out . . . She broke down and she started cryin' . . . she told me *she* was HIV positive. So I—I—I didn't get mad, uh, you know, 'cause we still have the children, you know . . . she passed [that] November, two days after Thanksgiving . . . We was teenage sweethearts. So when we decided to tie the knot, to find out . . .

Elijah described how during their 30-year relationship, "it was two breakups . . . I guess the second breakup . . . she had an affair. I had an affair." His narrative highlights the couple's multiple exposures to HIV, both through the syndemic amplification with the concurrent drug epidemic[35] as well as from their relationship breaks when they partnered with other people in a high-HIV-prevalence environment.

Forty-three-year-old Langston's narrative revealed the potential for concurrency to spread HIV across multiple sexual networks. He grew up in the western US, and after his "mother and father passed three months apart," he dropped out of college and moved to DC to join other family members. He met his first long-term girlfriend in the SE, and a few years later, had a concurrent partner. As he described:

I was 19 when I met [Girlfriend 1]. And I think I met [Girlfriend 2] when I was 25. I was cheating on both of them . . . me and [Girlfriend 2] . . . had a child together, me and [Girlfriend 1] never had a child together . . . me and [Girlfriend 1] would have been a better couple . . . But I, I fell in love with [Girlfriend 2] . . . I loved [Girlfriend 1] too, but I felt like, I fell in love with [Girlfriend 2].

His relationship with his second girlfriend was in the end a "love-hate relationship" because while they loved each other, they always argued. They had since moved on, and he suspected she "might have another friend," but he still called her his "wife," and they enjoyed their grandchildren from their son. Langston suspected that he acquired HIV from his friendship group and their collective concurrency. He described how he and his friends used to share sexual partners, then one by one they got diagnosed with HIV, which for some led to AIDS-related death:

[One of] my buddies [Friend 1], he would always have two or three women at his house. Every night, you know, we'd hang there and party . . . And I would have sex with some of these girls. And this went on for maybe like a year or two years, you know . . . although I was still messing with [Girlfriend 1] . . . My best friend [Friend 2] . . . he was the first one who was diagnosed with HIV, he passed, um then . . . my buddy [Friend 3] . . . he was diagnosed with HIV, and he died of complications of AIDS. Yeah. And that's what really, really made me go get, and get myself checked out . . . it was, unprotected sex, you know . . .

As each participant became newly infected, high viral load meant dramatically increased transmission probabilities, speeding HIV through the sexual network. Lack of HIV risk awareness meant late testing, diagnosis, and ART uptake, increasing the chances of dying from AIDS. Langston continued:

Once I found out, I stopped having sex with [Girlfriend 1] and um, [Girlfriend 2] we just stopped, period . . . and they, they questioned me. You know, "Why you don't want to do nothing?" "Oh I'm tired." [And then] I disappeared . . . I just left from around them . . . and I think I was more fearful that they found out that I had it, you know, and . . . thank God that they didn't caught it, they never had it, and I didn't pass it on to them.

Despite abstaining from sex after diagnosis, Langston's girlfriends had nonetheless been exposed during the years he was living with undiagnosed, and thus unmedicated, HIV.

CONDOM USE, DISCLOSURE, AND ONWARD TRANSMISSION

Condom use and HIV status disclosure to partners were critical in stemming onward HIV transmission. However, in interviews, prediagnosis condom use was low, and HIV status disclosure was inconsistent in part due to stigma. In men's interviews, condom use was primarily discussed in relation to postdiagnosis relationships. Despite its obvious protective value and preeminence in HIV prevention campaigns, in practice, condom use was imbued with ambivalence. It is a sign of a deliberate decision to not become a father, or of not trusting a partner, or a signal to a partner of one's involvement in concurrent relationships. This discouraged condom use.[36] Women had differential attitudes toward and abilities to negotiate safe sex.[37] In a study of DC women, Lisa Bowleg and colleagues found that while they wanted to use condoms, they felt that their male partners controlled initiation and could refuse using them.[38] For women I interviewed, prior to their HIV diagnoses, inconsistent condom use was the norm. As 49-year-old Hazel remarked, "We know HIV is out there, but we're also looking for it to be among guys who are gay." Like Alyssa, she did not consider herself at risk. Further, aging and economic insecurity complicated safe sex, as Hazel went on to note:

> You could say back then, "Because I don't wanna get pregnant." But now people know you're 43 or 45, you're menopausal, so you're not gonna have a baby anyway, so what do you want to use a condom for? So there goes our excuse. So then you have to have lots of self-esteem and not be in an economically low place, where when you meet a man you got to go with what he says.

Even vigilant people could be affected when they slipped up. Forty-eight-year-old Rita was one of the few respondents who reported regularly using condoms, "but not with everybody." She was fully aware that "AIDS had been hitting and we had lost a friend," so she would urge her friends to use condoms. "I would take them to the store and make them buy condoms and say, 'You don't go on a date without these.'" Rita nonetheless contracted HIV when she was 27:

> I had what I called a fuck partner ... Known him for a few years and whenever I was not in a relationship or just wanted to have a good time I would call him, 'cause that was just great, we made each other laugh, but um he was the one with the HIV. He didn't know. And I can tell you in '90 we did it, and that night I got infected. He was at my apartment, it was one of those nights I had a fight with the boyfriend that was away and I called him over, we were sitting around drinking some Hennessey [whiskey] ... and I had sex in the front room with my friend unprotected and I got HIV.

Rita's HIV acquisition highlights the challenge of being in a high-HIV-prevalence community; "folk epidemiology"—where condom use was for strangers and love and trust turned familiar partners, even if they were on again/off again, into people who were safe—became deadly as it led to both potential repeated HIV exposure and a lower likelihood of condom use.

Rita subsequently struggled with HIV transmission guilt and disclosure:

> And see, that's another thing you have to live with before you officially diagnosed. How many people did you sleep with unprotected that you passed it to? I go in my head and I know at least two ... I went to the health department. I gave their names, I gave their jobs, I wanted them notified. And one guy did get notified 'cause he got kicked out the military ... he got diagnosed

and he was out. And I felt so bad because he had a whole family to support, well an ex-wife, but still. So you live with the guilt with this thing. You don't know if you've killed somebody.

The fear of "killing somebody" also haunted her navigation of subsequent relationships. In one relationship, she described how "we having sex and the condom broke and I freaked out more than the guy did." She insisted he go to the doctor, "and then I couldn't have sex with him anymore, and he couldn't understand it. And I'm like, 'I don't want to kill you.'" She also experienced a lot of stigma when finding new partners. One guy "thought I should be grateful 'cause he wanted to date me," arguing that "nobody else would date your dirty ass." Indeed, her last relationship ended when she found out that her partner had married someone else without her knowledge but "thought that I should be grateful because he's married and still interested." When she felt a relationship might be going somewhere, "then you have to tell them, and then it's like 'Oh, you nasty.'" Reflecting on these experiences, she said, "I think it's tougher for me because I'm straight and trying to date in the straight world being HIV positive. I think in the gay community, it's not expected, but it's not a surprise."

While Rita was forthright in disclosing, many others struggled to disclose their status to partners, which could increase transmission. Forty-nine-year-old Cora was diagnosed in 1989 and started medication in 2006. She described condom use as a recent practice:

SANYU: Did you ever use condoms, like, during those years?

CORA: Now, now.

SANYU: Now. But not back then?

CORA: Uh...no. Mm-mmm...Maybe a few times...if you did, you did, you didn't, you didn't...but recently, in the last few years, yeah. Mm-hmm...[I] had to learn how to protect me, you know. Now the women's condoms is something I know about...my form of protection was the male condom, but I finally have gone for the female condoms now.

Regarding HIV disclosure, she said, "Never told any of them. Mm-mmm. Just started doing that recently, in the last few years. Mm-hmm. Last few years." Her condom use was motivated by having a woman-controlled option and self-protection from reinfection. Some nondisclosers felt people should take personal responsibility for their own sexual safety. When an HIV prevention professional explained to me why she had not had a direct conversation with her decade-plus cohabiting partner about her HIV-positive status, she noted, "I mean, this is *[pause]* an age where I would have to suspect everybody. And that's what I tell people who come and get tested about using condoms. I said you have to suspect that everybody has it, that everybody is infected in order to keep yourself negative."

An interview with a couple gave me a glimpse into the challenge of HIV status disclosure within a relationship. Fifty-year-old Wynton, who had spent his youth (22 years) in and out of prison, had three prior relationships before meeting his current partner, Lily, while dining at a restaurant where she waitressed. They had been together for just over three years. He found it easy to disclose to family members. However, among his previous partners, while one also had HIV, the other two "found out." I asked about Lily, and it turned out that she also "found out." When they met, Lily "kept asking and asking [him] to come take a test with me before we really started having sex," but he had told her he "didn't need a test." Because she "was in love with him . . . I believed what he told me." She felt there was no need for condom use since he "wasn't in the streets like that." They eventually moved in together, and one day, she felt God telling her to "get up, go Google his medicine on the computer," and "that's how I found out." They were still together because "I love that old cat . . . I'm gonna stay with him . . . if he gets sick, I'll be there for him." However, she was still angry that "he never gave me the chance to decide whether I wanted to be with him" and that he had left her fully exposed to HIV. Right now, "we working it out. And I know I'm taking a chance . . . but I got a God. You know what I'm saying. Mm-hmm *[laughs]*." Thus, love, God, and Wynton's medication, which reduced his viral load, were keeping her in the relationship, "working it out," and HIV free.

In sum, the HIV epidemic appeared to have caught many heterosexual Black people in Washington, DC, unaware. Racial homogamy combined with dramatic distortions in the sexual economy to produce shortages in the supply of heterosexual men, leading to their higher demand. This shaped community norms, leading to women's higher tolerance of men's concurrency and lower leverage to demand condom use. A partner's condomless concurrency in a racially contained syndemic zone, with multiple HIV exposures amplified by the drug epidemic, heightened HIV risk, even for those who were mostly monogamous or mostly used condoms. The framing of HIV as a racially and sexually contained disease, affecting only White gay men, contributed to decreased awareness of the need for HIV prevention through condom use or proactive HIV testing. The "sleeper" nature of HIV, combined with stigma that complicated HIV status disclosure, contributed to delayed HIV diagnosis and ART uptake, as well as a heightened community viral load, promoting onward transmission.

By 2022, the epidemic had become younger. While most people (over 93%) with HIV were 30 and over,[39] almost three-quarters (70.5%) of new cases were now among 20- to 39-year olds.[40] However, as Figures 26–29 showed, sexual economy distortions have remained in place, with continued low marriage rates, and Black people still comprise three-quarters of new cases (73.3%).[41]

THE HIV EPIDEMIC AMONG TRANSGENDER WOMEN

Transgender women, and Black transgender women in particular, are a small population, but they are at high risk of HIV acquisition.[42] National HIV-prevalence estimates from systematic reviews and meta-analyses of nonrepresentative samples suggest very high HIV prevalence rates among Black trans women that are more than 6.5 times higher than White trans women.[43] In DC, the HAHSTA surveillance reports did not provide estimates of the transgender HIV epidemic until 2016. In that report, the closest to the time of my interviews, while transgender people comprised a small proportion (1.9%) of city cases, Black transgender people were disproportionately affected.[44] They comprised 62% of the city's transgender population[45] and 83.8% of its transgender HIV cases.[46] My estimates of the city's 2022 transgender HIV prevalence are 0.67% for White transgender people and 9.1% for Black transgender people, more than 13.6 times higher than their White counterparts.[47] (For comparison, that year, prevalence was lower for Black [4%] and White [1.4%] cisgender men, and lower for Black [1.7%] and White [0.1%] cisgender women).[48] I conducted interviews with Black trans women who were living with HIV. While they are a highly select sample (as most Black transgender people do not have HIV), my interviews illuminated some of the reasons for their disproportionate vulnerability. They experienced similar relationship challenges to cisgender heterosexual women, including partner shortages and concurrency, and similar vulnerability to that of cisgender sexual minority men, such as higher-risk receptive anal sex. Racial containment in a syndemic zone, along with integrated sexual life, with intense community transphobia compounding HIV stigma, complicated transgender women's ability to prevent HIV acquisition and onward HIV transmission. I turn to the life stories of trans women to illustrate some of these points.

Transgender Life Course Pathways to HIV

Forty-three-year-old Cheryl, assigned as a boy at birth, knew early that she

> was different from all the other kids in my neighborhood. I was momma's boy, grandma's boy. I did everything that females did. I didn't play football. I didn't play sports. I didn't take gym. I played with doll babies . . . everything a girl did, I did. Um, so my grandmother informed my family members that if they would give me something, make sure it was for a girl, a girl's gift . . . I knew I was different. I felt different.

Unfortunately her difference was taken advantage of. She was molested by different teenagers in her early childhood, and when she was 13, a 30-year-old man

> end up having me. I guess he was ah pursuing me 'cause he's seeing that I was probably different. And um I used to sneak off with him . . . And he made me feel loved. He made me feel as though like he really cared about me, but really he was just ah taking advantage of me.

Her mother and stepfather "wasn't looking for me 'cause they was drinking." Substance abuse, including family alcoholism, was a major theme of many interviewees' childhoods (across gender); indeed, a syndemic zone feature (and syndemic amplifier) in many predominantly Black neighborhoods nationally is a saturation of liquor stores.[49] Cheryl's parents' alcoholism was profound enough that "we were one of the families in the neighborhood that the neighborhood kids teased because my mom and father used to drink, and you know, our lights used to get turned off here and there at times."

Her childhood of sexual abuse and parental neglect contributed to her transition to soliciting sex when was 16 because "I just wanted to be loved, you know, that's all. And I found that in the streets sleeping around with people . . . I felt love, yeah, being with someone for that moment of pleasure, I felt maybe that they loved me."

She first came out as gay, which her family accepted. Her gay cousin "took me to my first gay bar. And um I became, I guess, a newcomer the way as though I slept around in the bar 'cause I . . . wanted to fit in." However, she realized that her difference was something else. As she elaborated:

> I met another friend that was transgender and I loved it. I dressed up one day for Halloween, it was in '83, and, um, I never came out of it. I'm still that person that, um, I liked the attention. I liked the, I liked the illusion of being a woman. And, um, I felt complete, you know.

This feeling of completeness when she was 15 led to her transitioning to living as a woman, secretly. The outing of her womanhood to her family got her kicked out of home when she was 17 or 18. Her mother's friend

> see me on the bus dressed up in women's clothes. So told my mom, I seen your son dressed up on the bus . . . One night my mom was up waiting. So I got in the door, and she told me to get my shit and get the hell out. And I said, "For what?" She said, "Just get out 'cause I'm not gonna have no goddamned man here walking around with no women's clothes on. I want you to get your shit and get out." And I said, "Well where am I going to go?" And she said, "I don't give a fuck where you go, just get out.

Cheryl moved in with a friend who, along with her mother, supported her transition. However, drug addiction along with selling sex consumed her life. As she described:

> It was like a trick house. You know, me and her used to go out . . . and bring tricks in all night, 24/7. Then the addiction part kicked in and I got on drugs real bad. It was cool on drugs at first, you know, it didn't kick off. It was, this is what we were doing, and I was comfortable with it. But at the end it was ugly.

She eventually got out and into a "long-term relationship with this guy who took care of me for five years, and he was good to me." However,

> he also hit me, beat, you know, hitted me and stuff. And I, I knew he was a man to step around. I knew he was a man that been with many transgenders . . . I was young and vulnerable and, you know, I did what he wanted me to do, you know, because he was taking care of me. And at that time I became set in that way that if I had to sleep with someone to stay with him, I would. And I did on numerous occasions with guys, not only him. And, um, I do believe that he's the one who got me infected.

For Cheryl, as with several other transgender women I interviewed, HIV infection occurred as an outcome of a short lifetime packed with traumatic and challenging events. In her case, a childhood and adolescence of sexual abuse by several people and parental neglect by alcoholic parents was followed by eviction from the family home because of transphobia, which led her to a life of dependency, the cover story for a constant search for love. She lived in a "trick house" where she sold sex—an activity that made her feel loved—in exchange for a place to live, and then she also became dependent on drugs. She found a long-term partnership; however, there, caring provision that included housing stability meant tolerating her partner's physical abuse, his controlling of her, and the sex she felt coerced to have to keep him. She was diagnosed with HIV in 1995 when she was 27 years old. In the years leading up to the interview, despite help from a family member who provided accommodation, she had been living on and off the streets, selling sex, struggling with crack addiction, and not on HIV medication.

For 52-year-old Dorothy, "a Washingtonian, born and raised here in the District of Columbia," an HIV diagnosis also occurred after a short lifetime of condensed trauma. In her childhood, her constant refusal to wear boys' clothing led her parents to take her in for a medical evaluation when she was nine:

> The end result was that they said I had more female chromosomes than I did male chromosomes, and it was causin' effeminate appearance and feeling, but if not treated, at that point in time, back then, bein' that young, they said that they felt that male hormones could balance the genes. But my family was very religious and did not agree to that.

She began stealing women's underwear, and an arrest, combined with her family's transphobia, led her to a two-year incarceration at age 14 in a program for children called "People In Need of Supervision," which her family hoped would change her. Kids were "committed to DHR [the Department of Human Resources] care by the courts because of noncriminal acts such as truancy and refusal to obey parents" at the Maple Glen juvenile facility.[50] This was followed by a stint at Cedar Knoll, another juvenile institution.[51] Then came eviction from her childhood home at age 17 following release because her time at the two facilities had not succeeded in producing the change her family was seeking. Homeless and living on the streets, Dorothy nonetheless managed to graduate from high school. However, she sold sex to make ends meet:

> Some older transgender women kind of took me and showed me the way. The first thing I was introduced to was prostitution, drinking, all that. So that's

how the drugs and all that started in my life . . . we stayed out all night, and the goal was to at least try to make enough to provide for food and possibly a room.[52]

Dorothy did not think she needed to worry about HIV/AIDS until people around her started dying, when she was about 30. As she described:

The disease had already been talked about and we were hearin' about it, but the fact was, none of us thought, me or my [transgender] sisters, that it affected us, because they were talkin' about White gay men. But then suddenly we start hearing about little cases like, "Did you know so-and-so and so-and-so is sick in the hospital? They think they may have that disease." "That's impossible. You mean AIDS?" . . . And so it hit so quickly, and then after that we start hearing numbers, and people just start falling, just dying. "So-and-so died, so-and-so died, so-and-so died."

Dorothy got tested for HIV the following year, in 1990, and found out she had HIV. At the time of the interview, when she was in her 50s, she continued to face transphobia. As she observed, "Lesbian, gay, it's easier to make it. But when you actually fully transition from one gender outwardly, appearance, then society, it really starts. Family, everybody go off . . ."

In the course of her work, she encountered the continued eviction of children, four decades after her own:

The fact is, kids are gettin' put out so young, just like I experienced . . . When they get put out they're traumatized, and then they're traumatized more when they have to do the things that they would not normally do . . . Like, someone takin' you in at home and sayin', "Well, you can stay here, but we have to have sex every night." They get more and more traumatized. When we get 'em, they're fully traumatized . . .

At the time, she said that the city appeared to only have one emergency youth shelter, with 15 available beds. Persistent transphobia pushed transgender children into the cycle that marked many of the adults I interviewed, putting them at heightened intergenerational risk of HIV acquisition.

Indeed, Black transgender people, and women in particular, are the "truly disadvantaged"—they occupy the bottom sector of an intersectional "matrix of domination" when it comes to race, gender, sexuality, and often (but not always) as a result, social class.[53] Nationally, Badgett and colleagues estimated that Black transgender people have twice the rate of poverty (38.5%) of their White counterparts (18.6%). (This compares to poverty rates of 25.3% for cisgender Black people and 9.1% for cisgender White people.)[54] In the DC portion of a national survey on transgender people,

> 88% of those who were out or perceived as transgender at some point between Kindergarten and Grade 12 (K-12) experienced some form of mistreatment ... 67% ... were verbally harassed, 30% were physically attacked, and 18% were sexually assaulted in K-12 because of being transgender. 23% faced such severe mistreatment as a transgender person that they left a K-12 school."[55]

Further, a quarter (25%) "reported being fired, being denied a promotion, or not being hired for a job they applied for because of their gender identity or expression" in the last year.[56] A DC needs assessment additionally noted mental health challenges that could lead to suicide among transgender residents.[57] Thus, ironically and sadly, HIV was simply one among many challenges faced by transgender people in the city.

Partner Shortage, Concurrency, and HIV Risk

Black transgender women also shared the challenges of Black cisgender women—a partner shortage, given my respondents' preference for straight cisgender men, as well as their partners' concurrency—which compounded their HIV vulnerability. Forty-two-year-old Hannah, who transitioned at age 25 and previously had relationships as a gay man and then as a transgender woman, found that when she became a woman, the challenge with long-term relationships with straight men was that they wanted to have biological children. This was a theme and source of sadness among other transgender women I interviewed, as they felt that in the competition for already scarce men, they often lost out to cisgender women who could have children. Others found that straight men were ashamed of being in public with them, also limiting the length of their relationships. Mary's ex "identifies as a straight man" but "basically rejected me because I'm a transgender woman. And then he had the nerve to parade his new girlfriend in front of me, who is a biological woman." When I asked if finding relationships was hard, she said:

> I'm HIV and I'm a trans woman ... it's hard, it's hard ... I wanna be respected as a woman ... because I do meet guys, but they just want to have *sex,* you know. You're a trans woman, and you're beautiful, and you're beautiful enough for me to have sex with you, but you're not that beautiful to where I could be in a relationship with you, and I can walk, and I can introduce you to my friends, that's what I wanted *[pause]* ... I don't wanna settle. It creates

... a lonely existence, 'cause I know what I want. I just want them to love me, accept me, and profess, you know, and that's all I want, nothing else, ya know, and *[pause]* it's hard to find, yeah.

The shortage of straight men, the unique emotional needs of transgender women—for validation, acceptance, and affirmation as women—alongside the universal need for love, however, led to relationship compromises.

Cheryl, described earlier, stayed in a physically abusive relationship and tolerated her partner's concurrent relationships. For her and others, there were also compromises with HIV status disclosure and condom use. When I interviewed Cheryl, she was in a relationship where she had not disclosed her status and was having unprotected sex. She was living with AIDS, suggesting a high viral load; however she had started medication. She comforted herself with the fact that they now had infrequent sex and used condoms. She was worried he may become violent if he found out she had HIV:

> I end up meeting this guy who um adores me. Um, I can ... say that I adores him ... never thought that I would be with someone this way. [I've been] with him for two and half years and him not knowing my status. And that's been a big problem now. Um, at first I didn't think about it, but now as the years progress ... it gets harder and harder for me to tell him. And I'm making it worse and worse in not telling him. But he's one of them people that's not that accepting. You know what I'm saying, he's one of them. I don't know what he'll do. I wouldn't care if he left me alone, but, um, I do care if he can harm me, I care about that. But however he respond, he's entitled to respond that way, you know what I'm saying. But he's not gonna be hitting on me, I'm not gonna allow that. But um ... now I feel bad ... 'cause this person does everything for me, gives me the world. Um, I don't work nowhere, I just make work look good 'cause I don't have shit *[laughs]*, but, um, he really supported me in my recovery um. And I have had sex with him unprotected a few times, by his choice. He didn't want me to use them. "No, I don't use condoms, um fuck that," and I didn't. Which I did have the choice to say, "We're going to use one." But now we do use condoms. It's not sex no more, it's just, it's more love. He loves me. He don't have to have sex with me ... we may have sex five or six times. So that's good for me ... That ultimate secret ... I don't think he would take it well at all.

Overall, partner shortage, straight men's preference for cisgender women, and transphobia reduced leverage to demand safe sex. Further, prior trauma, neglect, abuse, and family rejection were compounded by fear of partner rejection if they disclosed their HIV status. These factors combined to heighten the premium placed on both condomless sex, which enhanced intimacy, and keeping quiet about HIV.[58] As 42-year-old Hannah explained about HIV disclosure:

> You have to earn that. You have to . . . it's not a conversation piece, "Hi, my name is and I'm sick, I have HIV." . . . No it's nothing like that. Even, even now, you know, you pick and choose . . . you have to trust the person, you have to know that they're not malicious.

However, when 40-year-old Mary started disclosing her status, she found that some men still wanted to have unprotected sex, leaving it up to her to decide. One partner

> knew about my status, and we still had unprotected sex, and I was like okay, that's one time. But after that he wanted it to be normal practice, and you know, I brought the subject up, and so now it's normal practice . . . he was really, really uncomfortable having the conversation, and he basically left it up to me where if you want to use condoms, we can, if you don't want to, we can.

Helen also found that as her relationship progressed, her partner wanted to have unprotected sex. Unfortunately, he acquired HIV even though she was on medication:

> I was telling him, you know, it's still a risk and stuff like that. But my numbers are fine, and I wanted it just as much as he wanted me to do it, and it was like, "Okay we're fine." So when he finally went into treatment . . . it was a whole big old thing, he started looking at me funny, then he wanted to think about the choices that *we made, we made* together. You a grown adult, you made that choice just like I did, ya know what I'm saying . . . So all of a sudden he ready to be worried about it. And at the same time, a sense of me kind of be like, "Damn, I wouldn't want nobody to feel the way I felt in the beginning of being diagnosed," you know what I'm saying, especially somebody that I cared about. No matter what we done been through, you know. But that's the choice that he made, that we made, and it ain't like he didn't know. 'Cause he knew, you know. So I had to look, think back on it and not be regretful because of the choices that we made, 'cause I made it too, ya know so.

Their mutual desire for condomless sex as people who loved each other, and especially for Helen, who had found that rare straight man who cared about and affirmed her as a woman, coupled with her assessment of her numbers (which she assumed indicated low infectiousness) overrode her worry about HIV transmission and his worry about HIV acquisition. However, even though he knowingly had unprotected sex with someone who had HIV, Helen did not escape the transmission guilt, a large price for the purest form of intimacy.

In sum, transgender women's desires to find partners who accepted their womanhood and HIV status, and who loved and cared about them, contributed to an even greater shortage of straight men for them compared to cisgender women. This led to more compromises around HIV disclosure and condom use. Because it was hard to find a partner, once found, it was hard to resist the kind of intimacy that condomless sex provided. In addition, they were having the highest risk sex with respect to HIV acquisition. This meant that the sex that conferred the most love also carried the most HIV risk.

CONCLUSION

This Part has examined the consequences of sex and love in a syndemic zone, in this case characterized by high HIV prevalence rates, which led to repeated exposures to HIV, combined with overlapping and amplifying drug epidemics. We like to think that getting HIV is solely about individual high-risk behaviors, such as having multiple partners and not using a condom. And this can lead to blaming people for not being rational and responsible about their sexual practices. In doing this, however, we forget the irrationality and messiness of human life, that love and intimacy often work against the logic of "safe sex," and that carrying an expectation of potential HIV infection into a long-term relationship is what is irrational. Indeed, in many instances, people are at greater risk from repeated exposure through unprotected sex with a long-term partner living with HIV than from a one night stand with a stranger. We also overlook the fact that in oppressed and stigmatized communities, the communion and comfort found in sex might mean more and matter more, and condomless sex may take on a larger premium in signaling true love and intimacy, especially for those who are the most marginalized.

Finally, as this Part has illustrated, we can easily ignore how racial containment and its historical legacies and institutions have created contemporary structural problems, which set social constraints and create microlevel dilemmas for African Americans navigating sexual life in a syndemic zone. For gay and bisexual Black men, racism in gayborhoods and Black community homophobia contributed to the creation of close-knit enclaves within a racially contained community—forging tighter links and denser sexual networks through which HIV quickly spread once it hit the city. Among hetero-sexuals, distortions to the sexual economy led to partner shortages and high rates of concurrency, which contributed to gender power imbalances shaping condom use and women's risky compromises to keep their man. Transgender women suffered not just transphobia but also the challenges of both gay and bisexual men—including racism, homophobia, and the highest-risk kind of sex—as well as the challenges of cisgender heterosexual women—including concurrency, partner shortages, and limited relationship power to demand condom use. This produced heightened HIV vulnerability. Across all sub-groups, the framing of HIV as a White gay man's disease led to a lag in HIV prevention and ART uptake among African Americans (which will be explored in-depth in Part 5). In Part 3, I examine the city's heroin and cocaine epidemics in greater detail, illustrating how they overlapped with and further amplified the HIV and homicide epidemics.

PART THREE

The SAVA Syndemic:
Drugs–HIV/AIDS–Homicide

Washington D.C. is engulfed by an alarming epidemic of heroin addiction. It is now estimated that there are 16,800 heroin addicts in the city, or 2.2 per cent of the total population. . . . Two thirds of the addicts are under 26 years of age, 91 percent are Black, 74 percent are male.

ROBERT DUPONT (1971:320)

The 1981 population-based HRD [heroin-related deaths] mortality rate . . . for the District of Columbia is the highest ever reported in the medical literature.

MORBIDITY AND MORTALITY
WEEKLY REPORT, CDC (1983)

IN PART 3, I EXAMINE the role of cascading waves of drug epidemics in amplifying the HIV epidemic in Washington, DC, and in creating spillover homicide epidemics, resulting in a drugs–HIV/AIDS–homicide syndemic, one iteration of the SAVA syndemic (see Introduction).[1] Both individual drug use and drug epidemics are the result of a complex interaction of factors related to the drug (e.g., chemical properties, short- and long-term neurological impacts, etc.), individuals (e.g., personality, genetics, etc.), relationships (e.g., peer networks), and to the social structure (e.g., drug availability, physical environment, sociohistorical period, legal regime, global geopolitical environment, etc.). These factors work together to create and entrench personal addiction and a national epidemic. This is equally true for drug recovery at an individual level and a waning epidemic.[2] As such, instead of a primarily drug–user focused discussion, I conduct an in-depth multilevel analysis attending to global geopolitical, sociostructural, relational, and individual dimensions of the syndemic, drawing on archival and contemporary materials, longitudinal health and homicide data, as well as interviews with Black people who lived with drug addiction and HIV in DC.

I focus on the heroin (Chapter 6) and cocaine (especially crack) (Chapter 7) epidemics, giving a historical context and describing the global and national supply chains to and drug economy within Washington, DC. I then show how individuals were drawn into this economy and how it, in turn, amplified HIV risk. I illuminate the amplifying roles of the commercial sex economy and the lack of drug treatment (Chapter 8) on the drugs, HIV, and spillover homicide epidemics (Chapter 9). I show how the city's drug epidemics thrived in racially contained zones of abandonment and disinvestment and created syndemic zones—socially and economically disadvantaged places with high levels of overlapping and interacting epidemics. I examine how the institutional ecosystem (including Congress and city entities) and related racialized policies enabled and sustained syndemic zones, and I show how poor health could cluster and metastasize among Black people living and dying in these places, exacerbating racial health inequality.

· · ·

PART 3 PLAYLIST

Jay-Z	BBC (2013)
The Notorious B.I.G.	Gimme the Loot (1994)
Stop the Violence Movement	Self-Destruction (1989)
Common ft. The Last Poets	The Corner (2005)
Nas	I Gave You Power (1996)
50 Cent	Many Men (Wish Death) (2003)
TLC	Waterfalls (1994)
Prince	Sign o' the Times (1987)
Wynton Marsalis	Find Me (2007)
2Pac	Dear Mama (1995)
Experience Unlimited	Peace Gone Away (1977)
Marvin Sapp	Never Would Have Made It (2007)
Fred Hammond	No Weapon (1996)
Kirk Franklin	I Smile (2011)
Tamela Mann	Take Me to the King (2012)
Donnie McClurkin	Stand (1996)
Wale	DC or Nothing (2011)
Nonchalant	5 O'Clock (1996)

SIX

First Comes Heroin

1960–2016

A CHANGING NATIONAL RACIAL AND GENDER PROFILE OF AND RESPONSE TO OPIATE-ADDICTED PEOPLE

In the late 1800s, the typical opiate-addicted American was "a middle-aged White woman of middle-class background"[1] whose dealer was her doctor. Doctors prescribed opiates, such as morphine or laudanum, extracted from opium legally imported by pharmaceutical companies, for "female complaints" and "diseases of a nervous character."[2] Women's opiate dependence was maintained by doctors long after the initiating ailment had passed. Addiction became even more acute when technologies enabling hypodermic injection of opiates were developed.[3] Declining opiate dependence, in part due to the aging out of the medically addicted population, was accompanied by a shift to narcotic conservatism and, by 1914, a law—the Harrison Act—which restricted prescriptions, reduced drug access, and supported a growing intolerance for addiction maintenance.[4] These developments were accompanied by a gendered, classed, and then racial shift in the typical opiate-addicted person. Indeed, by the 1930s, "the typical American addict was a thirtyish White male from a 'deteriorated metropolitan section' working at a menial job, addicted for 10 years, and engaging in petty crime to support his habit."[5] Strict new laws shipped people with addiction off to Lexington, Kentucky, to the first narcotic prison (opened in 1935) specially built for punishment and recovery.[6] World War II significantly disrupted drug supply chains, and opiate addiction was reportedly at an all-time low.[7] After the war, however, heroin came back with a roar, and for most of the second half of the 20th century, the typical opiate-addicted person was a young urban Black man,[8] and mass incarceration became a major response to drug epidemics.[9] A national study of opioid overdose death rates (1979–2015) found that Black heroin-overdose rates steadily rose between 1979 and 1995, before finally stabilizing. A racial crossover occurred in 2000 with White people beginning to die at higher, and then much higher, rates than Black people, especially from overdoses on opiates other than heroin.[10] Matching the statistics, the typical opiate-addicted person shifted to a (small town/often rural) young White man, and the national response began focusing on regulating pharmaceutical companies, interdiction of overseas drug supplies, and ramping up treatment.[11] (Another racial crossover occurred in 2020; Black overdose rates now surpass White overdose rates).[12] Shifting opiate use and abuse across race, class, and gender lines over the last 140 years highlight the fact that drug epidemics are not inherently about user characteristics, belying legislative responses. Rather, they are about the interaction of factors above and beyond individuals that shape their propensities, opportunities, and constraints in a given historical period.

WASHINGTON, DC, 1960–2016

In Washington, DC, there were at least three major heroin epidemics between 1960 and the mid-1980s, the first of which amplified the homicide epidemic, and the last of which amplified the HIV epidemic. In both cases, the homicide and HIV epidemics far eclipsed the preceding heroin epidemics. Figure 30, reproduced from Ruttenber and Luke's study, illustrates three waves of heroin overdose deaths in the city.[13] Heroin overdose deaths in the 1960s and '70s were rare events and represented the tip of the iceberg of the heroin addiction epidemic. The figure is especially useful in showing the shape and length of heroin epidemics in the city. As I will explore in more detail below, the first wave started in the mid-1960s, peaked in 1969, and kicked off a homicide epidemic, thus creating a heroin–homicide syndemic. It declined in the early 1970s, even while the homicide epidemic persisted. The second wave was significantly smaller and rose and fell between 1974 and 1976. Many of my heroin-using respondents began using during this wave. The third wave began in the late 1970s and continued into the 1980s, overlapping with and extended by the cocaine epidemic. It also coincided with the beginning of the city's HIV epidemic, making both new and established heroin users uniquely vulnerable to HIV, creating a heroin–HIV syndemic.

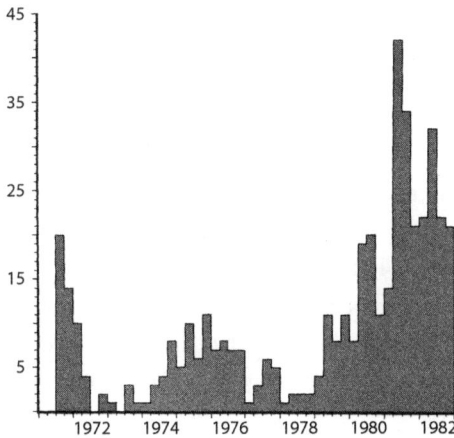

FIGURE 30. Heroin-related deaths, DC, 1971–82. Source: A. James Ruttenber and James L. Luke, 1984, Heroin-Related Deaths: New Epidemiologic Insights, *Science* 226(4670):14–20, DOI: 10.1126/science.6474188. Reprinted with permission from AAAS.

First Wave: The 1960s and Early 1970s

Global Supply Chain and Drug Distribution. Between the 1960s and early 1970s, DC's major heroin supply chain reportedly began with opium poppies harvested in China, Turkey, and India, transported to Aleppo, Syria, and Beirut, Lebanon, where it was reduced to gum, and then transported to laboratories in Marseilles, France (the so-called French connection). There it was processed into heroin. It then either came directly to New York or was transported to Montreal, Canada. It made its way to New York through the false luggage bottoms of unsuspecting European immigrants and through ambassadors exploiting their diplomatic immunity, among other means. At its height in 1969, an estimated eight to ten tons per year of high-purity heroin was flowing into the US. Overseeing the distribution of drugs within the US were the five Mafia families or the "Cosa Nostra," said to control 95% of the domestic illegal heroin trade. From New York, a variety of couriers delivered heroin to Washington, DC, by train, plane, or car, reportedly overseen by a "dozen local kingpin heroin-wholesale" dealers with connections to the Mafia who supplied a variety of smaller operators in DC. Lawrence "Slippery" Jackson, a major Black drug lord, for example, was supplied by the Genovese family (one of the five Mafia families) and had been running a "five-day-a-week, 24-hour-a-day operation" from his SE DC home until his arrest and conviction in 1970. Warren Robinson was supplied by the Lucchese family, running his Georgia Avenue operation until his conviction in 1974.[14]

Once heroin entered the city, it was diluted and put into capsules. In the early 1960s, it sold for $1.50 per capsule, or $1 each (about $10 in 2024 dollars) if a customer purchased 10 or more (an ounce of heroin yielded 400–450 capsules); by the mid-1960s, the price had risen to $2.50 per capsule.[15] The markups along the supply chain were "staggering," in journalist Dan Morgan's words. In 1966, he calculated that "10 kilos of opium, which produced one [kilo (2.2 pounds) of white] heroin, [sold] for $350 in Turkey," $700 in Syria and Lebanon, $3,500 in France, and $10,000 in Canada. A courier picking up one ounce of heroin in New York for $400 could sell it in DC for $1,000. The total value of that initial kilo by the time it was sold on DC streets, diluted to 5% purity, was $225,000 in 1966 dollars (about $2.1 million in 2024 dollars).[16]

The City Heroin-Homicide Syndemic. Heroin use in the city likely became epidemic sometime between 1964 and 1966. By then, heroin was said to be openly sold throughout the city,[17] which was estimated to house the "5th largest addict population in [the] United States."[18] The decade was marked not just by dramatic increases in heroin users but also increased drug purity (rising from 1%–15% purity to 80%–90% purity) and increased drug overdoses.[19] Mark Greene, a CDC official on assignment, conducted a study of city residents seeking addiction treatment (methadone). Figure 31, reproduced from his study, illustrates addiction incidence (new cases) peaking in 1969 before dramatically declining.[20]

In a special report published in *The New England Journal of Medicine* in 1971, Robert DuPont described the city's heroin epidemic in eerily similar terms to those used to describe the HIV epidemic three and a half decades later, when 3% of the city was found to be living with HIV. The city, he said, had been "engulfed by an alarming epidemic," with an estimated "16,800 heroin addicts in the city or 2.2 per cent of the total population." He went on to note, "the related crime rate is appalling."[21]

Washington, DC's, crime rates were national news, and Richard Nixon, then Republican presidential candidate, called it "one of the crime capitals of the Nation," further noting, "D.C. should not stand for Disorder and Crime."[22] The increase in heroin use and prices coincided with a sharp increase in property crime, such as house burglaries and shoplifting, to support the expensive addiction.[23] The increased violence, including drug-related assassinations, indicated that the drug epidemic had given birth to a homicide epidemic, thus creating a heroin–homicide syndemic. Federal

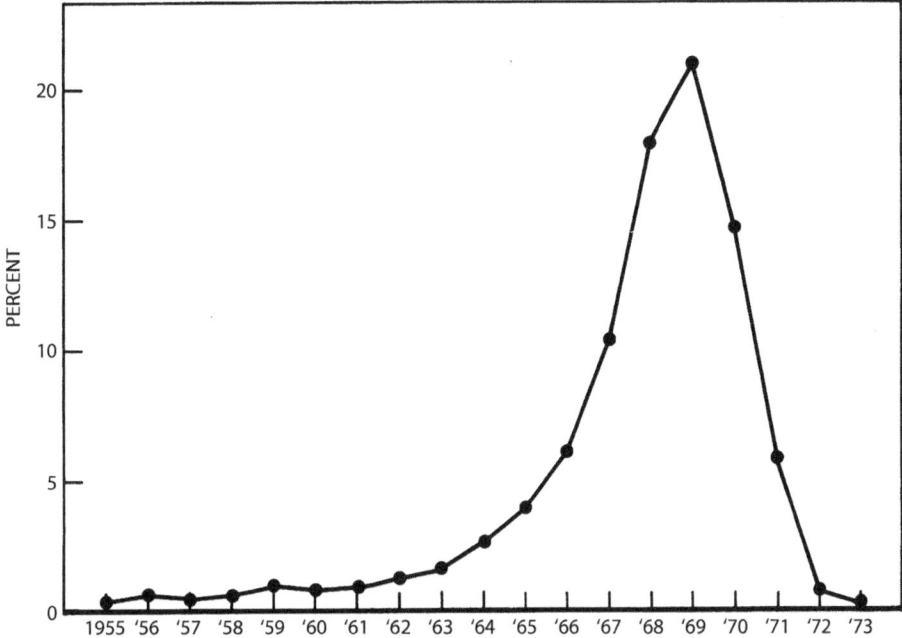

FIGURE 31. Heroin addiction incidence, 1955–73. Source: Mark H. Greene, 1974, An Epidemiologic Assessment of Heroin Use, *American Journal of Public Health* 64(12 suppl):1–10. Reprinted with permission from *American Journal of Public Health*.

officials at the time described "a self-proclaimed 'Black Mafia' . . . said to be attempting to gain full control of heroin distribution in Washington through threats of death to drug peddlers who refuse to kick in a percentage of their sales."[24] Since the appearance of the group, they said that "Washington has seen its first drug-related murders, many in the form of assassinations."[25] Figure 32 illustrates the annual and cumulative number of homicides between 1960 and 1973. The figure illustrates how closely homicides tracked with the incidence of heroin use (see Figure 31): stable until 1963, then rising to a peak in 1969. However, unlike the incidence of heroin use, which then declined (see Figure 31), the homicide epidemic continued, becoming its own free-standing epidemic divorced from the initiating drug epidemic. By the end of the first heroin wave, an estimated 2,445 people had died by homicide, far more than had died of heroin overdose.[26] In other words, the worst mortality outcome of the drug epidemic was the homicide epidemic it gave birth to.

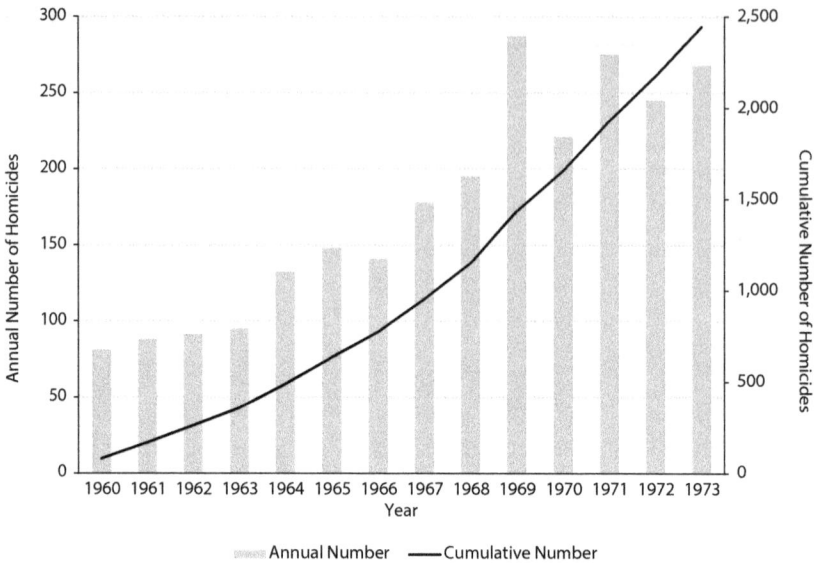

FIGURE 32. First wave—Annual and cumulative homicides, 1960–73. Data source: Disaster Center, District of Columbia.

Racial Containment, Heroin Use, and a Shifting Strategy. The heroin epidemic was also highly racialized and spatialized. White youth were initially perceived, across the nation and in DC, to be predominantly taking marijuana, LSD, and pep pills, while heroin was seen as "mostly a Negro problem in Washington."[27] Greene concurred, describing the racial and spatial profile of the city's heroin-addicted people:

> In Washington, D.C., the typical new user was a 17-year old, unmarried, unemployed, black male with a criminal record at the time of onset of heroin use ... As expected, users are not uniformly distributed throughout the city ... users are concentrated in the urban core area in those neighborhoods where other measures of social disruption (crime, low income, high unemployment, inadequate housing, broken families) are also high. This, then, completes the triad of person, time, and place by means of which epidemics are traditionally described.[28]

Robert DuPont noted that "the rates of heroin addiction range from less than 0.1 per cent for the relatively affluent Northwest section west of Rock Creek Park to 4.0 per cent in the Model Cities area."[29] A study focused on the Model Cities area,[30] which included some of the city's most disadvantaged communities, found an alarming heroin epidemic among Black youth: An estimated 20% of teenage (aged 15–19) boys and 38% of men 20–24 years old were addicted to heroin.[31] There was also little by way of help in terms of treatment. Morgan observed: "The 30 bed unit on the second floor of DC General [the city's public hospital] is the City's only non-punitive answer to the problem . . . Washington, in fact has responded to the narcotics problem with one answer only—tough relentless enforcement of the narcotics laws."[32] DuPont, then at the Department of Corrections, found that 44% of arriving prisoners in 1969 were heroin users.[33]

By the late 1960s, however, heroin had been discovered by reporters in White DC who noted that heroin was now said to have "found a new home among the area's White middle class young" who lived "within the safe White world of Northwest Washington and the suburbs."[34] What was framed as novel belied the fact that studies finding a predominance of young Black men addicted to heroin were not random samples of the city or its suburbs. The statistics were from prisons, Model City areas, and the city's Narcotics Treatment Administration clinics. Most clinic clients were young (under 26), Black (91%), and male (74%).[35] In other words, they were estimates of incarcerated people (heroin use was a crime), residents of disadvantaged parts of the city, and/or clients of publicly funded treatment clinics. They were essentially sampling on the dependent variable. Indeed, while poor Black areas and people with addiction are highly visible to public institutions such as clinics and the criminal justice system, "middle class addicts rarely are."[36] White middle-class youth copped heroin in Black neighborhoods to use or resell in the suburbs for a profit; they could afford private lawyers to avoid prison time and had insurance or family resources allowing them to "seek private medical and psychiatric care—nearly as expensive, in some cases, as a sizable heroin habit itself,"[37] keeping them off the addiction and criminal-surveillance books. This is not to say that Black people were not more affected but rather that the true extent of the racial disparity in heroin use and addiction was unknown.

What is known, however, is that government approaches to heroin addiction started to change with a series of national legislative and policy changes from the mid-'60s to the early '70s. A shift in perceptions of people with heroin addiction from being criminals to being people needing treatment occurred alongside the perception that heroin use had crossed the racial containment line to young White DC MSA residents (who might be legislators' children). Congress passed the Narcotic Addict

Rehabilitation Act in 1966, which amended a previous law. Section 2 of the act stated:

> It is the policy of the Congress that certain persons charged with or convicted of violating Federal criminal laws, who are determined to be addicted to narcotic drugs, and likely to be rehabilitated through treatment, should, in lieu of prosecution or sentencing, be civilly committed for confinement and treatment designed to effect their restoration to health, and return to society as useful members . . . in order that society may be protected more effectively from crime and delinquency which result from narcotic addiction.[38]

The Narcotics Treatment Administration (NTA), formed in 1970, began to provide the new medical treatment methadone hydrochloride, along with rehabilitative care, to the city's addicted population.[39] By 1971, an estimated one-fifth of that population was being treated at the NTA.[40] Describing the story of the NTA, DuPont, who talked to reporter Rebecca Sheir, said:

> [On] February 18, 1970, Walter Washington, the mayor at the time, appointed me head of a new agency to treat heroin addicts in Washington . . . And we started the Narcotics Treatment Association [sic] . . . In the next three years, we treated 15,000 heroin addicts in the city . . . the heroin overdose rate went from 70 people in a year to four in a year.[41]

There was another reason for the decline. DuPont, the NTA's first director, who later became the first director of the National Institute on Drug Abuse when it was launched in 1974 and later the White House drug czar, described "a new attitude . . . in the White House, in the Justice Department and in the police department. They're saying 'our job is not to arrest addicts but to disrupt heroin distribution.'"[42] The NTA opening coincided with the Nixon administration's efforts to shut down the French connection in the heroin supply chain, including through diplomacy and by prosecuting major traffickers "for income tax evasion," which led to a drop in drug supply and purity, a price increase, and a waning drug epidemic.[43]

In sum, the city's heroin epidemic ended not just because fewer individuals were inclined to use heroin but also because of mass provision of public addiction treatment in lieu of incarceration and because of global geopolitical and local actions to disrupt the city's heroin supply.

Second Wave: 1974–1976

An apparent lull after the first wave was followed by a resurgence in heroin use as supply chains shifted from white heroin sourced from the Middle East and Europe to brown heroin sourced from Mexico (Mexican mud) via LA and white heroin sourced from the Southeast Asian Golden Triangle (Burma, Laos, Thailand) via New York or via Amsterdam, and from there, directly to DC.[44] The Mexican supply chain began in the mountains of Durango, Mexico, where opium was harvested, refined into heroin, and transported to Mount Pleasant, DC. Heroin retailers then packaged it into tin foil and sold it for $100 (about $640 in 2024 dollars) per packet.[45] Drug distribution had shifted from a kingpin setup to one comprised of "younger independent wholesalers," who supplied retailers, who in turn supplied peddlers across at least seven drug markets spread across the NW, NE, and SE quadrants of the city.[46]

Wynton, born in 1961, was one of these peddlers. He began using drugs in 1975, when he was 14. He first started smoking marijuana and drinking, and his curiosity "about what it [drugs] was doing" to different people he saw at parties led him to try out different things:

> Then I started shooting, shooting drugs. *[Sanyu: Oh heroin?]* Yeah heroin. And when I started shooting heroin . . . all of a sudden it hit . . . I'm snorting it and then I started shooting it . . . once I started shooting it, I liked the high, how it made me feel, and the way that it was getting money. And I was selling it on the street, and I was getting so much money a day.

Wynton described sales of about $500–$600 a day, suggesting he was supporting about 50 people who had $10-a-day habits, or many more people with smaller habits. He dropped out of high school in 11th grade to focus on selling full time "'cause it wasn't nothing in high school . . . school was keeping me from getting money, getting, using drugs." He sold drugs throughout the city, "standing on corners, from place to place, southeast, northeast, northwest, you know every time I was standing on a different place." As he elaborated:

> Back then, you ain't had no territory . . . it's all about who you knew. If you knew somebody in the northwest or southeast, or you been selling drugs around there for, for a long time, you can always come back and sell . . . it wasn't a whole lot of fighting about, "You can't come over here," 'cause that's,

that's how they do now, but they don't do that when we, when I was coming up. You sell drugs, you sell drugs. Everybody was out to do the same thing, it's making money.

He worked long hours, accommodating customers' varied work and drug habit schedules:

I used to go out like . . . early in the morning . . . to catch the early people that . . . wanna buy drugs before they go to work or get high before they go to work, or some people might wanna come out there during lunch time and then go back to work. Some people might wanna get it in the evening time, when they get off work and just go home . . . I'd stay out there all day . . .

His description is telling, characterizing his customers as high-functioning, regularly employed heroin users, and illuminating of their role in underwriting the lucrative DC heroin economy. Wynton found out he had HIV in 1992, attributing it to his injecting drug use. His addiction lasted 25 years; he finally quit after a year in a drug rehabilitation program in 2000, when he was 39. And since then, "I haven't turned back or had a desire to use no drugs not, uh, at all. My health then got a whole lot better, my HIV got a whole lot better."

Lengthy heroin careers are typical of people addicted to heroin.[47] As has long been recognized, many people who use illegal drugs do not become addicted.[48] However, prolonged opioid use transforms brain functioning, promoting both drug dependence and addiction. When combined with enabling social contexts, it can result in a decades-long, chronic relapsing brain disorder.[49] Forty-nine-year-old Cora began using heroin around 1974, when she was 12 or 13, to escape the pain of sexual abuse by her mother's partners, and she ran away from home at 14. Heroin "took away the pain, didn't have to feel, you know, and I stayed in that addiction for 30 years. Mm-hmm. Off and on, off and on, off and on, but still in it. Mm-hmm." After years of being in and out of methadone clinics, she finally got clean in 2006, when she was 45. Like Wynton, she was diagnosed with HIV in the middle of her addiction, in 1989.[50]

As Sam Friedman, Don Des Jarlais, and many others have comprehensively documented, injecting drug use, prolonged drug use leading to multiple potential exposures, and addiction were a deadly combination once HIV began to circulate in drug networks.[51] Sharing used "works," such as needles, carries an estimated 63/10,000 per-act HIV-acquisition probability.[52] This is a low probability. However, multiple years of repeated exposure, in an epidemic with newly infected people with high HIV viral loads, dramatically increased this probability. Cornelius described how heroin addiction warped individuals' decision-making around HIV prevention:

> I sat in a car with some people, with this girl that I know who's HIV positive. And, and, heroin [addicted people], they, they get sick, they need the dirt right away. They knew this girl was HIV positive. They didn't want to ride all the way home to get bleach 'cause she only had one pair [of] works, she was spending the money, she was gonna do her first . . . They wanted to get the dope in themselves right then and there. And I watched that decision-making going on. I could watch it in their heads, them thinking about this . . . and I watched them pull over in this car . . . I watched them use that needle, all of them, even though she's HIV positive. They did clean it out, tried to rinse it out with water, but the virus is still in there . . . And um, so stuff like that happens, um, um, people figure it's not gonna happen to them.

The Heroin-Homicide Syndemic. The second, smaller heroin epidemic was perceived as more racially mixed. The market was seen to be dominated by marijuana users; however, compared to the first wave, the heroin was of a higher purity, contributing to overdose deaths, was sold at a lower price, and was available in plenty.[53] Even as the heroin supply and addicted population were on the rise again, the NTA stopped receiving new patients and was folded into city programming after city budget cuts that accompanied controversy about methadone use.[54] The epidemic died down in part due to global geopolitical actions, including a crackdown on the Mexican supply chain through border control and poppy field destruction.[55] Unfortunately, the homicide epidemic kicked off by the first heroin wave continued, though at lower levels. As illustrated by Figure 33, homicides were high in 1974, before a slow decline and stabilization over the next four years. Nonetheless, 1,081 people died by homicide, many more than died by drug overdose over the same period.

The Third Wave—Enter HIV: 1978–2016

The third heroin wave dwarfed prior epidemics. Starting in late 1978, heroin use became epidemic again, and this time it was "pouring into Washington"[56] as production increased in the Middle East and Southeast Asia and as Cold War politics combined with political turmoil in Afghanistan, Pakistan, and Iran to reduce interdiction and provide cover for smugglers.[57] Drugs came to DC from

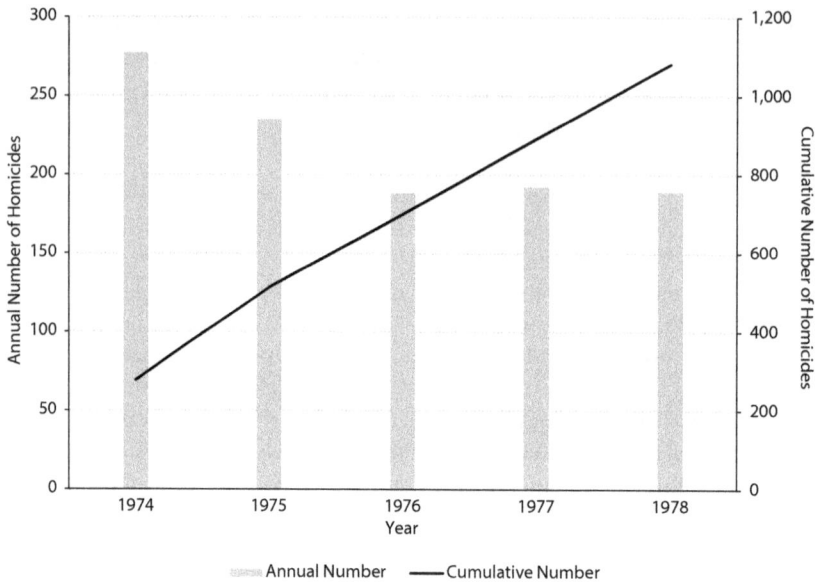

FIGURE 33. Second wave—Annual and cumulative homicides, 1974–78. Data source: Disaster Center, District of Columbia.

Turkey, Thailand, and Amsterdam.[58] The market glut of heroin led to the price declining from $7.71 per milligram in 1978 to $2.64 in 1979.[59] Drugs were distributed by independent dealers who "all got their own connection" either within the US or in Europe.[60] Shooting galleries, where people could rent works, proliferated in abandoned houses near open-air drug markets.[61] Middle-class White suburbanites were served through "drive-up drug markets," incentivized by a bag of heroin in DC costing $35–$40 compared to $100–$200 in Virginia.[62] By 1981, the "quality and quantity of the heroin available in Washington [was] on a par with what it was 10 or 12 years ago."[63] The city's abundant heroin supply led to dealer competition to offer users purer heroin, contributing to a dramatic rise in heroin overdoses, led by middle-class users.[64]

By 1981, Washington, DC, led the nation in heroin-related overdose deaths.[65] Indeed the CDC's *Morbidity and Mortality Weekly Report* stated that, "the 1981 population-based HRD [heroin-related deaths] mortality rate of 17.4/100,000 population for the District of Columbia is the highest ever reported in the medical literature."[66] Overdose deaths continued to climb for several years after, in line with national trends.[67]

By the mid-1980s, reporters documented at least 20 drug markets, four of which were 24/7 markets, operated by "makeshift clusters of addict-dealers" organized into a hierarchy of "crime captains, lieutenants, sergeants and crew members."[68] From them, the city's estimated 12,500 heroin-addicted people, along with their suburban counterparts, could openly purchase heroin. Many then went to "oil joints" (the local name for shooting galleries) in nearby home basements and apartments to shoot up or hired a "hit doctor" for $5.[69] Fifty-six-year-old Alexandra, who attributed her HIV acquisition to utilizing used works, "had traffic going in and out, in and out [of the apartment she shared with her boyfriend], 'cause I used to hit people, and I sold drugs and stuff, people were hollering up at the window." She learned how to "hit" working as a health aide. Forty-nine-year-old Ruth attributed her HIV to shooting up in an oil joint:

> They had like oil joints [where you] shoot heroin . . . So you come in, you get a seat, you do your little thing right there, you know, that's why I know I probably contracted pretty much from the needles, from exchanging, you use each other's needles, you use each other's water, you use the cookers, you know, so. When I hooked up, I was infected.

By the early 1990s, of an estimated 39,100 people who injected drugs (PWID) in the DC MSA, 14.5% had HIV.[70] Within DC proper, in 1990, there were an estimated 16,000 people with drug addiction (about 2.6% of the city), and in drug treatment settings, PWID HIV prevalence was 22.2%.[71]

Injecting drug use was also racialized. Nationally, the Bureau of Justice Statistics reported in 1992 that three-quarters of heroin users were White (74.5% White, 14.8% Black, 10.7% Hispanic).[72] And like sexual networks (see Part 2), drug networks are also largely racially homogamous (same-race injecting partners).[73] Thus, once HIV enters racialized networks, it will spread in racialized ways. This reflected racial containment, which created predominantly same-race neighborhoods (see Part 1) and thereby predominantly same-race friend and peer-group networks. Todd Pierce, who conducted ethnographic fieldwork in DC in the early 1990s, found racially homogamous drug networks among the Black and White PWID he studied.[74] Black PWID tended to be DC natives, lived in neighborhoods and family environments saturated with drugs, and had "histories of [drug-related] incarceration." Oil joints reduced Black users' visibility to the law and provided heroin and needles for rent but carried significant HIV risk. For Black PWID, drugs were easy to find, but the main challenge was finding money to purchase them. White PWID were suburban middle-class youth, who had few run-ins with the law. They easily procured syringes through posing as patients at local pharmacies and had resources to buy drugs. As such, while they shot up together, they did not need to share needles or go to oil joints to rent works, which completely eliminated their HIV risk from injecting drugs. The main challenge for White PWID was copping drugs, for which they had to leave their neighborhood unless they had a supplier.[75] A supplier made heroin use less visible to the law compared to Black PWID.

Pierce also found that this setup made quitting easier. Once White PWID ran out of resources or lost their supplier, they faced "hard limits." Continuing to use meant engaging Black neighborhoods and streets where "they were not part of that scene and they didn't know how to act or play the role when there."[76] This, along with "fear of losing friends, family and social status," made it easier to quit after a much shorter drug career than Black PWID, who lived in enabling environments. In this way, even if White PWID injected more, racial containment kept them safe and contributed to racial HIV inequality among PWID.

THE ROLE OF THE CITY AND CONGRESS IN THE HEROIN–HIV SYNDEMIC

Amplification and spatialized racial containment of the heroin–HIV syndemic as well as the unequal life outcomes that followed were the product of a web of interrelated local and federal government policies. Abandoned physical structures in poor Black neighborhoods (discussed in Part 1) served as venues for drug markets and shooting galleries. This was in part the result of not rebuilding or maintaining buildings in burned-out and destroyed areas after the Martin Luther King Jr. assassination riots in 1968.[77] In addition, the city neglected to maintain their own buildings (see Part 1). Reporter Loretta Tofani's article, with the headline "City Owns a Heroin 'Shooting Gallery,'"[78] described a boarded-up city-owned building used by a squatter who had been running a shooting gallery business there for two years, with the city's knowledge and complicity. The article noted that "homeowners along the block say they have complained repeatedly to the police and Department of Housing about the rowhouse junkies—with no results." The response to the reporter from a city representative was, "I know there's lots of drug activity in there . . . we keep nailing boards up, and they [heroin users] keep pulling boards down . . . we're just waiting for the City Council to approve a nonprofit sponsor." The city hoped the sponsor would rehabilitate the place, followed by a sale. In other words, the city expected homeowners to tolerate the drug use and hope for benevolence from a nonprofit.

Shooting galleries were a response to drug paraphernalia laws.[79] Following the 1979 creation of a model act capable of withstanding constitutional challenges, developed at the request of states by the DEA during the Carter administration, several states and the District of Columbia passed drug paraphernalia laws banning their "manufacture, advertisement, sale and possession" and that directed police to arrest people caught with works for consuming drugs.[80] Specifically, the model act suggested that states and the District make it

> unlawful for any person to use, or to possess with intent to use, drug paraphernalia ... [to] introduce into the human body a controlled substance in violation of this Act. Any person who violates this section is guilty of a crime and upon conviction may be imprisoned for not more than ( ), fined not more than ( ), or both.[81]

Washington, DC, followed the model closely in drafting its own law, which was signed by Black mayor Marion Barry in 1982 and sent to Congress for a 30-day review before being passed into law that year. DC residents could be charged based on their statements, "proximity of the object in time and space," "the existence of any residue of a controlled substance on the object," and circumstantial evidence, among other means. Violation would result in up to 30 days in jail, up to a $100 fine, or both.[82] Indoor shooting galleries, located close to open-air drug markets, were thus a perfect solution for heroin users—there, they could rent works rather than being arrested with them on the streets.

A consequential congressional action was related to syringe/needle exchange programs. While in many American cities, these programs were set up to limit HIV spread,[83] Washington, DC, was the only major city without a syringe/needle exchange program because of a congressional ban,[84] upheld by both Democratic and Republican administrations, that prohibited the use of DC's own municipal funds for exchange programs. The ban persisted until December 2007 when it was finally lifted by the Bush administration.[85] Perhaps not coincidentally, the city's first HIV surveillance report, released in November 2007, announced that the city "had the highest AIDS case rate nationally."[86] The contribution of the congressional ban to this status is evident in Figure 34, which shows an exponential climb in PWID HIV cases up until 2007, a subsequent tapering off between 2008 and 2011 after the ban

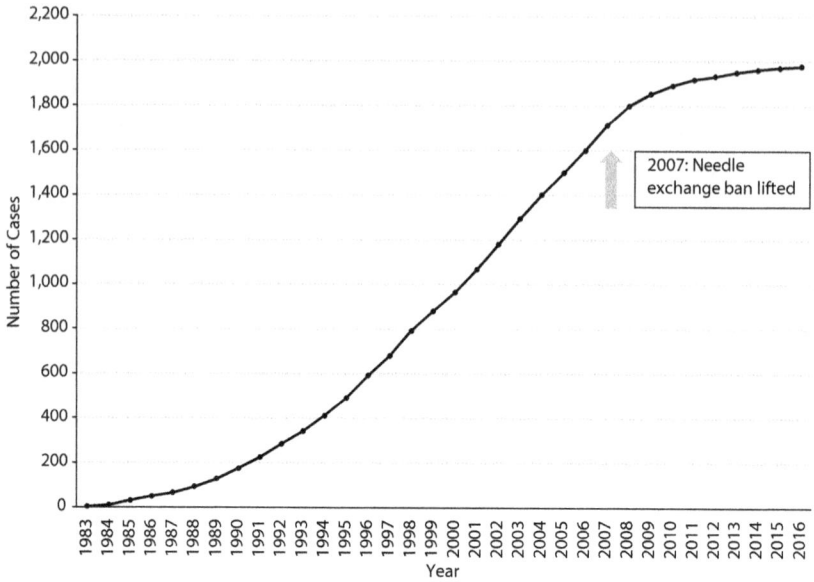

FIGURE 34. Cumulative number of people who inject drugs with HIV, 1983–2016. Data source: DC HAHSTA HIV/AIDS Surveillance Unit.

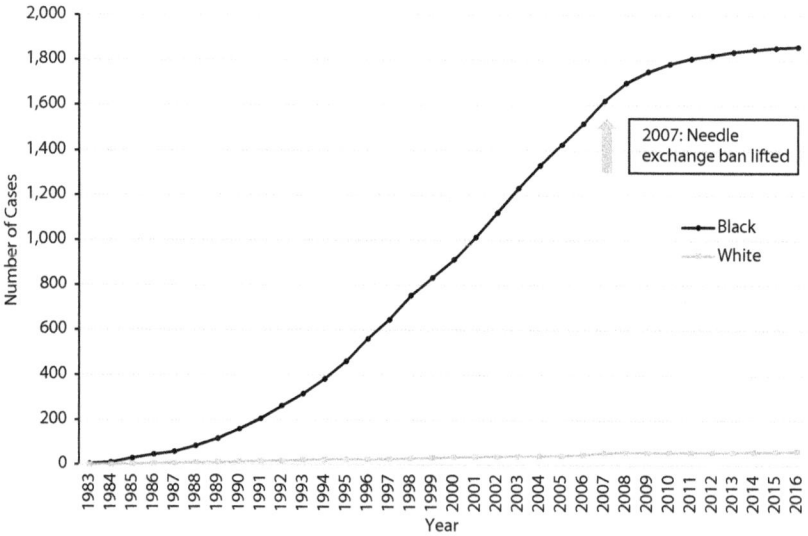

FIGURE 35. Cumulative number of people who inject drugs with HIV, by race, 1983–2016. Data source: DC HAHSTA HIV/AIDS Surveillance Unit.

was lifted, and a stall in the number of new cases after 2012. After the ban lifted, the city, under Mayor Adrian Fenty, poured more than half a million dollars into syringe/needle exchange programs,[87] and George Washington University's Monica Ruiz and colleagues calculated a 72.7% decrease in PWID HIV cases.[88] However, Figure 35 clearly illustrates the racial consequences of the ban. Throughout the epidemic, a disproportionate number of PWID with HIV were Black.

In sum, heroin addiction and HIV acquisition were not purely a function of individual choices and decisions; rather, they were deeply intertwined with congressional and city policies that facilitated both the heroin and HIV epidemics, as well as interactions between the two epidemics. Underscoring the entrenchment of the racial containment principle, this outcome was shaped by racialized responses to global geopolitical dynamics and perceived characteristics of addicted people, as well as actions and policies from both White and Black, Republican and Democratic leadership. However, heroin was not the only illegal drug fueling the HIV epidemic in the city.

SEVEN

Then Comes Cocaine

LATE 1970S–2010S

CASCADING COCAINE EPIDEMICS were another major means through which the city became vulnerable to syndemic-driven disease and mortality. Cocaine (and its derivative, crack, in particular) led to significant illness and overdose deaths, amplified the HIV epidemic, especially through its fueling of the commercial sex economy[1] (Chapter 8), and amplified the homicide epidemic to a level that far eclipsed the heroin epidemic (Chapter 9). In this chapter, I examine the national and local cocaine epidemic, the global supply chain to DC, the local drug economy, and how users became addicted.

TRACKING THE EPIDEMIC

Cocaine use is an endemic feature of American life; however, there has been significant variation in when use becomes abuse, is considered epidemic, and/ or produces mass life-devastating addictions. Over the last 140 years, cocaine has been widely available in the US; in the late 1800s, it was used in beverages such as Coca Cola, added to whisky, and smoked in cigarettes and cheroots. It was also an ingredient in over-the-counter and mail-order patent medications, ointments, and sprays for children and adults; and it was a surgery anesthetic.[2] An addiction wave associated with widespread usage led to the 1906 Pure Food and Drug Act, which required patent medicine producers to add ingredient labels to products.[3] Since then, cocaine's use has waxed and waned, and as several scholars have shown, each rediscovery of cocaine begins among society's elite, who are enthusiastic, glamorize it, and consider it harmless. Once it trickles down into middle and lower classes, widespread use leads to more visible addiction, a moral panic ensues, the drug is then banned and/or criminalized, and users, at that point often the poorest and most marginalized citizens, bear the most punishment.[4]

As Ansley Hamid documented, the rediscovery of cocaine in the late '70s followed exactly this trajectory.[5] Beginning in after-hours clubs and among the political and Hollywood elite, powder cocaine served as a party appetizer and social lubricant. The use of cocaine then spread across social classes. Journalists described freebasing (which involves inhaling cocaine vapors) taking off as a "rich man's drug that causes 'extreme euphoria,'" while "rock cocaine [was] selling like crazy, heralding a marketing break-through that furnishes this middle-class drug to the poorest neighborhoods."[6] (Using rock or crack cocaine involves directly smoking cocaine.) Increasingly large numbers of youth reported cocaine use to survey researchers. The national survey on drug abuse from the National Institute of Justice of 18- to 25-year-olds found 9% reporting having ever used it in 1972, 19% in 1977, and 28% in 1979.[7] In a 1985 National Institute on Drug Abuse (NIDA) household survey, 25% of 18- to 34-year-olds reported trying cocaine.[8] In terms of racial trends, the NIDA-funded Monitoring the Future survey, which included over 70,000 high school seniors, found that between 1985 and 1989, White boys and girls were two and three times more likely to report cocaine use than their Black counterparts, respectively.[9] The Bureau of Justice reported in 1992 that White people comprised the highest proportion of cocaine (62% White, 23.4% Black, 14.6% Hispanic) and crack users (49.9% White, 35.9% Black, 14.2% Hispanic).[10]

The period was also marked by a significant escalation in several metrics tracked by the CDC. Between 1976 and 1981, they found a threefold increase in cocaine-related ER episodes, a more than sixfold increase in treatment program admissions, and a fourfold increase in cocaine-related overdose deaths, increasing from 4.5/10,000 to 19.1/10,000 in medical examiner reports.[11] In 1986, data from NIDA's Drug Abuse Warning Network from 21 metropolitan areas showed that cocaine was "the leading drug related to ER episodes since the second half of 1986, and in ME [medical examiner] cases since the second half of 1987."[12] Across all metropolitan areas, between 1987 and 1989, about two-thirds of cocaine-related ER episodes were among men and among Black people, and about three quarters were among people aged 18–34.[13] Powder cocaine accounted for about half of cocaine-related ER episodes while crack cocaine accounted for about a quarter of episodes; about a third were cocaine in combination with alcohol.[14] Cocaine-related deaths also continued to escalate, with a more than sixfold increase in cocaine overdose deaths between 1983 and 1988.[15] As cocaine-related emergencies grew and high profile overdose deaths of athletes, such as Len Bias, raised alarms, the user profile changed. Richard Miech, utilizing data from the National Longitudinal Survey of Youth, found a class reversal between 1984 and 1998, from greater use among higher-SES teenagers (White and Black) to greater use among poorer teenagers.[16]

Within DC, before 1986 the main illegal drug was purportedly PCP (phenylcyclohexyl piperidine, a synthetic drug also called "angel dust" or "love boat").[17] A controversial program that tested trial defendants enabled tracking the transition from primarily PCP to cocaine use in the city. In 1984, 22% tested positive for cocaine use.[18] By 1985, it was 30%.[19] By November 1986, it was 48%, and reporters noted that "crack has made its first significant foray into Washington."[20] By 1988, most arrestees (57%) used cocaine,[21] and by 1989, 63%–66% used cocaine.[22] The first steady drop in arrestee cocaine use occurred in 1990.[23] While testing tracked escalating cocaine use, another data source indicated a cocaine-abuse epidemic. Data from NIDA's Drug Abuse Warning Network showed that while the DC metro area had 3,032 cocaine-related ER episodes in 1987, it had 4,930 such ER episodes in 1988 and 4,451 such ER episodes in 1989.[24] This was the fourth highest number of episodes across all 21 metropolitan areas covered in the system in 1987 (following New York, Detroit, and Philadelphia), and it was the third highest in 1988 and 1989 (following New York and Philadelphia).[25] Considering the relative size of the New York metro area (19.8 million in 1990) compared to the DC metro area (4.1 million in 1990),[26] this suggests a relatively high level of DC MSA cocaine overdoses. By 1989, three-quarters of DC cocaine-related ER episodes were due to smoking cocaine; the overdose death rate was 4.5/100,000 (1990) and 11.3/100,000 (1997).[27] In the ensuing decade, nationally and within DC, the cocaine epidemic began to wane, age, and concentrate in poor minority neighborhoods;[28] nationally, youth transitioned to marijuana and meth, before the opioid epidemic took center stage again.[29]

GLOBAL COCAINE SUPPLY CHAIN TO DC

The ebbs and flows of the national and DC cocaine epidemics were shaped by global geopolitical dynamics—with a mass exchange of drugs and billions of dollars between Latin America (primarily Peru, Bolivia, Colombia, and Mexico) and the US—and the futility of US government efforts to control the exchange through interdiction efforts.[30] The journey of cocaine into Washingtonian bodies began with leaves growing on coca shrubs in Peru and Bolivia.[31] The Colombian Medellín and Cali cartels, the so-called kings and queens of cocaine,[32] flew coca base from Bolivia and Peru to laboratories hidden in the jungles of Colombia for processing into cocaine powder and then packaging for shipment to the US. The transition in the US from powder cocaine to its more addictive derivative, crack, was precipitated by declining demand among powder users as well as cocaine overproduction as Colombian cartels began to control the levers of the state. The "narco-state" neutralized resistance to production and created efficient distribution systems within the US, earning billions of dollars each year.[33] As the Colombians began to ease out of direct distribution within the US and shifted towards expanding their European markets, Mexican cartels took over, coopting banks and creating narco-towns and narco-cities and controlling parts of government, bringing in billions of dollars.[34]

Once in the US, major cocaine distribution centers were in New York (especially New York City) and Florida (especially Miami), as well as in California, Texas, and Arizona, which border Mexico. From these states, tons of cocaine were disseminated across the US through compartmentalized franchise-style drug-distributor cells.[35] As markets in major transshipment cities became saturated and less lucrative, cities such as Washington, DC, became especially profitable for selling drugs. From New York and Miami, major Jamaican posses moved westward across the US, while LA Bloods and Crips (gangs) moved eastward to distribute cocaine and its derivative, crack.[36] Couriers from New York, Florida, and California brought cocaine to DC using planes, trains, buses, and cars (that had hidden compartments).[37] Drugs also came directly from Bolivia and Peru on a plane landing in Dulles airport nicknamed "the Cocaine Express," as well as from Panama.[38]

THE DC POWDER AND CRACK COCAINE ECONOMY

The global glut in cocaine in the early '80s gave DC a special draw. As the national supply increased, prices in south Florida dropped from $55K–$60K per kilo to $25K–$35K per kilo; in New York, the drop was from $75K per kilo to $30K–$40K per kilo, while in LA, the drop was from $45K–$55K per kilo to $10K per kilo.[39] Meanwhile in DC, the drop was from $55K–$75K per kilo to $50K–$60K per kilo, reflecting an economy supported by an affluent DMV (DC, Maryland, and Virginia metro area) clientele.[40] The markups were significant. A dealer could cut pure cocaine down to 22% purity and sell it for $100 a gram (about $350 in 2024 dollars), thus making "nearly a half million dollars [on] a kilo of undiluted cocaine" (about $1.7 million in 2024 dollars).[41] Because of the glutted market, even as cocaine demand increased, the price of powder cocaine plummeted and purity increased; a gram of cocaine that cost $125 with 12%–15% purity in 1985 was selling for $60–$70 at 35%–40% purity in 1986.[42] It was also sold in "quantities small enough to cost only $10, $15 or $25," prices to facilitate a mass market.[43] There was also a bustling suburban market, with sophisticated cocaine rings among the "preppies" of Alexandria,[44] in Montgomery County, "whose reputation for affluence provided a ready market for 'fashionable' drugs such as cocaine," in Prince George's County[45] and Fairfax County, where teens experienced long waits for treatment,[46] as well as in more rural suburbs.[47] As the market transitioned from powder to crack cocaine, crack became highly lucrative. The area cost for crack packets and vials weighing 5–10 milligrams between 1986 and 1988 ranged $10–$30 each, compared to crack vials bought for $5–$10 in New York or Miami.[48]

Nationally, as crack became more lucrative, selling became more hierarchical. Major gangs and crews set up production lines to transform cocaine into crack and package it, and they organized sellers to disseminate it privately, at outdoor markets, on street corners, in crack houses, and/or to set up bases in public housing projects and other venues to disseminate it more broadly.[49] As many, such as Elijah Anderson and Terry Williams have documented, the illegal drug industry became a critical part of inner-city economies across the country, providing jobs and steady and lucrative income against a backdrop of declining economic opportunities for unskilled workers.[50] Waldorf and colleagues described how "the crack industry has been 'investing' in inner-city neighborhoods precisely when legitimate industries have been moving out and taking jobs with them. Unlike most legal industries, the illicit drug business is an equal opportunity employer offering good pay to the unskilled."[51] For young unemployed or underemployed minority men, selling drugs earned them money for their own personal consumption, as well as to support families and friends.[52]

While nationally, high unemployment was a key driver of young Black men's involvement in the drug economy, in DC, many who sold drugs also had legitimate jobs. In a survey conducted among arrestees between 1985 and

1987, Peter Reuter and colleagues at the RAND Corporation found that two-thirds of the mostly young, unmarried Black men had not completed high school but were employed in legitimate jobs making a median hourly wage of $7.[53] "Eighty-eight percent lived in a private house or apartment" with multiple household members. Unlike in other cities, like Chicago,[54] drug-selling in DC was a "high paying supplement" to legitimate jobs. While arrestees made about $800 per month legitimately, daily drug-sellers made about $3,600 per month. As Reuters and colleagues noted, "A tax free $40,000 per year is much more than such persons might reasonably expect to earn from working hard at unskilled or semiskilled jobs." They also found that DC served as a distribution center for suburban residents, with a "substantial middle class demand for [cocaine]." They concluded that these "high earnings [were] only explainable by the existence of a large middle class market."[55] Richard Broughton, a DEA intelligence specialist, estimated the DMV (DC and its MD/VA suburbs) cocaine trade at $24 million per day,[56] supporting Reuters and colleagues' conclusion that middle-class and affluent buyers had a role in underwriting the DC drug economy.

City Collusion and DMV Drug Sacrifice Zones

Indeed, DC was a central hub of DMV-area drug distribution, with open-air drug markets hosted in public housing projects, as well as on streets and street corners in poor neighborhoods, which constantly shifted from block to block, neighborhood to neighborhood, as police conducted drug sweeps. As I describe below, clientele came from throughout the DMV, and middle-class White and Black suburbanites would drive in and out of the city to procure drugs,[57] leaving the community to deal with the severe immediate and intergenerational consequences that came with living and growing up in a syndemic zone—including drug addiction, spillover epidemics, attendant under- and overpolicing,[58] and overincarceration.[59] In this way, racially contained poor Black neighborhoods became "sacrifice zones" (see the Introduction) for the DMV's drug habit. Further, decades earlier, housing projects had been sited in the middle of stable middle-class Black neighborhoods (see Part 1). Thus, the class containment barrier was crossed, and they also experienced spillover effects from housing projects taken over by drugs.[60] Black reporter Courtland Milloy described the intraracial complexity of the drug epidemic, noting:

It appears that the young crack dealers, usually boys from poor households, have instigated a redistribution of wealth that has them living better, materially, than many of their middle-class customers whose wallets and brains are being drained by drugs . . . In Washington, the Black community is being burned at both ends of its class spectrum.[61]

As he observed in an article a year later titled "Insulation on the White Side of Town," "the impact of the crack explosion has been contained in predominantly Black neighborhoods of Washington . . . It appears that as long as you stay west of 16th St NW, your chances of getting assaulted, raped, robbed or burglarized are greatly reduced."[62]

Reflecting historical continuity, drug markets were facilitated by the city government's inadvertent enabling of the DMV drug-economy infrastructure. A good example is the story of Hanover Place, described by reporter Linda Wheeler in 1985:

For five years, day and night, cars with Maryland, Virginia and D.C. tags have created traffic jams there as their occupants negotiated to buy $50 packets of exceptionally pure cocaine from the many willing vendors who lined the narrow street [which] met all the requirements for a thriving drug market. Like many of the 50 other neighborhoods in the city that support such bazaars: It is near major thoroughfares—North Capitol Street and New York Avenue—allowing quick and easy access for buyers from Maryland, Virginia and D.C. Many buildings are abandoned. Therefore, there are fewer neighbors to object. Also, dealers have places to hang out, hide from police, and store the drugs. Garbage is allowed to accumulate . . . the trash in turn provides thousands of hiding places for small quantities of the drugs the dealers are holding . . . but Hanover Place didn't commit suicide; it was helped to its death bed by an indifferent city government including the police department.[63]

Indeed, while city neglect contributed to the creation and maintenance of this market, city attention contributed to its closing through a combination of continuous police presence, the public works department clearing garbage, the housing department enforcing code violations, and the city installing high-intensity lights.[64] Previously upscale middle-class Black apartment complexes, such as Mayfair Mansions, a 600-unit complex comprised of 17 three-story buildings, and the Paradise Gardens complex that had run down due to poor maintenance,[65] also became ground zero for DMV drug distribution operations. In the mid- to late '80s, the complex was described as hosting "one of the biggest open-air drug markets on the East Coast [with] as many as 100 dealers."[66] Reporter Sari Horwitz, drawing on interviews and the court trial transcript of one gang, "The Committee," who operated there and were convicted, described a gang of six to ten people stationed at the complex making about $25K per day through selling $25 bags to Black customers, $50 bags to White customers, and dealers coming from throughout the metro area, "some buying in bulk orders of 100 bags or more."[67] Frustrated by city police, who were trying to put out multiple fires, residents eventually called in the Nation of Islam, a Black Muslim nationalist group, to help restore order.[68]

The city also owned several drug havens in both scattered sites (unmarked and unclustered public housing units)[69] and in regular public housing buildings. In 1987, *The Washington Post* published an editorial titled "Where Drug Dealers Prey" describing the challenges faced by the city's public housing complexes.[70] Gangs and drug lords began to move into and take over complexes characterized by deterioration and city abandonment, and in which a concentration of poor Black people lived (see Part 1). Empty apartments were used for drug production. Residents were preyed upon as their apartments were co-opted for both drug production and to use as crack houses.[71] *Post* reporters conducted monthlong observations and interviews at Potomac Gardens, one of the complexes, and reported that "to a large degree, the market at the Gardens is fueled by outsiders, some of them White residents of Maryland and Virginia, who park their cars outside the complex, hurry into the courtyards, purchase their drugs and leave," heading back to areas with relatively limited surveillance to use or deal discreetly.[72] However, as DC's drug-related violence and police surveillance increased, drug markets expanded to the suburbs in counties such as Fairfax, Montgomery, and Prince George's (PG).[73] Police identified numerous outdoor suburban drive-up drug markets, as well as less visible distribution in cocktail lounges and hotel rooms.[74] A RAND Corporation report found that the DC suburbs "had worse drug abuse problems with cocaine and PCP than any other suburban area nationwide."[75]

This was striking as the DMV was the home of US presidents, Congress, the Supreme Court, and the national headquarters for the FBI, DEA, and NIDA. FBI director William Sessions said that "the FBI has not targeted the drug trade in the District for special emphasis because it is dominated by low-level street dealers rather than major narcotics trafficking organizations active in other cities."[76] However, when drug use was perceived to have crossed racial containment boundaries, such as Rock Creek Park and Fairfax County, William Bennett, the new drug czar, declared DC the "first 'high intensity' drug trafficking city . . . to make the city a 'test case' in the federal drug war."[77] Yet despite the city's crime prevention efforts and despite hosting "thousands of people [who] are paid a lot of money to figure out what's gone wrong in urban America,"[78] "the drug's price . . . remained stable, its potency high and its supply plentiful."[79]

DRUG ADDICTION IN DC

Racial and class containment obviously did not mean that people were immobile. However, it did reflect on the nonaccidental nature of the places they came home to, where they socialized, the institutions they encountered, such as schools, those they patronized, such as clubs, and the social and physical environments in which they grew up and felt comfortable, even if they were dangerous.[80] For many Black District youth growing up in the 1980s and early '90s, while the vast majority stayed away from drugs, they were nonetheless common, especially among the most disadvantaged. An Urban Institute survey of predominantly Black (96%) teenage boys from the poorest neighborhoods in the city found that about one in ten (9%) reported using crack or powder cocaine, and one in six (16%) reported ever selling drugs.[81] Multiple exposures to drugs—at home, in friendship groups, and on the streets—within contained neighborhoods—whose boundary lines were enforced by police, but whose efforts had not succeeded in stopping the flow of drugs—increased the chances of trying, regularly using, and for a smaller proportion, becoming addicted to drugs. Reflecting epidemic-style incremental and then exponential growth, many respondents who became addicted experienced a gradual saturation of drugs, first in their neighborhoods, and then in their networks and friendship groups, within their own families, and with romantic partners. This multilayered exposure of their social worlds to illegal drugs made the drugs hard to escape, and eventually they succumbed to use—and subsequent abuse—of crack cocaine.

Many trans women I interviewed had struggled with crack addiction (see note).[82] Forty-three-year-old trans woman Maggie grew up "very depressed. I was in a dysfunctional home, watching my mother get abused . . . my stepfather used a lot of drugs, and he beat my mom *[long silence]*." Unfortunately school was not a refuge. Starting in elementary school, as a gay boy, she "was teased a lot in school because of my gay lifestyle . . . school was terrible, my grades suffered, I ran into drugs." In addition to emotional eating, when she was 12 or 13, weed helped her to "escape the reality." The constant teasing became intolerable, and after attempting suicide at 16, she dropped out of school and went to live with her grandmother in Richmond, Virginia. Unfortunately, while there, she was raped and almost killed. She moved back to DC to live with her mother and started working odd jobs to earn money. However, her mother's intolerance towards her sexuality (as a gay boy) led her to eventually leave home at age 21. She "went to the streets in DC, and that's where everything spiraled downhill from, there."

Maggie was a late crack adopter in part because she was using PCP. After a late night party with her brother, she went to her mother's house the following morning and found

> my brother was still up. I was like "You been up all night?" He was like, "Yeah." He was like still smoking crack ... So he said, "You wanna try it?" And I tried it. I really didn't get it at first, I didn't understand it, so I let it alone ... When I went to the streets, everybody was doing it. So I'm like, maybe there's something I'm missing. Maybe I'm not doing it right. So I kept trying it and I kept trying it and then someone explained to me that "you're looking for the same thing you're getting from this and it's not gonna happen. This is a whole different concept." So when they told me that and I knew what to look for, I got it. And when I got it, it was instantly addictive. It held me down for so long, it did, it held me down.

The multiple exposures she had are striking in this account, as is the role of members of her family and her street community doing crack, which contributed to her multiple attempts to "get it." Twenty-two years later, at the time of the interview, despite efforts to get and stay clean, she had just had a relapse. She paid a heavy price for "getting it," and it was still holding her down. As several scholars, such as Howard Becker, have demonstrated, and as I found in this and other respondent accounts, drug initiation was a social process—familiar people introduced respondents to drugs, taught them how to use them, and how to look for the high of a particular drug. Multiple exposures thus combined with social networks and personal ties to spark and then normalize regular use.[83]

For those who became addicted, crack then seemed, as neuroscience confirmed, to take hold of their brain and not let go.[84] Maggie described what the addiction felt like when I asked her about the price of crack:

SANYU: So how much is crack?

MAGGIE: Very expensive, for a little piece, and it goes just like that.

SANYU: How much is that?

MAGGIE: For $20. For $50 you might get a size like that, and you break it into pieces and you smoke it, and the high lasts for a few minutes and then you go into a geek. And the geek is what makes you chase it and want more and want more until you're constantly going, constantly going, and you're wearing your body down, you're losing yourself spiritually, mentally, physically, emotionally, all of that, you just lose yourself in that.

SANYU: So the $50 lasts for how long?

MAGGIE: 30 minutes . . . at most 30 minutes . . . [then] you want more, you constantly want more, it's a mind controlling drug. And it makes you do anything. It makes you have unprotected sex, makes you sleep with nasty old men, and makes you do things with dirty people, it makes you do things you never thought you would do.

Forty-two-year-old Hannah was introduced prior to her gender transition, when she was a 22-year-old gay man:

Um, I went to school, got good grades, went to college, graduated, um, and then that's when I started . . . I dated this guy, who was a um [local DC university] student . . . We used to go to parties and crack was like an appetizer for everybody. So um, that's when I was introduced to it. Then the gay life in DC, you know, I met some friends, then that became, you know, something that we did.

She was able to use and hold down a company job until her use became abuse and addiction during a relationship in which "he was enabling me and he wanted me . . . instead of going to the movies, let's get high." By the time her relationship ended, she was addicted. It was 16 years before she got clean.

Once respondents were addicted, it was hard to sustain an intimate relationship that was not centered on drugs. Many described losing relationships with non–drug using partners in the course of their addiction. Relationships that worked involved a partner who was an enabler—supplying drugs, money, or an apartment—or a partner with whom to get high. Maggie described one such relationship she had a year before the interview:

MAGGIE: The last relationship I had was a crack relationship, and I lied to myself thinking it was more. It wasn't more. Same scenario.

SANYU: What's a crack relationship?

MAGGIE: Built on drugs, built around drugs. We were just basically get-high partners, good sex partners. When I wasn't around he did whatever he wanted to, with whoever he wanted to do. And I went out and tricked and prostituted to get more crack so that he would stay around me. That's basically all it was. Like I said I had a very low self-esteem and he made me feel good. He made me feel wanted and accepted. So I kept him there. And he was fine as hell. I have to put that in. *[We both laugh.]*

Describing one of her drug relationships, trans woman Henrietta illustrated the complication when love entered the picture:

When he did drugs and I did drugs, he was really nice ... he was so good in bed. He would kiss me and love me. His sex was like love. He was only doin' it for the drug, to get more and more and more, and when the drugs would be gone, he would be gone. And I would do anything and everything to keep him there, even if it's not paying my rent ... I didn't pay my rent. That's when I lost the house, just to keep him there with me. But it still didn't work. When the money was gone, he was gone.

Family Entanglements

Friend, intimate partner, and family use created a thick web of overlapping networks through which drug use and abuse became normalized and reinforced; as Eloise Dunlap, Leon Dash, and others have illustrated, drug use spread across extended families.[85] My respondents described how a family could be clean except for one relative who "still had an effect on the household if [they were] still coming around, ya know." In other cases, entire families could be involved. Forty-year-old Benton was caught in a particularly dense family web—with multiple crack users in different locations and generations. Born in DC, he moved to North Carolina when he was 12 to live with his father and was introduced to crack by friends in his teens. His use was reinforced by family in both North Carolina and DC when he returned. As he explained, in North Carolina, he was "smokin' a lot of crack, because my grandmother and them—a lot of my family members used to smoke crack, so my grandmother was already, like, selling, bootleggin', and she was selling it and stuff."

It was family drug use that led to his HIV diagnosis at age 17:

I started smokin' with them, and it was just like a thing, we was just doin' it, just gettin' high in the house ... I couldn't get high off the crack no more, so I started shootin' up crack, and I think that's how I caught the HIV, 'cause I shared needles with people in a circle, 'cause I was shootin' between all those people that died of AIDS ... I caught HIV, but I'm still here.

When he moved back to DC,

> I was stayin' with my mother [and then] my sisters. They were tryin' to show
> me the ropes about DC. And my sister was on crack in a big way ... She was
> always with somebody that was sellin' it and doing stuff like that. She had
> access to it all the time and everything ... I just got strung out on it again.

Thus, family entanglement made it hard for Benton, stymying his efforts to
stay off drugs.[86]

Drug use and abuse sometimes shifted at the family level. For 42-year-old
Ida, except for one sister, "my whole family used drugs all the time," noting,
"It's like this was our recreation for our family ... This is what we do." She
described how

> at that time it wasn't nobody using crack. Like early on, we just smoked mari-
> juana, we might smoke a little hash or some [other drug] every now or then
> ... then it was like everybody, drug habits changed. 'Round the late '80s, early
> '90s ... Everybody kinda escalated from one thing to another.

Recovery similarly spread through her family as "they was one by one getting
theyselves together, you know quit[ing]."

Interviewing 40-year-old trans woman Mary, it was clear as she described
her first time "getting it" how intoxicating crack still was, even though she
was now four years clean. On her way to a club, she stopped to pick up her
friend whose mother was "like *the* crack lady" in the neighborhood:

> So I went in the house to see what was going on, and her and her mother was
> in there smoking. And um, *[sigh],* that was when I [was] first exposed. And
> I took a hit and that was *it*. I stayed in there for about thirty minutes ... she
> told me how to *[breathes in]* inhale and burn it, and do it right, and hold the
> smoke. And we went out to the club, but that's all I thought about. And that
> night was *[Sanyu: When's the next one?]* the next one and I went the next day,
> and the next night I went back at it with a vengeance. I wanted to have the
> taste of it and the feeling that I had, the smell of it, the smell of the things
> that was involved. I was romanticized by it *[breathless sigh]*. Caught up in it.

Her romance with crack lasted about two decades. Mary's use was reinforced
by her mother:

> Um, I come from, um *[pause]* a single mother who was an IV drug user ... I
> wish that she could see me now, you know, um, because I was in my addiction
> when she died ... She was a heroin addict, but you know, crack came and she

smoked crack too, and we smoked crack together. And she used to give me money to go buy crack, and we would get high together.

Born in DC in 1971, Mary had been living with her grandmother because she had been disowned by her father (for several years, lasting until a few months before he died) when she transitioned from being a boy to being a girl, and her mother was addicted to heroin. As she described it, crack use became a bonding activity for mother and daughter. What followed affected the course of her life: "My father died in '88, and my mother died in '89, and she died from complications of HIV. *[Sanyu: Oh, your mom also had HIV?]* Um hm, yeah, so ya know, and it's like maybe two or three months later that I tested positive." Having buried her father at age 17 and her mother at age 18, she was 19 when she was diagnosed with HIV:

> I uh thought my life was over, 'cause it's like, ya know, I knew she was HIV, and then maybe a year or later she was dead, you know, so I'm thinking that this is how my life is gonna be. You know, um, and that's how I lived life. Like, it's gonna be over tomorrow. I'm gonna use drugs, I'm gonna continue to engage in unsafe sex, and um, I didn't die, for a lot of years, I didn't die. I don't know why, but I didn't die, so . . .

Her story reflects the multilayered, intergenerational transmission of syndemic disease from mother to daughter against the backdrop of cascading drug epidemics. Beyond the sociohistorical and environmental factors at play, genetic-epidemiological studies find a range of about 30%–80% heritability of the propensity for cocaine addiction.[87]

Spiraling to the Bottom

Across my interviews, a recurring phrase when respondents with addiction described their lives after beginning drug use was "spiraling down." For 51-year-old Cornelius, "[when] the drugs and stuff became involved . . . it spiraled downward from there." It was a source of deep regret that a decision made 30 years ago had shaped his entire adulthood:

> It's such a, um, strong addiction . . . I regretted that, you know, the first time I tried it. Um, that was my fault, that was something I had control over, making the decision to try, start it. After that, it was like I had no control over relapsing and doing it again and again . . . I have been going through meetings for like 30 some years. I could not get a year for nothing . . . It's so strange.

Sixty-one-year-old Gordon described how comprehensively crack consumed his life, how it could "change your whole outlook, um, your appearance, your behavior, your thinking" and how life became "a total, *nightmare*. Because I would, um, use the drug until I would run out of money . . . so far as my personal hygiene upkeep. I wouldn't take baths, I wouldn't eat, I lost a lot of weight, um. Ashy, dirty, smelling . . . " It was, "nearly, literally, destroying." Henrietta simply described all she lost: "I had a house, I had two dogs, I was very successful. And when I started doin' it, I lost it all. I lost my house, I lost my dogs, I lost everything to drugs."

They had somehow moved from the "sweet spot" of "going with the flow" to everything spiraling out of control, wanting more and more drugs, and seeking higher highs by shifting mediums of drug intake. Further, drug addiction affected their financial status; savings could only support a habit up to a point. Their work and ability to hold a job steadily declined, and they began selling possessions to support their habits. Catching and/or passing on HIV often happened in the middle of that spiral down and at the cycling around at the bottom.

In sum, my respondents' addictions were not just the results of their individual decisions and choices but also the products of family, social network, and neighborhood dynamics that structured their multiple drug exposures, as well as the city's drug economy and the wider DMV clientele who made it lucrative, along with city government and congressional actions and inactions, and global geopolitical dynamics, which drove the shift from powder to its more addictive derivative, crack. On the ground, people with addiction had a key daily challenge—how to pay for drugs, a topic I take up in the next chapter.

EIGHT

Paying for a Habit

COMMERCIAL SEX AND
DRUG ADDICTION TREATMENT

THIS CHAPTER EXAMINES HOW drug users paid for their expensive habit, with a focus on the commercial sex industry. It then more briefly examines local and federal government attempts and budgetary allocations to treat DC's and the nation's collective drug habit. Handling the escalation from crack use to crack addiction without further engaging in criminalized activity became impossible for many. While coming from a higher social class and having a better paying job gave some, such as Henrietta and Hannah, a longer runway on the spiral down, eventually addiction began to overtake even the more well-off respondents' financial ability to acquire enough drugs to satisfy their addiction. Several respondents turned to the illegal economy to support their habit through selling drugs[1] and engaging in a wider range of criminal activities. Fifty-one-year-old Cornelius, for example, was a broker connecting White suburban drug dealers to product.

> SANYU: So, um, so how were you uh, paying for the drugs at that point? Did you have a job or . . . ?
>
> CORNELIUS: . . . I met people from Virginia, Maryland, um, these White guys would come in and spend all this money buying for their friends, and they would pay me to help them find something . . . I didn't really commit a lot of crimes, my thing was meeting people. And that's how I supported my habit, I knew a lot of people . . .

Forty-two-year-old Ida was involved in a number of drug-related hustles including "sell[ing] some drugs so we [she and her friend] could get high" and laundering money in exchange for drugs. As she described:

A guy came there [to the crack house where she lived]. And I believe he had robbed a bank or somewhere where the money had spilled, so he had all this marked money. And we ... got rid of the money for him, for drugs. You know we would carry it to hustlers, drug dealers, we would carry some to gasoline stations, different places.

Fifty-eight-year-old Hiram's apartment was a base for drug operations:

SANYU: Did you, so did you get addicted to crack?

HIRAM: ... I could say yes because I was doing it and I was turning my apartments into, what I call, um, drug dealer service centers. I had the drug dealers come in, they would cut the product up ... sometimes it would be between, between five and ten thousand dollars' worth. So, I would let them sell it out of my house, out of my apartment and everything, so I got in like really deep. And, because I was getting so much from them, I didn't have to go nowhere to get it 'cause they came to me. Yeah I was, I was, yeah, I, I think that I was addicted to it. And um, I had to make a conscious decision after a certain time that this is not for me.

Other respondents engaged in robbery and shoplifting to support their drug habits. (As I describe in Part 4, drug-related criminal activities were a common pathway to incarceration for my respondents).

People needing to acquire fast money to support their addiction, however, confronted a gendered economy. Both men and women faced financial strain from drug addiction, but women faced lower pay in the legal economy, and they had fewer assets and other wealth buffers to run through. The illegal drug economy was uniquely able to provide cash that could come fast enough to keep up with the pull of crack addiction; however, it was also gendered. Researchers find that in many settings, drug sellers are often men, while women often serve in auxiliary roles, earning less money.[2] Thus, for many women, selling sex is the most lucrative and reliable way to generate as much (or more) money as men with the same rapidity as selling drugs.[3] As a result, both nationally and in DC, there was a gendered symbiosis between the drug economy and the commercial sex economy, with each enabling the other.[4] The symbiosis also worked to amplify the national HIV epidemic[5] and, as I will illustrate, the DC HIV epidemic.

*The Social Organization of Sex Work:
Stratification and Sexual Containment*

The US capital's commercial sex industry has long been highly stratified, with sex workers servicing elite, middle-, and working-class clientele. Tamika Nunley examined the city's 19th-century commercial sex economy, drawing on court and police records as well as news reports and other archival documents.[6] During the Civil War (1861–65), Nunley notes that there were an estimated 7,500 area sex workers: "2,500 in Alexandria and Georgetown" and 5,000 in DC. A third were Black women. Nunley also notes that there were "450 registered bawdy houses," of which 12 were "coloured [sic]."[7] Black women also sold sex in houses run by White madams.[8] Indeed, there were both inter- and intraracial commercial sex economies. Black women's "clientele primarily included White men and immigrant and free Black laborers who could afford the services of more inexpensive prostitutes and bawdy houses."[9] While many madams were White, Black women were also stratified across statuses such as "madams, prostitutes, slaves and servants in bawdy houses."[10] Sex work provided not just accommodation and food but also highly lucrative employment. As Nunley found, "although madams made the most money and often paid the highest fees in court, it was not uncommon for prostitutes to earn more than wage earners and laborers in other industries."[11]

The lucrative, war-driven expansion of the commercial sex economy led to a move to spatially contain it. As the city's population swelled with well-paid military clients, vagrancy laws to police sex work (as it was not illegal) became insufficient. Nunley described how "Brigadier General Joseph Hooker made plans to geographically contain the sex industry to monitor the whereabouts of Union soldiers. Named after Hooker, Hooker's division became the cordoned hotbed of sex commerce in the District, located near what is today referred to as the Federal Triangle."[12] The stratified and spatially contained nature of the city's commercial sex economy then also characterized the scene in the 1980s–2010s, over a hundred years later. At the higher end of the economy, DC was rocked by a scandal involving the White "DC madam," who started her business in the early 1990s, employing young, college-educated women to service the city's elite at fancy hotels, such as Four Seasons and The Mayflower. Her lengthy list of 10,000–15,000 clients serviced between 2002 and 2006 included a US senator and high-level government and military officials.[13] While the DC Madam and some of the call girls were arrested and charged, many male clients were not, and a judge barred the release of most client names. High-class call-girl sex work often operates quietly, the DC Madam case notwithstanding, and commands the highest amounts of money. However, the most visible, cheapest, surveilled, and prosecuted sex work is among street workers, who comprise an estimated 10%–20% of the sex work industry.[14] An estimated 15%–18% of men in the US have ever paid for sex.[15]

While many factors attract workers to the commercial sex economy, including its highly lucrative nature, for my respondents, drug addiction was a common initial motivation. About a third of my sample who used or were addicted to drugs (especially to crack) sold sex at some point in the course of their addiction. In exchange, they gained free drugs and/or money to support their habit. As they entered this economy, they sorted themselves into its stratified and spatialized economy. Forty-three-year-old Sidney sold sex from his home. As he described: "I had my own place. And I had a cell phone, and I had like regular dates that would spend money on me, like, so . . . I didn't really necessarily have to go on the street." Forty-two-year-old Ida sold sex while living in different crack houses, places where she would "only pay three dollars a month for rent, low income housing" and where you could "get high, sell sex, and then go . . . about your business." Among street sex workers, there was a highly stratified system based on both looks as well as drug use, as forty-eight-year-old trans woman Henrietta observed among the estimated 100 street sex workers she knew:

> Everybody pretty much knew everyone, but it was kind of divided. The pretty girls went on Seventh Street, the mediocre girls stayed on Fifth Street, and the crack heads were in the back, the back street. We called it the Back Street Girls. I was one of the Back Street Girls, the not so popular. Every once in a while I'd walk up to the mediocre girls and get a trick over there, but most of the time when I got high and I knew I looked kind of on the dusty side, I would go back with the crack girls . . . [The pretty girls] didn't use drugs, pretty much . . . some of the pretty girls . . . were on snorting coke . . . it is addictive, but your high is longer. So therefore you don't run like the crack heads. Crack heads, your high is so instant that you have to go back and get more . . . You're always running gettin' more. But the girls who snorted, their high was a little bit longer, where they could do stuff a little bit longer.

My respondents, many not on HIV medication (which reduces infectivity) for several years while they sold sex, also described a range of clientele, revealing the potential for HIV spread across race, gender, sexual orientation, social class, and marital status throughout the DMV area. Ida's clients included "polices, uh correction officers. I had a clientele of people that had work. The mens that worked. Productive members of society." For Sidney, "well, a lot of 'em would be straight or gay men . . . married and single." Trans woman Lisa described both Black and White clients and noted that not all were hiding the fact that they paid for sex from their partners: "I had clienteles that had wives, where they would take me home to meet their wives and all that, and we would threesome." For trans woman Hannah, clients were "straight, uh straight men, White men, young boys who sell drugs. All types of clients . . . straight men with family and kids."

While clientele came from across the DMV area,[16] street sex work was spatially contained and surveilled in another form of sexual containment (see Part 2). There was a clear geography of sex work, not only in terms of who worked where but also the role that drugs played in their work.[17] In the 1980s, among gay and bisexual men, DC was apparently "becoming known 'in a lot of gay circles as the boy-whore capital.'" Reporter Joann Stevens described male sex work occurring in front of the Cafe Naples on New York Avenue NW near 13th Street, near the Chesapeake House, and on Dumbarton Avenue in Georgetown, with a "stream of late model Mercedes, El Dorados and other luxury cars" even at 2:30 a.m. Police estimated 30 or more "dial-a-date agencies" where men charged "anywhere from $45 an hour to $500 a night for house calls."[18] There was also a thriving heterosexual sex work industry conducted in massage parlors throughout the DC area,[19] with "sex related businesses [that had] become so common that suspected prostitution houses advertise in newspapers and the telephone book and flourish within blocks of the White House."[20]

Sex work also thrived on the city's streets, albeit more heavily policed and surveilled. In the late 1980s, the third police district, including neighborhoods such as Cardozo-Shaw, Columbia Heights, Dupont Circle, Logan Circle, and Mount Pleasant, was nicknamed "Valley of the Dolls"; the red-light areas for cisgender women were in Logan and Thomas Circles, while trans women worked on K Street and near 10th and M Street/Blagden Alley, within the Shaw area.[21] The separate spaces were in part to avoid violent confrontation of those who might mistake trans women sex workers for cisgender women sex workers.[22] Sex work geography was also a function of policing strategies, which paralleled drug sweeps and sometimes moved sex work zones from one place to another. For example, in 1988, police launched

STOP squads (Stemming the Operation of Prostitutes) with four patrol units assigned to ridding the third district of sex work.[23] In 1991, a Department of Public Works survey of traffic patterns on L Street in downtown DC apparently found that at 1:00 a.m., "there were over 1100 cars backed up which is double the amount of cars during rush hour in any part of the city."[24] Soon after, the police began "mass arrests of streetwalkers" and issued "at least 5,000 tickets [to drivers] during the first six weeks of the crackdown."[25] In 2006, city council lawmakers passed the Omnibus Public Safety Emergency Amendment Act. This legalized "prostitution-free zones," which were operationally located by police near gentrifying parts of the city.[26] As such, the social organization of sex work and its containment retained many of the same patterns established in the city's early history. The crucial difference, however, was the way drug addiction and HIV fueled the commercial sex economy at both structural and individual levels.

The DC Drug Economy–Commercial Sex Economy–HIV Symbiosis

In commercial sex economies driven by drug addiction, the price of sex often falls to the price of a session of drugs. For example, a study of DC's economy conducted by Meredith Dank and colleagues at the Urban Institute found a significant decline in the price of sex after the onset of crack.[27] They described a range of $50–$300 among street sex workers in the '70s and early '80s that declined to a range of $20–$150 in the mid-'80s to '90s. With the onset of crack, more sex workers—especially younger, addicted women—flooded the city's economy, creating a supply surge.[28] The period also coincided with the shift from a predominantly heroin addiction epidemic to a predominantly crack addiction epidemic. This had a significant impact on the city's HIV epidemic. Howard University professors Ernest Quimby and Arvilla Payne-Jackson's study of sex work in a DC neighborhood is instructive. They observed how properties of heroin and crack differentially affected the pace of sex work among users. While heroin gave users a longer high, crack users, with quickly fading highs, kept "coming back frequently to buy or use sex to trade or earn money for more crack."[29] It is worth noting the historical contingency of these two trends—the shift to crack and the drop in the price of sex—for the course of the HIV epidemic. In combination, they created the need for sex workers with crack addiction to have more partners to support their habits at precisely the time that the city's HIV epidemic was expanding.

A perfect storm was thus created by this unique amplifier to HIV spread within the city's drug and sexual networks.

It was also startling to hear in interviews that an HIV diagnosis itself was a driver to sell sex (or sell even more sex), with consequences for transmission. Sixty-one-year-old Gordon, diagnosed when he was 46, said sex work "started right after, you know, the HIV came in, 'cause that's when everything started to like, really get um, overpowering me." Helen said that "after I found out [I had HIV], it was like a death sentence. I was just tricking, prostituting real hard, smoking drugs real hard because in my mind I was gonna die." Mary also found that an HIV diagnosis pushed her into a more intense cycle of sex work, as she "used drugs and prostituted, and used drugs and prostituted, and used drugs and prostituted . . . I did that for like 15 years." (She began medication seven years into the cycle). Indeed, for her and others, sex work continued postdiagnosis, with or without condoms, with or without medication when available.

Forty-eight-year-old trans woman Henrietta had lived a full life before beginning sex work at age 32. She had grown up as a much loved and long-awaited only child of working-class parents who "did very well in life." Assigned as a boy at birth but feeling different, she endured insults in school and tried hard to "hide it and mask it." After graduating high school and completing some college before dropping out, she worked at a large store, rising to a supervisor role. She moved into a house, got pets, and began a long-term heterosexual relationship that became serious. However, her life took a turn after the relationship ended, her beloved mother got Alzheimer's and went into a nursing home, and she found out her father had another partner:

> So I started doin' the drugs and I started spiraling down . . . Then I started doing the prostitution on Fifth and K, back when it was popular . . . for all of the queens, for the drag queens. We would all go down there and prostitute . . . And there's where I met a lot of people that were just like me, but they were just like vampires. They would come out in the night and hide during the day because you weren't accepted during the day, but at night you were accepted. So it was like, "Lights, camera, action!" in the nighttime, you were all excited, men wanted you, you could get money and all of that. And I did that for eight years . . . And there's where I contracted HIV is when I was prostituting. Condoms would burst, guys with big penises, things like that.

She was diagnosed after three years of selling sex. Before HIV began to "combat my body" she commanded a lot of money, especially after she learned to perform the kind of femininity that would fetch the highest prices:

I did get lots of money, 'cause new girls on the block get money. You're new, you're a new hole to fuck. It's not necessarily that you're just pretty, it's just that you're a new one to try out . . . you make lots of money. I made lots of money when I went out there . . . The first night I made, like, $200. And then after that, when I started you know, getting better at it, because I wasn't really good at the makeup or anything else, I didn't have all the stuff that I really needed, but then after I got all the heels, this, that, the other, I started makin' $300, $400 a night. Some nights I made, like, $600. Yeah, I would make lots of money on the stroll, lots of money.

For forty-two-year-old trans woman Hannah, "the money was really easy and fast and plentiful doing that . . . You know you get a hundred dollars, two hundred dollars for like a half an hour . . . So back then it was really, really easy." However, a recurring theme in interviews was that while they made a lot, they also spent a lot because of their addiction. Forty-three-year-old Sidney described making hundreds of dollars a night selling sex to feed his drug habit. He was diagnosed at 17, began sex work at 35, and started medication at 42.[30]

> SIDNEY: I started doin' that [selling sex] for my drug habit. And a lot of times I felt ashamed about doin' it, but I did it . . . I can remember how I transitioned into it because I didn't have any money at the time, and I knew that if I did it that way, I would get money to support my habit.
>
> SANYU: So how much were you getting?
>
> SIDNEY: Anywhere between $500 to $800 a night . . . For various clients.
>
> SANYU: So would all that money go to—
>
> SIDNEY: —drugs. Not all of it, but the majority of it.

The cash flow created a clear disincentive to stop selling sex after an HIV diagnosis, especially if it supported an addiction. Further, even though, as Henrietta described, "everybody used condoms. We all used condoms. There was a condom truck that came around," clients paid more for condomless sex. Additional money was hard to resist if addicted, regardless of HIV. As Henrietta described:

> Some guys would pay you more for not using a condom . . . Like, my price was $40 for head, $80 to fuck, but that's because I never used the front part of me, but guys wanted for some queens to use their penis. I never did, so I never got as much as those girls . . . my price was $80, and if I didn't use a condom, they would give me $100 more . . . I always said no. But I did say yes for head. If you want to not use a condom for giving head, I said OK. It would pay $30 more or $40 more.

This pricing system was problematic when combined with drug addiction and the nighttime commercial sex economy. As she explained:

> The guys knew that the time was ticking, that the prices would start to go down by morning, because it was time for you to go in, and the drug dealers were goin' in ... they would offer you $100 more at the beginning of the night, but then the prices would go down, and then your addictions would be so fierce ... that you could take $25. You would take $10. You would take whatever it was, because your addiction was so bad by then, because you were drugged throughout the night. It wasn't like you would wait until morning to make all your money and then you'd go get your drugs.

As Cheryl, diagnosed in 1995 and on medication in 2009, described it, "In your addiction, you don't care, you don't care, you don't care, you do anything for it, and clients would say, 'Yeah, don't use a condom, baby. I'll give you a tip if you don't use a condom,' and I'm like, 'Okay.'" Ida, who started taking medication seven years after diagnosis, pointed to how gender exacerbated things:

> A lot of times women leave it, that option up to a man. They didn't have female condoms where you can just put a condom in and say "We're doing it, I don't have a choice." He has to put the condom on or you have to put the condom on, so like a lot of times with me, I would stand my ground a lot of times, and then sometimes it depend on how far, when the last time I had a hit. Yeah. When the last time I had some drugs.

Drug addiction thus skewed condom-use incentives, even when a sex worker had HIV.

Continual sex work took its toll, and as the clients piled up and the addiction wore on their bodies and lives, it became "a world with no faces, basically." Drugs became the solution to the problems they had created—they enabled sex workers to continue to sell sex, to overcome fear and the feeling of selling one's body, and to live with HIV. Henrietta described how in her experience,

> most girls would go get drugs, get high, and that would give you enough feeling to not be afraid of getting in cars with people you didn't even know that could kill you ... You don't know who you're getting in a car with, if you're getting in the car with a mass murderer or you're getting in the car with somebody who's really gonna date. But the drug gave you the power to get in the car ... And I've gotten stabbed and I've gotten hit in the head and busted my head with a pistol. I've gotten robbed twice by gettin' in the car. Yeah. I also

had a gun put up to my head while I was out on the stroll and asked me for my purse ... some things have happened.

Sex workers, in DC and elsewhere, are especially vulnerable to violence and homicide.[31] Many also died of AIDS. Fifty-two-year-old transgender woman Dorothy, who sold sex when she was younger, reflected, "When I talk about my circle of friends today, there are very few of us that are still here." She estimated that 80% of them had died.

In sum, the DMV-wide commercial sex economy hosted in DC amplified the drug–HIV/AIDS syndemic by providing a market where people could exchange sex for money to fund addictions. Market norms also incentivized condomless sex, amplifying HIV risk for both sex workers and clients. Long periods between HIV diagnosis and treatment, when it became available (discussed in Part 5), further amplified transmission and AIDS deaths among sex workers.

"THE ROAD LESS TRAVELED": ADDICTION TREATMENT

Both the nation and its capital spent considerable funds paying for the epidemics and associated spillovers that resulted from its residents' drug habits. The big debate was whether to treat addicted people as ill or criminals, and it was clear which side won. Despite acknowledgement of the need for addiction treatment, this was not reflected in the policies on which the nation or city spent the most money between the 1980s and early 2000s. Interdiction, law enforcement, and criminal justice, with a special focus on mass incarceration, were the nation's largest response in the War on Drugs (discussed in Part 4), and criminalization and court orders were often the surest path to securing long-term state-supported (and especially medication-free) substance abuse treatment.[32] It was not until the Mental Health Parity and Addiction Equity Act (passed in October 2008 during the Bush administration) and the Affordable Care Act (passed in March 2010 during the Obama administration and with provisions in force from 2014) that health insurance companies were mandated to cover drug addiction treatment.[33] Examining federal drug-control budgets between 1981 and 2008 shows what these budgets prioritized: At the end of the Carter administration, 33% was spent on treatment and 8% on prevention, with the balance spent on criminal justice, law enforcement, and interdiction. Under Reagan, 24.4% was spent on treatment and 10.3% on prevention. Under George H. W. Bush, 17.4% was spent on treatment and 16.3% on prevention, while under Clinton, 18.9% was spent on treatment and 16.2% on prevention. In 2003, under George W. Bush, 19% was spent on treatment and 14% on prevention. (During the opioid epidemic, Obama evenly split supply- and demand-side policies; in 2015, 43.4% was for treatment and 4.6% for prevention. Under Trump, in 2017, a complete reversal had occurred, with 7% for criminal justice, 8% for law enforcement, and the remaining 85% spent on treatment, recovery, and prevention.[34])

In Washington, DC, the need for treatment was acknowledged early on but continually underfunded in the ensuing decades. In 1984, city officials proposed a bill to establish "the first city funded residential drug treatment center," giving city residents the right to get treatment "regardless of their income."[35] City officials had "estimated that there are more than 12,000 heroin addicts ... 60,000 who are dependent on cocaine, PCP and other illegal drugs, and 88,000 who are chronic alcoholics."[36] Given the population size at the time—625,000[37]—they were basically estimating that about a quarter (26%) of the city was enveloped in the substance abuse epidemic, with about 10% addicted to cocaine and other drugs. (The city's inclusion of alcoholism underlay the recognition that it is the most destructive, but legal, type of substance abuse, which in 1982 was said by the US Health Secretary Joseph Califano Jr. to be "involved in more than 66 percent of the nation's homicides, 50 percent of its rapes, up to 70 percent of its assaults and 80 percent of its suicides."[38] As noted earlier, a feature of racial containment was the overconcentration of liquor stores in poor Black neighborhoods.[39]) However, there were no designated funds to support the efforts described in the bill, and previous attempts to get drug treatment covered by health insurance plans were unsuccessful.[40]

The need for treatment beds was dire. A 1989 report ordered by the city's Commissioner of Public Health Reed Tuckson indicated that "the District's network of drug clinics is better suited to treat the heroin junkies of the 1960s and 1970s than the crack and PCP addicts of the 1980s."[41] The city had limited beds and long waiting lists, and the $31 million treatment budget was often subject to funding cuts and personnel freezes to deal with the city's budget deficit (see Part 5).[42] In early 1988, for example, the city had 3,600 outpatient and 400 inpatient slots. However, there were 1,304 people on the waiting list, with many waiting for six weeks. Many could not afford to pay for private treatment.[43] The gold standard was inpatient residential treatment, and Colburn reported on one such facility which had a 300-person capacity and a three- to four-month wait, and turned 2,500 away.[44] In DC General, the city's only public hospital, a 20-bed program, had a 200-person waiting list in 1989.[45] By 1991, the city waiting list had grown to 2,000, and some programs had stopped accepting new applications. At DC General, the waitlist was now 500 people, and the city's budget had been cut.[46] It tried to add capacity, but residents did not want halfway houses or treatment facilities in their neighborhoods.[47] The city was thus faced with a Sisyphean challenge—its efforts and successes were swallowed up and made invisible by rapidly rising demand; its treatment capacity was never enough and could not expand fast enough to accommodate the demand. As one commentator noted, it was "much easier to get drugs that it is to get treatment."[48]

Part of the challenge was that treatment was on the losing side of national and local budgetary battles, especially as the city went into deficit in the next decade. Between 1994 and 1996, the city lost a third of its treatment capacity due to budget cuts,[49] and between 1996 and 1998, "federal funding for District drug programs [fell] by more than 50%. Among the casualties of the parallel cuts: 890 outpatient treatment slots, 820 methadone maintenance slots, 70 detoxification beds and 220 residential treatment beds."[50] Reporter Sari Horwitz highlighted the ironies of the city's priorities: "The city spends $43 per capita on drug prevention and treatment, compared with $1257 per capita on criminal justice," yet "nearly 70% of all arrestees test positive for drugs, while fewer than 10% receive drug treatment, and two-thirds of DC homicides appear related to alcohol or drug use."[51] Indeed Congress and the city were focused less on dealing with addiction or its root causes and more on punishment through mass incarceration. Yet ignoring policies to reduce the demand for drugs contributed to syndemic amplification and the worst homicide epidemic in the nation, as I explore in the next chapter.

NINE

Homicide Redux and Life in a Syndemic Zone

IN THIS CHAPTER, I EXAMINE how the crack–homicide syndemic developed, the spatial organization and racialized impact of homicides, and how individuals and families experienced life in a syndemic zone.

THE CRACK–HOMICIDE SYNDEMIC

As with the heroin epidemic (see Chapter 6), the crack epidemic was a less significant cause of mortality than the homicide epidemic it gave birth to. Along with the dramatic increase in drug use, and in particular the shift from PCP to crack, there was also a dramatic increase in homicide,[1] and there was a syndemic relationship between the two. Observers chart the rise in homicides to a number of simultaneous changes in the organization of cocaine distribution. Following the arrest of Cornell Jones in 1985, a major DC kingpin who had controlled one of the city's leading cocaine markets in Hanover Place, posses began travelling to DC to take advantage of the profits to be made. At the same time, the city had begun its transition from powder cocaine to its more lucrative derivative, crack.[2] These three factors drove a shift in the city's drug market ecology, marking the beginning of a violent homicidal decade. Crack began to flood drug markets and turf wars began among posses from New York and Miami.[3] Local DC crews also got involved. As Tanya Golash-Boza and others described, the city was divided up east and south of Rock Creek Park into territories marked by street intersections, which lent them their names (such as the P Street, R Street, and Newton Street crews).[4] Drawing on police records, reporter Brad Wye graphically depicted in *The Washington Post* (reproduced in Figure 36) how homicides

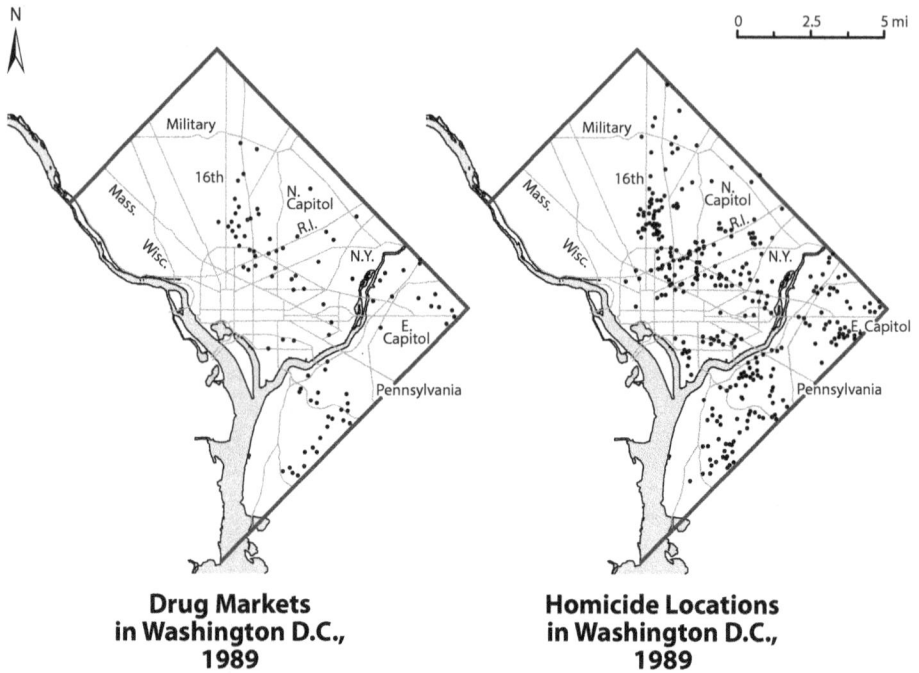

**Drug Markets
in Washington D.C.,
1989**

**Homicide Locations
in Washington D.C.,
1989**

FIGURE 36. How drug markets compare with homicide locations in DC. Source: Brad Wye, *The Washington Post*, Jan 13, 1989. © 1989 *The Washington Post*. All rights reserved. Used under license. https://www.washingtonpost.com/.

occurred in the same locations as drug markets, underscoring their spatialized syndemic relationship.[5]

As arrests of outsider gangs picked up, drug distribution and its associated violent turf wars transitioned more fully to local DC street gangs, in battles playing out in residences and on city streets, sometimes spilling over into prominent nightclubs such as Chapter III and the East Side Club, with commentators noting, "It's the locals who are doing the killing now."[6] Aiding the killings was the widespread presence of guns. Entrepreneurial brokers flouted the city's strict gun laws and procured guns from Florida and neighboring Virginia, selling them for a significant profit to local gangs and crews.[7] While the initial driver of the homicide epidemic was the drug epidemic and its associated carving up of and defense of territories and markets, drug-related killings gradually declined, dropping from accounting for 70% of homicides in 1988 to 39% of homicides in 1990, suggesting that homicide had become its own independent epidemic.[8] And as Andrew Papachristos has demonstrated, like other epidemics, gang-related homicide can be contagious, spreading across social networks through interactional dynamics of establishing dominance, saving face, and retaliation.[9] Additionally, as Laurence Ralph richly illustrated, "Social bonds between gang members [were] so often solidified through violence."[10]

Another driver of the homicide epidemic was low conviction rates, reaching a low of 25% in 1993, and low case-closure rates, reaching a low of 37% by 1999.[11] By the end of the 1990s, as reporters put it, "In the District of Columbia, more and more people are getting away with murder. Fifteen hundred homicides have gone unsolved over the past decade. Nearly two-thirds of the homicides that occurred in 1999 remained unsolved at that year's end, the poorest performance in the last 10 years."[12] A contributor to slow case closure was the medical examiner's office. By 1989 Abramowitz reported that the office had not had a permanent chief for six years, and had only one certified pathologist; five had quit within an 18-month period a few years earlier, and the budget had been cut.[13] Without autopsies, it was hard to move homicide cases forward. Office turnover was still apparent in 1996, with no permanent medical examiner and multiple pathologist vacancies.[14] These outcomes were compounded by an overwhelmed and underfunded police department and court system, as well as overcrowded prisons, even as the city was cutting budgets.[15] In combination, these factors may have contributed to residents "taking matters into their own hands." This was highlighted by a smaller proportion of homicides being drug-related and more being linked to revenge and street justice. It was also reflected by the code of silence maintained in communities who could not count on police or courts to bring justice.[16]

HOMICIDE CAPITAL OF THE US

And the scale of the homicides was profound. As Figure 37 illustrates, the crack–homicide syndemic far eclipsed the two heroin–homicide syndemics of the previous eras in number of deaths. Between 1960 and 1968, annual homicides were below 200; between 1968 and 1982, annual homicides fluctuated between about 200–300. Between 1986 and 1995, there were at least 3,832 homicides with over 400 per year between 1989 and 1993.

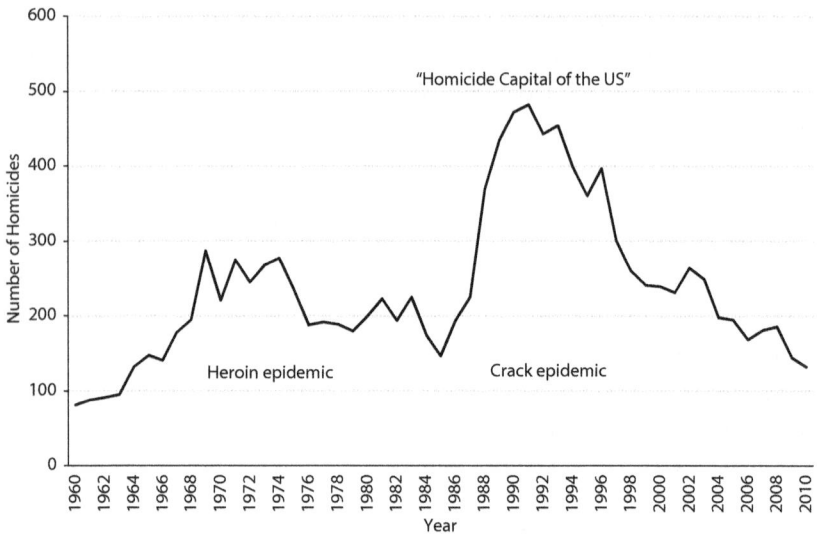

FIGURE 37. Annual homicides in DC, 1960–2010. Data source: Disaster Center, District of Columbia.

Further, even while "438 people were killed in 1989, 1,879 [were] wounded."[17] Reporters described "ambulances ... pulling up regularly, like planes taking off at LaGuardia" to DC General, the city's only public hospital.[18] The Army was even "send[ing] doctors to [DC hospitals] to learn how to treat gunshot wounds."[19] While there was an ongoing national drug-homicide syndemic for four years in a row, Washington, DC, stood out as having the nation's highest homicide rates (80.6/100,000 in 1991).[20] It took another four years before the epidemic waned[21] and another 15 years before rates returned to 1960s levels.

Many city and congressional officials were concerned about the global image of the US portrayed by its capital city leading the nation in homicide. For example, Assistant Police Chief Isaac Fulwood Jr. commented, "I don't think the federal government can afford to have the capital of the free world portrayed as the nation's murder capital."[22] Republican Senator Warren Rudman of New Hampshire stated, "We can't have people killed and blood running in the streets like some Third World capital run by a despot."[23] Indeed congressional members' personal experiences living and working in the homicide capital, some with staffers among the dead, arguably contributed to the extreme national legislative response that resulted in world-leading mass-incarceration rates (see Part 4).

The Spatial Distribution of Homicide

Homicide, however, did not affect city residents equally. It was both racially as well as spatially disparate. Nationally, in 1990, Black men were "six times more likely" than Black women, "nine times more likely than" White men, "and 26 times more likely than" White women to die of homicide.[24] The city's racial disparities were more extreme—that same year, at the height of the city's epidemic, Black men's homicides were seven times higher than Black women's, 27 times higher than White men's, and 82 times higher than White women's.[25] Spatially, as illustrated in Figure 36, homicides were contained east and south of Rock Creek Park, in many of the city's poorest, predominantly Black, neighborhoods. Between 1986 and 1991, the highest homicide rate occurred in Ward 8, comprising on average about 20% of the city's homicides, while almost no homicides occurred (on average less than 1%) in Ward 3.[26] Figure 8 (see Part 1) illustrates that the spatial distribution had not changed two decades later.[27]

This geography of homicide reflected the dramatically different lives lived on either side of Rock Creek Park. As reporter Courtland Milloy put it:

> On the right side of town, parents think of sending their kids to college. On the other side, kids go to hospitals and morgues. Wakes and funerals are as common as summer camps . . . but you don't have to worry about that. And when a murder rate can skyrocket unabated in the backyard of the president of the United States, you obviously are not alone.[28]

Importantly, the epidemic did not arise on its own. It was the result of insufficient federal interdiction of drugs into the city, inadequate treatment for addicted people, city government–owned infrastructure that enabled drug use, and many DMV area residents participating in and financially underwriting the drug economy. These actions were all crucial in facilitating and fueling the spillover epidemics that ensued, and these, by design, were contained within many of the neighborhoods hosting drug markets.

RACIAL CONSEQUENCES OF THE SYNDEMIC

The cover of a 1992 federally financed homicide report, published at the epidemic's height, featured names of those who had been killed between 1986 and 1991 (Figure 38). Ninety percent were Black (77% men, 13% women), and

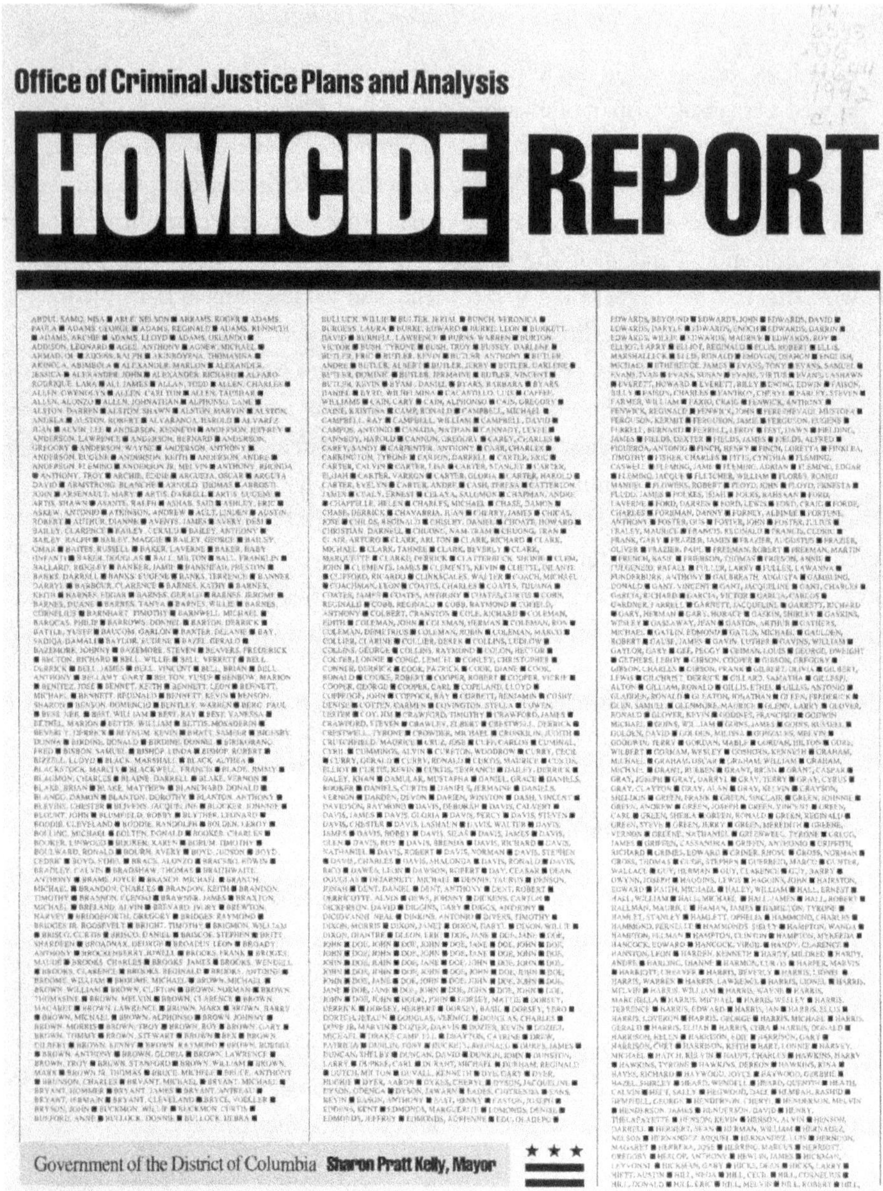

Office of Criminal Justice Plans and Analysis

HOMICIDE REPORT

Government of the District of Columbia Sharon Pratt Kelly, Mayor ★ ★ ★

FIGURE 38. Cover page of DC homicide report, 1992. Source: Office of Criminal Justice Plans and Analysis, *Homicide Report* (US Department of Justice, National Institute of Justice, 1992).

by 1991, most (65%) were under 30. Most (60%) alleged assailants were under 25, and most (62%) had not completed high school.[29] Many of these names represent not just a dead young Black person but also a grieving family, grieving friends, a wounded neighborhood, and a traumatized generation of children.

Sharkey and colleagues found that living in a neighborhood when a homicide occurred there is associated with children's lowered cognitive performance, attention spans, and impulse control.[30] Further, homicide epidemics create their own spillover epidemics. Ralph described the oft-ignored epidemic of long-term disability among the wounded.[31] Adolescents exposed to community homicides have amplified anxiety and depression.[32] Homicide exposure is associated with small gestational age and low birth weight, which contribute to infant mortality.[33] Chronic stress and inflammation, which might be produced by multiple years living in neighborhoods with frequent homicides, may have a role in chronic diseases such as heart disease, kidney disease, and diabetes.[34] In this way, syndemic zones produce multiple drivers of illness and premature death across the life course.

As the homicide epidemic gradually became divorced from the drug epidemic, it was easier for Congress, the city, and DMV area residents to forget their own roles in enabling it and focus on victim blaming and assailant punishment. Indeed, as class and race reversals in drug use began to occur and the concomitant spillover epidemics began to unfold, attitudes towards drugs began to harden, and "America seem[ed] ready to go nuclear in its war on drugs,"[35] as was typical when drug use was perceived to have shifted towards minorities.[36] This punitive turn also occurred within the Black community. As James Forman Jr. comprehensively detailed,[37] Black residents, the primary victims of the city's syndemic, were a critical part of the city's and nation's shift towards mass incarceration (see Part 4) to end the tragedy and its severe toll on the community.

Living and Dying in a Syndemic Zone

As illustrated by Figure 39, while the nation and city were focusing on homicide, AIDS deaths were climbing and by 1990 surpassed homicide deaths. By 1995, annual AIDS deaths reached a peak of almost 900, more than twice the number of homicide deaths. Notably, without life-saving ART medication, AIDS deaths would have been significantly higher. AIDS deaths dramatically declined between 1994 and 1998, falling to about 400 annually between

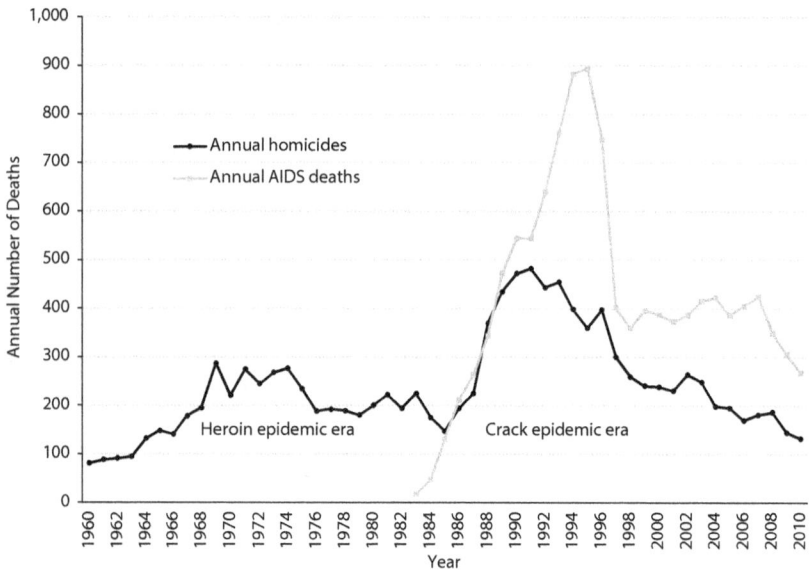

FIGURE 39. The DC SAVA syndemic, 1960–2010. Data sources: Disaster Center, District of Columbia, and DC HAHSTA HIV/AIDS Surveillance Unit.

1998 and 2007, before declining to under 300 annually by 2010. The most severe impact of the syndemic—with its cascades of worst-in-the-nation drug, infant mortality, homicide, and AIDS epidemics—was concentrated in predominantly Black wards of the city, illustrating the predictable outcomes of racial containment, which spatially clustered economic and social disadvantage on top of racial segregation. Containment meant that the full effects of the DC syndemic ricocheted and reverberated through Black neighborhoods, families, and individuals over generations.

Forty-eight-year-old Kayla, born in 1963, grew up as one of eight children in a middle-class DC neighborhood, with a father in construction and a stay-at-home mother. She graduated high school but was unable to complete further education due to lack of finances. An early pregnancy led to an early marriage that became physically abusive, as her husband "used to hit on me all the time." She began taking a variety of drugs when she was 18 and began mainlining heroin when her marriage ended 10 years later. She was a mostly functional heroin and cocaine user, holding down a variety of government and private sector jobs. As is typical of a syndemic zone, she had multiple potential exposures to HIV throughout her life. HIV may have come from an infected syringe due to her heroin use or from her four blood transfusions, which she received as she was losing her babies due to hemorrhaging (HIV screening of blood banks began in 1985, after she had begun childbearing). However, she thought that she got HIV from a relationship she began after her divorce; her partner had an affair with a woman with HIV. Her life of pain was compounded by the clustering of premature deaths that is a common experience among Black families nationally.[38] Her interview was punctuated by descriptions of deaths, some mentioned in passing and some in detail. Not yet 50 years old, in addition to her pregnancy losses, she had buried three siblings, her father, her daughter, and her granddaughter. She was undetectable (HIV virally suppressed) until three years before the interview when her father, and seven months later her daughter, died.

SANYU: What did she, what did she die of?

KAYLA: Everything. All her kidneys, they were deteriorating. It was eating her up. The E pills and the, and the angel dust and the drinking, and she had got stabbed, the girl gutted her up like a pig. Oh God, they jumped her, everything.

SANYU: She was jumped and just . . .

KAYLA: Got stabbed up. They cut her, I mean she was gutted like a pig. They called me. They said your daughter dead. And she died . . . But, they got, they found the girls, they got them. The ones who stabbed her . . . they finally prosecuted a couple of them, a couple of them are dead now.

Her daughter's homicide threw into her a mental health crisis or "an episode" as she described it, which drove her back to seeking drugs.

And I said I know what, I'm gonna get high. I'm gonna go get high, gonna go get high. I say, where you gonna get high at, you don't get high no more, you ain't around no type of people. Where you gonna go, where you gonna get it from? I said, oh, her friend was over there. And I'm serious. I was an awful mess.

She eventually recovered:

I was doing great. Undetectable . . . but last year was a major break down . . . I was at a 298 [close to the 200 CD4 count threshold for an AIDS diagnosis]. Oh God, my viral load was in the millions . . . I went everywhere I could go but they would not help me. They kept telling me if we can't put you in a, a psych ward, we can't help you. But I couldn't let them do that. 'Cause I was raising these boys. I said, "Oh my God, if I sign those papers . . . they gonna come to my house and take the children." So, with the help of God, it worked out.

She was thus unable to receive desperately needed mental health care because she was now "grandma daycare." At the time of her interview, she reported that "my viral load at 64. I'm . . . undetected again." However, she was still struggling to stay off drugs, though fully committed to completing the task of raising her teenage grandchildren. I asked her if she had stopped taking narcotics. She told me:

> I stopped now, I've been off . . . for like . . . 14 weeks. Everything. Oh yeah, I smoke cigarettes, and I drink sometimes that's it. That's it. I learnt my lesson, and I have my grandsons, and I have to be mom for them, right, because they be hearing what I did, I be telling them about this. And I can't, I can't mess my life up. You know what I'm saying. I got to raise them. And uh, I promised my daughter when she died, I was in the bed with her at the hospital when she died, and I promised her . . .

Trans woman Maggie described her mother's pain as the city's syndemic similarly tore through the family.

SANYU: Are you still in touch with your siblings and grandparents?

MAGGIE: My oldest brother is dead. He got killed in '92, and my little brother is doing life without parole. He got arrested in '92. And I think that was about the same time when my mother found out that I was HIV positive. So you can understand how devastating it was for my mother that year.

SANYU: Wow. So life without parole for your younger brother; and what was he in for?

MAGGIE: My younger brother, um kingpin status . . . drug lord, which consists of a whole umbrella of things . . . murders, kidnappings, major drugs, weapons, all that.

SANYU: And then your older brother?

MAGGIE: He was stabbed in his neck in the streets because of his addiction.

SANYU: And when was that?

MAGGIE: '92.

SANYU: Wow, so all that happened in '92.

MAGGIE: That's when my mother found out I was HIV positive, so that was a terrible year for her.

The drug and spillover epidemics had affected all three of Maggie's mother's children. Maggie's mother had already dealt with a physically abusive drug-using husband (see Chapter 7). Now, her daughter was caught up in the crack–HIV syndemic—becoming addicted, selling sex, and acquiring HIV, a death sentence without medication. Her son was a perpetrator in the drug–homicide syndemic and was socially dead because of it, with life in prison without parole. And her other son was a victim of the drug–homicide syndemic and was physically dead because of it. Racially contained life in a syndemic zone could indeed be terrible.

CONCLUSION

Overall in Washington, DC, while drug use and abuse occurred throughout the city and its suburbs, the design and social organization of the city, as well as the conjoined congressional and city responses to its epidemics over the last several decades, worked to contain and then amplify syndemic disease within Black neighborhoods and families. As I have illustrated, this occurred in a multilevel, cascading, and reinforcing fashion. During the multiwave heroin epidemic in the late '60s and '70s, some city residents began lifelong injecting drug habits, placing them and their connected others at risk for HIV acquisition when it appeared in 1981. HIV circulation within racialized injecting drug and sexual networks (see Part 2) was further amplified by the transition from powder to crack cocaine in the US in 1980s, which fueled a growth in the commercial sex economy, as well as a dramatic increase in homicides. Crack addiction led to an increase in the number of people selling sex in the city, and disincentive structures around condom use undermined safe sex, making commercial sex an important HIV epidemic amplifier. The explosion of violence and homicide in the city following each of the drug epidemics gave birth to significant spillover illnesses and deadly epidemics.

Crucially, each of these developments was not just the result of individual drug users' characteristics and propensities. Rather they were also enabled or facilitated by congressional and city laws, policies, and institutions related to housing, drugs, crime, and health care, among other areas. Further racialized spatial containment of drug distribution and homicide meant that the most severe consequences of the city's syndemic—illness and death—were concentrated and contained within the city's poorest Black neighborhoods, thus widening racial health inequalities and reproducing them for the next generation.

As I will illustrate in the next part, another form of containment—mass incarceration—was employed to try to contain the syndemic; however, instead it ended up further amplifying syndemic disease in Black communities.

PART FOUR

Mass Incarceration and Syndemic Amplification

What more do you want us to do? . . . We arrested 43,000 people last year. . . . What the hell is the police department going to do?

MAURICE T. TURNER JR., DC POLICE CHIEF
(*Washington Post*—Mar 25, 1989—Pianin)

THE PRIMARY NATIONAL RESPONSE to the cascading drug and spillover epidemics was the War on Drugs, an offensive waged against the nation's "public enemy number one."[1] Launched from Washington, DC, in 1971 by President Richard Nixon and pursued by subsequent presidents, it unleashed the full force of the federal government's executive, legislative, and judicial arms, along with several national agencies over the following 50 years. The most significant component of this national response was mass incarceration.[2] And so vigorously was this aspect of the war waged that the US has for a number of years had the largest number of incarcerated people of any country on earth. In "one of the most spectacular social experiments in American history,"[3] at its height in 2008, 2.3 million people were in US prisons and jails, with an additional 824,834 on parole and 4.24 million on probation.[4] Between 2006 and 2008, the US "incarceration rate peaked at 1,000 per 100,000" people.[5] Mass incarceration has been costly. Michael McLaughlin and colleagues estimated its aggregated (government and public) annual economic burden to the nation at $1 trillion.[6] A less expansive definition of costs from the Bureau of Justice estimated annual inflation-adjusted governmental (federal, state, and local) justice system expenditures at $305 billion per year.[7] Though still a world leader in incarceration trends, two laws—the Fair Sentencing Act (passed under Obama in 2010) and the First Step Act (passed under Trump in 2018)—have contributed to a 25% decline in the prison population.[8]

The war was conducted particularly intensely within DC itself, which once again led the nation, this time in drug-related arrests.[9] An estimated 70,000 people (about 1 in 8 DC residents) were under criminal justice supervision by the mid-1990s, one of the highest rates in the nation,[10] and Eric Lotke calculated that by 1997, half (49.9%) of the city's young Black men aged

18–35 were under criminal justice supervision.[11] Ten percent were in jail or prison, and 21% on probation or parole, while 19% had warrants or were awaiting trial. He noted that while the national Black-White disparity in custodial populations was seven to one, in DC, it was thirty-six to one. While at the extreme end, this racial disparity was nonetheless emblematic of national trends in mass incarceration. Black boys and men are disproportionately more likely than their White counterparts to be killed or injured in police encounters, more likely to be arrested and incarcerated, and serve longer prison sentences relative to White men for the same crime.[12] This has translated into disproportionate numbers of US prisoners being African American men. Currently, while comprising 14% of the US population, they make up a third (33%) of the prison population and almost half (46%) of people spending more than a decade behind bars.[13] Sarah Shannon and colleagues estimated that 5.6% of all US adult men had been to prison; among African Americans, it was one in six (15%) men.[14]

Many scholars, such as Loïc Wacquant and Michelle Alexander, have observed that the disproportionate mass incarceration of Black people is merely the latest data point in a trend line beginning with slavery.[15] The contemporary treatment of prisoners is instructive. A study by the American Civil Liberties Union (ACLU) and the University of Chicago Law School found that US prisoners, who constitutionally lose the right to refuse to work, earn on average 13–52 cents an hour, and sometimes nothing at all, despite producing "more than $2 billion a year in goods and commodities, and over $9 billion a year in services for the maintenance of the prisons where they are warehoused."[16] In addition to earning what is essentially slave wages, prisoners' treatment once they leave is also instructive. While 13% of all US adult men have a felony conviction, 33% of Black men have a felony.[17] A felony conviction, from crimes as varied as homicide, illegal drug possession, or stealing a car, carries significant and lifelong consequences. As Alexander described, "Once you're labeled a felon, the old forms of discrimination—employment discrimination, housing discrimination, denial of the right to vote, denial of educational opportunity, denial of food stamps and other public benefits, and exclusion from jury service—are suddenly legal."[18]

Further, these consequences are not dealt out in a race-neutral fashion. For example, in an audit study, Devah Pager found that while presumed White felons were half as likely (17%) to get jobs as presumed White non-felons (34%), they were nonetheless more likely to get jobs compared to presumed

Black non-felons (14%), and three times more likely to get jobs than presumed Black felons (5%).[19] Indeed, the "old forms of discrimination" amount to a multilayered exclusion from public life, a sort of social death, in addition to limitations in the ability to eat, legally work, and live under a roof, even after their debt to society has been paid. In the case of DC, criminalizing half its young Black men, many arrested on drug charges in the prime of their lives, created, in historians Chris Asch and George Musgrove's words, "a generation of felons."[20]

As I have argued so far in this book, health crises in alleys and slums were important rationales for urban renewal, the expansion of public housing, and racial containment (see Part 1). I have shown how racial containment served to create, concentrate, and amplify syndemic disease within Black neighborhoods, including the sexual spread of the HIV epidemic (see Part 2), drug epidemics, and their associated homicide and other spillover epidemics (see Part 3). In this Part, I show how instead of a massive public health response to control the syndemic, the response to which Congress and city government committed the most resources in terms of legislation, funds, personnel, and infrastructure, was mass imprisonment of Black people, and young Black men in particular. Thus, while the War on Drugs was conducted under a "tough on crime" rationale, through another lens, with historical continuity, it was once again utilizing another form of racial containment to deal with the era's health crises.

Moving back and forth between the national and local stories to place Washington, DC, in context, and drawing on archival material, literature reviews, and interview data (two-thirds of my respondents, all of whom lived with HIV, reported ever being incarcerated), I illustrate the multiple mechanisms through which racial containment operated to incarcerate Black people (Chapter 10). I then describe the racially contained prison-community dynamics that worked to amplify the city's syndemic (Chapter 11). This is ironic because theoretically prisons should and could ameliorate illness;[21] US prisoners, unlike most Americans, have a constitutional right to health care.[22] However, I show how while prison could provide drug rehabilitation, HIV testing, and medication, it also exacerbated negative health outcomes through facilitating high-risk drug and sexual economies, which both enabled drug addiction and heightened HIV vulnerability. I also discuss the implications this had for syndemic amplification in the community.

. . .

Coolio	Gangsta's Paradise ft. L.V. (1995)
Nas	Cops Shot the Kid (2018)
J Cole	Be Free (2014)
Kendrick Lamar	The Blacker the Berry (2015)
Common	Letter to the Free feat. Bilal (2016)
DMX	Slippin' (1998)
Childish Gambino	This is America (2018)
Akon	Locked Up (2004)
Ice-T	The Tower (1991)
Ludacris	Do Your Time (2006)
Andraé Crouch	Through it All (1972)
Cece Winans	Mercy Said No (2003)
Mary Mary	Shackles (Praise You) (2000)
Donnie McClurkin	We Fall Down (2000)
Huck-A-Bucks	Get Down (1995)
Backyard Band	Sick of Being Lonely (2002)

TEN

Creating Mass Black Incarceration in DC

THE RACIAL CONTAINMENT PRINCIPLE operated to bring about the mass incarceration of Black people through a range of institutions, including the police, Congress, judicial and legislative systems, schools, and the prison- and political-industrial complexes. I discuss these in turn.

POLICING PRACTICES: TARGETING BLACK NEIGHBORHOODS

Throughout the 1980s and 1990s, Washington, DC, the home of the War on Drugs' architects, undertook a series of vigorous campaigns. So prolific were the arrests that "the city outranked all other US cities and states in per capita drug arrests in 1985."[1] This zeal was especially evident in the prominent Operation Clean Sweep (1986–89), led by Mayor Marion Barry (who was himself "swept" for crack possession and use[2]), which produced numerous arrests of both buyers and dealers of drugs.[3] To implement sweeps, police predominantly focused on poor Black neighborhoods, and young Black men in particular, even though, as described in Part 3, while these neighborhoods hosted drug markets, users and dealers, White and Black, came from around the DMV area. In the 1990s, George Washington University's William Chambliss observed that the Rapid Deployment Unit "does not patrol the predominantly White sections of Washington D.C. . . . there are no 'rips' and no vehicular stops unless there is a clear violation."[4] Instead, there was "intensive surveillance of Black neighborhoods" and intense and brutal policing of young Black men, who were "defined as a criminal group, arrested for minor offenses over and over again, and given criminal records which justify long prison sentences."[5] James Forman Jr. similarly highlighted pretext policing in Operation Ceasefire in 1995, as well as "stop and frisk" in poor Black neighborhoods, noting that the second police district (including neighborhoods such as Woodley Park [Ward 3], Foggy Bottom, and Georgetown [Ward 2]), the city's wealthiest and Whitest areas, were officially exempted.[6] In surveys conducted between 1998 and 2000, George Washington University's Ronald Weitzer and colleagues found that "in the span of just one year, 61 percent of young Black men in Washington, DC, reported being stopped by the city's police either in cars or as pedestrians—and this figure is about 3 times higher than that for young White males."[7] There was also Black intraracial class containment. Weitzer found that while outside their neighborhood, the middle class experienced similar police mistreatment as the poor, *within* their neighborhood, "middle class Black respondents had more in common with middle class Whites than with disadvantaged Blacks," with almost no experiences of unwarranted stops, creating a "safe haven effect."[8]

Poor Black neighborhoods were subject not only to disproportionate arrests but also to excessive violence and brutality. This was in part the result of external pressures on police. By the end of the 1980s, the retirement eligibility of 60% of the police force[9] and the intensifying syndemic, despite Clean Sweep, led to considerable congressional pressure to hire more police officers.[10] Describing what turned into a disastrous process, Flaherty and Harriston reported:

> D.C. Police Chief Fred Thomas said the chief motivation for cutting corners on recruiting, background checks, psychological testing and training during that period was money . . . the nearly $500 million federal appropriation for the District for fiscal 1989 was made contingent on the city's bolstering its police force to nearly 4,000 officers. To reach that goal, the department hired 2,125 officers in about two years . . . at the peak of hiring in 1990, background investigators were directed by supervisors to clear 50 officers every two weeks, a task that normally took two months.[11]

The normal rejection rate of 20% in 1987 dropped to 4% in 1989.[12] In the following five years, the consequences of this pressured and rapid hiring process began to be seen and felt, reflected in rising complaints of police brutality and corruption. In 1991, the city's Civilian Complaint Review Board "had a backlog of more than 900 cases, a 50% increase from 1990."[13] Allegations of police officer crimes led to the FBI's Operation Broken Faith. "Of the 201 DC police officers arrested," more than half were recent hires.[14] The District police also had high rates of fatal shootings, including of unarmed people, even as city homicide rates had started declining.[15] As Jeff Leen and colleagues reported as part of an eight-month investigation by *The Washington Post*:

> The District of Columbia's Metropolitan Police Department have shot and killed more people per resident in the 1990s than any other large American city police force . . . Washington's officers fire their weapons at more than double the rate of police in New York, Los Angeles, Chicago or Miami . . . From 1975 to 1983, New York averaged 1.36 fatal shootings annually by police per 1000 officers, and Washington's rate was nearly identical at 1.44, according to a study by the International Association of Chiefs of Police. By 1995, New York's rate had dropped below 1 and Washington's had risen to nearly 4.[16]

The cohort of new recruits accounted for half the shootings in part because "50 to 60 percent of the force had not properly qualified with their firearms."[17] However, they went on to observe that "none of the police shootings of civilians has occurred in the more affluent areas west of Rock Creek Park, according to police records from 1994 through May 1998," and they illustrated this in a map. Figure 40 (a version of this map) clearly shows the spatial containment of police brutality.[18]

Mass arrests were highly incentivized. Clean Sweep was popular among street cops because they could "double their salary through overtime pay," on track to costing the city $19 million ($43 million in 2024 dollars) by the end of the operation.[19] Performing dragnets through poor Black neighborhoods, "sacrifice zones" of the DMV's drug epidemic, was an efficient way to rack up thousands of arrests in a short amount of time among people with the least resources and social capital to push back. Indeed it was a strategy that depended on spatialized racial and class containment. However, these practices had significant consequences on the everyday lives of many Black residents. They created a "pre-criminal" status[20] where Black people were presumed guilty by virtue of being in a particular space,[21] leading to the need to "spend an extraordinary amount of energy—through careful attention to dress, behavior, and speech—to mark yourself as innocent."[22] The saturation of arrests from particular Black neighborhoods essentially created "prison zip codes"[23] and transformed neighborhoods into "social prisons" and prisons into "judicial ghettos,"[24] where "ghetto and prison [had become] kindred institutions of forced confinement."[25] Indeed, in "DC's other neighborhood," a Lorton prison survey found that most prisoners were from a handful of zip codes in SE Washington, with a few from the NE.[26]

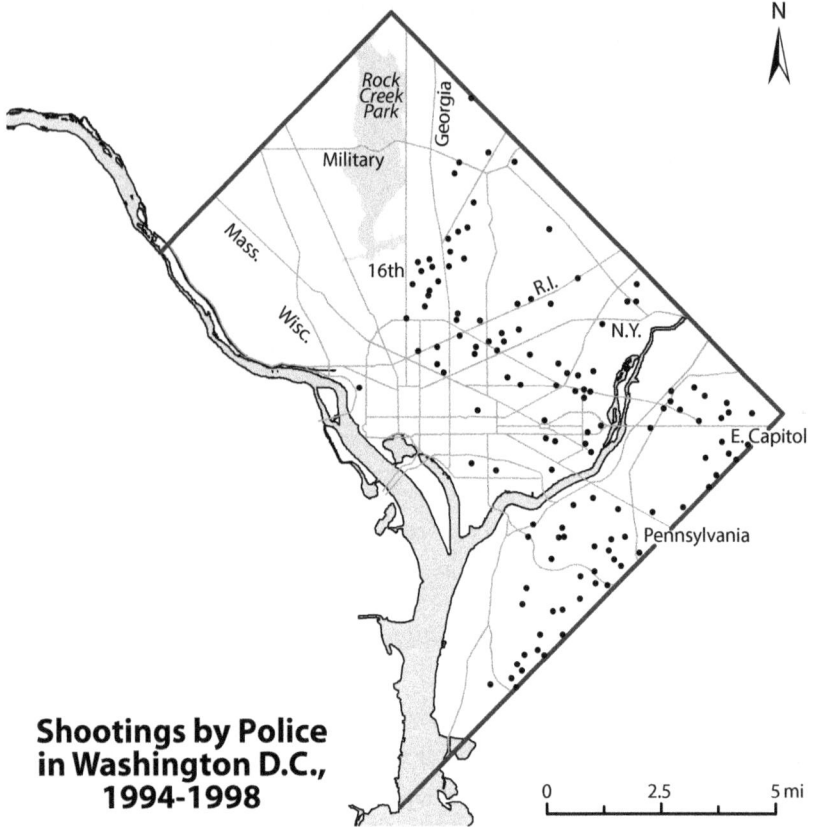

**Shootings by Police
in Washington D.C.,
1994-1998**

0   2.5   5 mi

FIGURE 40. Spatial distribution of police shootings in DC, 1994–98. Source: Jeff Leen, Jo Craven, David Jackson, and Sari Horwitz, District Police Lead Nation in Shootings, *The Washington Post*, Nov 15, 1998. © 1998 *The Washington Post*. All rights reserved. Used under license. https://www.washingtonpost.com/.

This concentrated spatial pattern of arrests was reflected in my respondents' experiencing jail and prison as a neighborhood or community.[27] As Wynton, age 50, described, "It was like, a, a playground . . . it was a lot of guys that you was in the street with, they was there, in there too 'cause they was locked up . . . It was like, you just went to a different place but you was behind bars." Theo, age 49, similarly observed, "It was kind of like bein' in the project, but no women there, just all guys. 'Cause everybody kind of knew everybody. You had people from north, west, south, east [DC]. People were brothers, cousins." Family and friends were thus not just on the outside "doing time together" with incarcerated loved ones, as Megan Comfort and

Donald Braman so powerfully described,[28] but also doing time together with other family members on the inside.

INTERSECTIONAL POLITICS

There were both racialized and classed politics at play in DC's War on Drugs. On the one hand, a predominantly White Congress controlled the financial strings, exercised veto power over the city's bills, used it as a policy playground, and put considerable pressure on it to pursue certain policy goals. On the other hand, as pointed out by Weitzer and colleagues, as well as by Forman in his Pulitzer prize–winning book, the key implementers were predominantly Black. They included DC's mayors, several police chiefs, most of the police department, with Eric Holder, a judge on the Superior Court of DC (1988–93) and US attorney for DC (1993–97), serving as the city's main prosecutor.[29] As Forman observed, with "racism shap[ing] the political, economic and legal context in which the Black community and its elected representatives made their choices," the Black community led the charge on mass incarceration in the city.[30] And most of their fire was directed at lower-class Black men. Reuter and colleagues found that most DC arrestees had less than a high school education.[31] This mirrored national trends. Bruce Western found that in the cohort born between 1965 and 1969, among those with less than a high school education, 11.2% of White men and 58.9% of Black men were at risk of imprisonment by their early 30s. Among those with some college education, 0.7% of White and 4.9% of Black men were at risk of imprisonment.[32]

In the decades before the civil rights era, racial containment united Black people across the economic spectrum as the full effects of discrimination were broadly felt; after civil rights laws ushered in Black mobility, widening class inequality contributed to a delinking of Black lives.[33] However, the persistence of housing discrimination and the placement of public housing in or near stable, middle-class Black neighborhoods following the racial containment principle (see Part 1) meant that in DC and elsewhere, as scholars such as Mary Pattillo and Nelson Kofie illustrated, middle-class Black people were less able to separate themselves from their poorer counterparts.[34] Many suffered from the consequences of living in or near drug-ridden neighborhoods with their attendant high rates of violence (see Part 3). Black families were both devastated by and financially benefited from drugs, had loved ones in prison or went to prison themselves, and caused and grieved deaths due to drugs and drug-related violence.[35] And families experiencing none of these nonetheless dealt with the fallout of living in or near a syndemic zone.

As noted in the Introduction, racial containment perniciously turns a community in on itself. In this case, it occurred through a foreclosing of alternatives to mass incarceration. There was an absence of a massive addiction-treatment campaign to stem the initiating epidemic, no softening of laws for addicted people, and no effective interdiction campaign to stem the flow of drugs (all of which occurred during the city's heroin epidemics when perceived to be affecting White youth; see Part 3). Further, there was an absence of substantial efforts to invest in the city's sacrifice zones—neglected and abandoned infrastructures and neighborhoods which hosted drug markets—and their residents. Thus, the only apparent recourse to ending profound Black suffering that had bipartisan and biracial congressional and city government support was the criminal justice system. This is why, as Forman documented, DC's Black community, which had understandably ambivalent attitudes about that system, nonetheless ended up "locking up our own."[36]

LEGISLATION AND SENTENCING:
AN INVERSE JUSTICE SYSTEM

Racial containment logics also expressed themselves through legislation and sentencing guidelines on cocaine, with higher jail terms for crack cocaine dealers and users—which, given the higher rate of White powder cocaine use, was a racialized policy that contributed to more widespread and longer imprisonment of Black people.[37] In the so-called 100-to-1 ratio, a series of acts established mandatory minimum sentences for drug offenses; in particular, the sentence for carrying five grams of crack cocaine was equivalent to that of carrying 453.6 grams of powder cocaine: a minimum sentence of five years in federal prison.[38] Once set up in this way, sentencing could proceed in ostensibly race-neutral ways, with attendant disproportionate consequences for Black people. As US District Judge Clyde S. Cahill of St. Louis put it:

This one provision, the crack statute, has been directly responsible for incarcerating nearly an entire generation of young Black American men for very long periods ... [it] has created a situation that reeks with inhumanity and injustice. The scales of justice have turned topsy-turvy so that those masterminds, the kingpins of drug trafficking, escape detection while those whose role is minimal, even trivial, are hoisted on the spears of an enraged electorate and at the pinnacle of their youth are imprisoned for years while those most responsible for the evil of the day remain free.[39]

The quote appeared in an article about a 20-year-old Black DMV resident with the headline "This Small-Time Dealer is Doing 20 Years. He Might Be Better Off if He'd Killed Somebody."

Disproportionate Black arrests were compounded by racial inequalities in sentencing. As Mary Flaherty and William Casey reported, "Nationally, Blacks got 2 percent longer jail terms than Whites . . . But the difference was greater in some regions, including the District of Columbia where Blacks got sentences longer by 12 percent in 1994 and 9 percent in 1995."[40] Thus, Black people had a higher likelihood of both getting arrested and getting more severe punishments for the same crimes compared to White people. The cumulation of racialized arrests and sentencing produced extreme racial inequalities. By 1992, Lotke noted that 42% of the city's Black men aged 18–35 were under some form of criminal justice supervision and, as described earlier, calculated that by 1997, it was 49.9%. Overall, Black people comprised 96% of those in custody that year, and just over half were young Black men.[41] Braman noted, "If these conditions persist, over 75% of young Black men in the District and nearly all those in the poorest neighborhoods can expect to be incarcerated at some time in their lives."[42]

The city's war on drugs ultimately failed in its ostensible justification of ending the drug epidemic; however, that did not stop the continued mass incarceration of young Black men for drugs, which had taken on a life of its own. As early as December 1988, the police chief, Maurice Turner (quoted in the epigraph), publicly admitted that Clean Sweep "has done nothing to curb drug use in the District . . . we must reduce the demand side of the drug business."[43] Nancy Lewis and Victoria Churchville commented that "it is the first time Turner openly has denied the efficacy of Clean Sweep, which has been the expensive centerpiece of Mayor Marion Barry's crackdown on drugs and has produced more than 43,000 arrests, 60 percent of them drug-related, since it was begun in Aug 1986."[44] However, Turner's attempts to shut down Clean Sweep were prevented by the city council and mayor.[45] As a result, DC's jails and prisons became severely overcrowded and the thousands of monthly arrests ran into the limits of the criminal justice system. Eugene Robinson observed early on that while police could make thousands of arrests, no other part of the criminal justice system can come close to handling this influx of new cases. Prosecutors can't possibly take all these cases to court; courts can't possibly find space on already crowded calendars to determine the guilt or innocence of all these people; and the District's prisons were already overcrowded and groaning under court orders to improve conditions before Clean Sweep began. The result is a kind of revolving door in which Clean Sweep officers run into the same people over and over again, released on bail or a plea bargain from the previous arrest.[46]

It was "like trying to mop the floor when the faucet is still running."[47]

CREATING A GENERATION OF FELONS:
THE SCHOOL-TO-PRISON PIPELINE

The process of criminalizing half the city's young Black men started early, and a primary mechanism through which racial containment worked was through the so-called school-to-prison pipeline.[48] Black DC youth in the prison-boom decades of the 1980s through the early 2000s were subjected to poorly funded and physically deteriorating schools, which had unconscionably poor educational outcomes, high dropout rates, and discriminatory deployment of zero-tolerance disciplining, which combined to push them out of school and thus placed them at risk for juvenile delinquency and a subsequent criminal career. I examine these factors in turn.

Public School Underinvestment

Poor funding for DC public schools (DCPS) was a perennial and congressionally created problem. In 1967, urban education scholar A. Harry Passow, examining DCPS, observed that "virtually the same fiscal problems have been cited in every major survey of the Washington schools for the past century."[49] He drew at length from the 1938 report of the President's Advisory Committee on Education, presumably to save repetition. For example, he quoted:

> By making appropriations for detailed items and by insisting that the expenditures within the items conform closely to the budget estimates, the Congressional [House and Senate] committees constantly determine educational policy, frequently in considerable detail. This procedure ... may prevent the adjustment of the educational system to needs and changing circumstances ... That Congress should control educational policy in such detail when the

schools are intended primarily to serve the residents of the District rather than a distinctly national purpose, and when seven-eighths of the financial support of the schools is derived from local taxes, cannot be regarded as in keeping with the democratic American way of providing school facilities.[50]

The "triple screening of school budgets—by the [DC] Board of Education, the [presidentially appointed DC] Commissioners, and Congress"[51] had "acted . . . to exert a conservative influence on school budgets."[52] He noted that between 1953 and 1966, for example, schools requested $82.3 million, DC Commissioners approved $64.5 million, and Congress appropriated $54.7 million.[53] The overarching problem, he noted, was that "the school lacks independent taxing authority. Consequently the school system must compete for funds with every other city agency."[54] Congressional budgetary oversight, triplicate budget screening, and DCPS's competition with other city agencies for funds, which continued into the twenty-first century,[55] was especially consequential when the criminal justice system commanded increasingly large chunks of the city's budget.

While among education scholars, a debate launched by the influential Coleman Report[56] challenged whether school funding made a difference to educational outcomes, in DC, there was a dire need for funds to improve public school buildings. Maureen Berner described DC Committee on Public Education studies, which found $30 million worth of "deferred expenditures . . . both capital outlays and deferred compliance with federal and state health and safety requirements" in 1983. By 1989, "the total repair cost of deferred maintenance exceeded $150 million."[57] The same 1989 study

found that the system was in poor condition . . . leaking roofs, ceiling and walls with significant water damage and crumbling plaster, heating systems whose controls did not function, bathrooms with missing partitions, and electrical systems that did not work . . . Between 1986 and 1989, of an estimated 21,295 work orders placed by the schools, only 3,559 were completed, with an average of 3 to 6 months of response time needed.[58]

Berner's own DC study found a significant association between poor building conditions and poor student achievement scores.[59] Poor school conditions continued into the 1990s and 2000s. As the Washington Lawyers' Committee for Civil Rights and Urban Affairs reported:

In 1998, a U.S. Army Corps of Engineers report found that 84% of D.C. school facilities were "in poor physical condition." Five years later, a 2003 Parents

United report explained that D.C. schools facilities had not improved: "roofs were leaking, windows needed to be replaced, boilers were failing, plumbing, wiring and heating systems were old and unreliable. Many of the floors, walls and ceilings were in poor condition, and people often avoided the use of the bathrooms altogether. There were very few schools in the District of Columbia with working science laboratories."[60]

Thus, most children growing up in the nation's capital during the 1980s, 1990s, and early 2000s, along with their teachers, were enduring freezing classrooms, unusable bathrooms, and were unable to properly teach or learn science. These conditions also likely compromised teacher effectiveness, quality, and retention. The Lawyers report noted that an earlier 2005 report had concluded that 50 years after *Bolling v. Sharpe*, a Supreme Court case prohibiting segregated public schools in DC, the DCPS was still "separate and unequal."[61]

Indeed, DCPS was deeply segregated; it was over 90% Black between 1980 and 1997, 86% Black by 2000, and 80% Black by 2010 (while comprising 69.7%, 65.4%, 59.5%, and 50% of the population in 1980, 1990, 2000, and 2010, respectively). White public school students remained 3%–7% or less of the school population during that period (while comprising 25.2%, 27.6%, 27.9%, and 34.8% of the DC population in 1980, 1990, 2000, and 2010, respectively).[62] These trends reflected White flight to the suburbs and/or non-DCPS city schools. Consistent with area studies on housing discrimination, while White and wealthier Black families were able to move their children to better schools, many, especially poor, Black families were "stuck in place."[63]

The 2005 report observed that "with no single entity accountable for both budgeting and policy making, each entity was able to deflect blame for the school system's failures."[64] It was not until 2007, they noted, that through the Public Education Reform Amendment Act, it was finally attempted, controversially, to put the system under the mayor's control (Mayor Adrian Fenty at the time, while the school chancellor was Michelle Rhee), creating "a single point of accountability."[65] Whatever its subsequent merits, this reform came too late for the generations of youth who had aged into and through the prison-boom era.

Poor Educational Outcomes

DCPS also produced very poor and widely unequal educational outcomes.[66] Mid-1980s reports found that the city's worst schools were more than a year below the national norm, while the city's best schools were up to "five years above their grade level."[67] In 1988, overall, DC 11th graders were scoring in the 30th–37th percentiles in reading, math, and language, and in the 27th percentile in science.[68] Poor outcomes continued into the 1990s. In 1990 median test scores for 11th graders were in the 40th–42nd percentiles.[69] Education Watch reported that "[in] 1998, the National Assessment of Educational Progress [found that] 28% of D.C.'s 4th graders performed at the basic level or above in reading, while only 10% performed at the proficient or above level."[70] Education Watch also examined racial disparities, noting that "the District of Columbia does not currently report state assessment results disaggregated by race/ethnicity." They found that 76% of Black versus 27% of White children performed below basic levels in reading, while 17% of Black and 21% of White children performed at the basic level (remaining students were proficient—meeting grade level standards—or advanced—above grade level).[71] By 2007, scores had improved, though wide racial disparities remained: 21% of Black and 3% of White children were below basic level, while 48% of Black and 10% of White children were at the basic level.[72]

DCPS also had high dropout rates. In 1992, *The Washington Post* reported, "About one in five D.C. residents from 16 to 19 years old is a high school drop-out, a rate that is among the worst for the nation's cities, according to a federal study of 1990 Census data."[73] By 1999, "one out of every three students who entered ninth grade in the District in 1994 dropped out by 1998."[74] A decade later, in 2007–8, the Black graduation rate was 58.8% compared to 88.9% for White students.[75] Unfortunately, leaving school without a high school diploma put students at high risk for delinquency and criminal careers. Becky Pettit and Bruce Western found that nationally, dropping out of high school was significantly associated with Black incarceration.[76] This was reflected in my respondents lives; two-thirds of those incarcerated dropped out of high school.

Racial Containment and the Opportunity Structure

Dropping out and performing poorly in school also set DC youth up for a lifetime of low-income legitimate jobs, long stretches of unemployment, and limited opportunities for upward mobility. These outcomes were due to a number of factors. Young Black people were born into the city's spatialized racial and class containment, or its "intense double segregation,"[77] by both poverty and race, which placed them in the wrong place at the wrong time. George Galster and Maris Mikelsons, Urban Institute scholars, compared the opportunity structures for Black and White youth, drawing on 1990 DC census-tract data. They found that compared with White youth, Black youth face the following in their "average" census tract—seven times the rate of out of wedlock births; six times the rate of drug use; six times the rate of drug arrests; five times the rate of public assistance; almost three times the rate of violent crime; almost three times the rate of poverty; two and a half times the rate of high school dropouts, [and] one and a half times the rate of male nonemployment.[78]

They found that all these factors were exacerbated if Black youth were in a single-mother household. As illustrated in my respondents' narratives (see Parts 2–3), the multiple waves of substance abuse epidemics in DC swept up many parents (recall the city's 1980s estimate of 26% of its residents being alcohol or drug dependent). This led to parental absence and neglect in part due to addiction, incarceration, premature illness and death, single parenthood after spousal absence or due to marriage market distortions (see Part 2), and the need to be away from home working multiple jobs to support the family. Galster and Mikelsons went on to note, "Our findings here suggest that urban space is organized in such a fashion that it encourages youth of different races and ethnicities to make different life decisions—decisions that ultimately perpetuate racial-ethnic social inequalities."[79]

While several crucial factors beyond the budget and deteriorating school conditions played important roles in low school achievement and premature exiting, such as teachers, parents, and educational practices,[80] a major feature shaping the opportunity structure of Black youth was the slow but steady infiltration of the drug economy into the school system. This is not surprising as most schools are not like airports, located outside the city, in the middle of nowhere, but are integral parts of neighborhoods. They are not total institutions[81] but porous, influenced by the surrounding community. Thus, as the drug epidemic swept through neighborhoods, it was inevitable that it would start to make its way into schools.

The Saturation of Drugs in the Community and in School

As described in Part 3, some neighborhoods were saturated with drugs, and they amplified both the HIV/AIDS and homicide epidemics, creating syndemic zones with dangerous neighborhood ecologies of illness and death for kids to grow up in. Many youth were involved in the drug economy. An Urban Institute report focusing on the city's poor Black boys aged 14 to 17 found that 18% had used illegal drugs, 16% had sold drugs, and 31% of drug sellers had also used drugs in the past year. The report found that "the heaviest drug users began in elementary school."[82] The primary city response to youth drug involvement was juvenile detention. Indeed, among many respondents, drugs led to both a first arrest and dropping out of school. A first arrest often kicked off a multidecade incarceration cycle. Forty-year-old transgender woman Mary described how she slowly transitioned out of school, onto the streets, and into incarceration:

> I was born and raised here in Washington, DC, I was educated in DC public schools. Um, I come from um *[pause]* a single mother who was an IV drug user. I was raised by my grandmother and a, um, somewhat emotionally and physically abusive environment ... I was basically just, just a feminine little boy that went to school and got good grades and stuff, and then I began to use marijuana and PCP and sleeping with random strangers, um, and then you know I became less interested in school and more interested in the street life ... and then um criminal behavior at a early age. I was arrested as early as 15.

She subsequently dropped out of school and began going back and forth to correctional facilities[83] for 21 years. Forty-nine-year-old Theo similarly described a pathway beginning with drugs, arrest, and dropping out in the 10th grade.

> Well, I grew up in Washington, DC, mostly in SE. When I was born we lived ... right across from the Marine barracks ... Around 7 or 8, we moved to far SE to the projects. Um, around 13, I started usin' drugs, marijuana, PCP, LSD, experimenting with drugs. I wound up gettin' in trouble. The first time I been on probation, I was 12 years old ... And I continued to go in and out of jail basically up until the last two years. I've used every kind of drug there is. I ... I just kind of—kind of lost touch with everything since my mama died in the first 10 or 12 years of my life, you know.

Theo's incarceration career lasted 30 years. He began by stealing bread, donuts, and milk for himself and his siblings after his mother died, and he graduated to robbery and burglary as well as selling drugs.

The number of District children and youth arrested for drugs climbed rapidly. By 1987, Victoria Churchville reported that almost 1,400 had been arrested as part of Clean Sweep over the past year; 38% were aged 15 years or less, 62% were 16–17 years old, and almost a third (30%) of those arrested tested positive for drugs. Police had targeted areas containing "the highest number of children and of public housing projects in the city," and Clean Sweep "operate[d] in every section of the city but Georgetown and upper Northwest where street sales of drugs [were] rare."[84] The arrest rate in 1987 showed a "456% increase in the number of juveniles arrested for the sale of illicit drugs" compared to 1986, a reflection of the increasing reliance on youth by drug dealers because youth got lighter sentences than adults.[85] By 1998, the city "maintained one of the highest juvenile incarceration rates in the nation."[86]

Zero-Tolerance Crime Policies: Pushing Kids into the Pipeline

The city was also "one of the most deadly places in the country for children and teenagers."[87] The 1997 Kids Count study by the Annie E. Casey Foundation found that rates of child death "nearly doubled, rising by 91 percent from 1985 to 1994," and violent death rates "increased by 669 percent from 1985 to 1994."[88] Teen homicides began to decline towards the end of the 1990s.[89] As the drug and violence wave escalated and started penetrating schools, there was a downward drift of zero-tolerance criminal-justice frames to the treatment of delinquent children and youth nationally, as well as in DC. These further served to push children out of school and into the juvenile justice system. The 1984 Comprehensive Crime Control Act, passed under Reagan, was a new federal law targeted at "drug dealers congregating near schools and pressuring students to buy drugs."[90] It increased sentences to "up to 30 years for each count of selling drugs within 1000 feet of a school."[91] Joseph diGenova, the DC US Attorney, referring to the six 18- to 19-year-old DC high school students who were being tried under the new law, said that they were "more than adults within the view of the law" and "if they can sell drugs, they can do the time."[92] The new law had thus transformed even a one-time transaction of drugs between fellow students into a potential 30-year sentence.

In the 1990s, scholars observed an increasing resemblance between school discipline and crime management as schools and prisons began to mirror each other, with similar policies (mandatory punishments, zero tolerance), personnel (police or "school resource officers"), and enforcement methods (dog sniffing, personal searches, metal detectors).[93] This shift was facilitated by congressional laws in the 1990s, passed under Clinton, including the Gun-Free Schools Act (1994) and Safe Schools Acts (1994, 1998). These acts provided funding for police presence in schools and mandated school expulsions and justice system referrals for students who brought guns to school.[94] Hirschfield found that "as of 2000, 41 states mandated law enforcement referral for school crimes including drugs, violence, and weapons violations."[95] Zero-tolerance policies limiting teacher discretion expanded to other disciplinary issues, such that as Johanna Wald and Daniel Losen observed, even while juvenile crime dropped, commitment to secured juvenile facilities for nonviolent offenses increased.[96] Policies created environments where students were increasingly treated as "pre-criminals," with an "anticipatory labeling . . . as future prisoners in need of coercive control or exclusion,"[97] and students were excluded for their "perceived potential to be dangerous, rather than for any overt act they may have committed."[98] Mallett found that between 1996 and 2013, at least 75% of schools had zero-tolerance policies,[99] and Wald and Losen reported "a near doubling" in annual student suspensions during the 1990s, when compared to rates in 1974.[100] In addition, the "nearly one billion dollars spent by federal agencies"[101] that provided funding for, among other things, more than 17,000 school resource officers, resulted in "increased student arrests on school grounds between 300 and 500% annually since the establishment of zero tolerance policies." [102]

The use of these kinds of policies was evident in DC as early as 1986, when, as reported by Linda Wheeler,

> the D.C. Board of Education unanimously approved stringent disciplinary rules for students yesterday that include automatic suspension for possession or use of drugs, alcohol or weapons in or around school buildings. The board also endorsed the establishment of a separate school for these problem students to attend, though no decision was made on where the school will be located or how it will be financed.[103]

The proposed alternative school for suspended students, PAUSE (Providing Alternative Unique School Environment), would "cost the school system about $1 million a year."[104] Zero-tolerance policies continued into the 2000s, and Black students were disproportionately more likely to be suspended.[105] A 2012–13 DC Equity report, for example, found that overall 12% of DCPS students were suspended for "at least one day"; however, there were wide racial disparities: 16% of Black students and 1% of White students had been suspended.[106] The report found that some DC schools suspended large numbers of their students; 37 schools "suspended at least 25% of [their] students," and 8 schools "suspended at least 50% for at least one day."[107] The report noted that these numbers translated to "nearly 10,000 DC students . . . suspended at least once during SY 2012–2013" and found that "out-of-school suspensions and expulsions" were four times more likely than in-school suspension.[108] Overall, Black students were 5.9 times more likely to be disciplined compared to

White students. They also had higher discipline risk factors. Discipline was higher among low-income students (1.3 times more), especially TANF or SNAP eligible students (1.5 times more), levels 1–3 special education students (1.4–1.75 times more), students with multiple disabilities (1.81 times more), and emotionally disturbed students (2.67 times more).[109] In other words, the students in most need of extra assistance—poor Black children with special needs and/or disabilities—were also the most likely to be pushed out of school, putting them on a pathway to a criminal career. And this was known early on—a 1980s General Accounting Office report found that 46% of DC's juvenile detainees needed (and were not provided) special education classes.[110]

DC was not unique. Nationally, Wald and Losen found that between 1983 and 1997, 80% of new juveniles were minorities. They also found that "Black students [were] 2.6 times as likely to be suspended as White students ... [and that] Black [students] with no prior criminal records were six times ... more likely to be incarcerated than White [students] for the same offenses."[111] They also estimated that "70% of the juvenile justice population suffer from learning disabilities and 33% read below the fourth grade level."[112] Scholars argued that these trends were exacerbated, inadvertently, by the Bush administration's No Child Left Behind Act (2001), whose effect was to "narrow ... educational instructions—thus, teaching to the test—and encouraged the removal of low-performing students"[113] in order to improve school ratings. In DC, this occurred long before the law was passed, with commentators linking high dropout rates to schools pressured to show improved student educational out-comes. As Athelia Knight, investigating Washington area dropouts, reported:

> In many cases, faculty members have given up on the at-risk students and they have given up on themselves. It is often felt that these students (1) reduce the grade point average of the schools, (2) contribute to low standardized test scores, (3) lower attendance rates, and 4) take away instructional time from students who are ready to learn. Now, we say, the school would benefit if these students quit school.[114]

Creating a Criminal Career:
The Back-and-Forth of Incarceration

Overall, as observed by Robert Sampson, John Laub, David Knight and others, and as was clear in many of my interviews, early involvement with the criminal justice system initiated a lifelong cycle of going back and forth to and being biographically shaped by juvenile detention and adult jail and prison.[115] Wynton, age 50, was one of five children, with a single mother who worked two jobs as a caterer and a housekeeper to support the family. He dropped out of a local DC high school in 11th grade. He started experimenting with drugs and became addicted to heroin. As he described,

> I didn't really start doing a lot of stuff until like 13, 14 years old. You know I started getting into the street life, you know I started selling drugs . . . I was in jail as a juvenile [for selling drugs] . . . I was 16 . . . it was only like 6 months.

However, that initiated a 22-year cycle to and from prison (1977–99):

> The next time I went back it was adult . . . I think I went in like I was 21, I think I came out like at 23 . . . And then I went back in when I turned 24. And I didn't come back out again till like, 28. That was the long stretch . . . then I went in again like . . . 30 years old . . . when I got out . . . I was like, I think it was like . . . like . . . 38 . . . and then after that I just started trying to do better, you know.

What changed was an opportunity to spend a year in a drug rehab program directly after leaving prison.

Sixty-year-old Kevin was addicted to cocaine. In contrast to several other respondents, he grew up in a stable, two-parent "hard worker" household with three older siblings. But he nonetheless also turned to crime, influenced by peers. His parents

> didn't have the best education, but they worked and they provided for us. But I always wanted to have the best of things and they weren't able to provide the best of things. They could just do the basics. So what I did was I got caught up in peer pressure and started hustling you know . . . to earn my own keep . . . buy my own clothes, you know buy what *I* wanted to buy.

He was incarcerated for pickpocketing, stealing, and bank robbery. His career began at age 14. As he describes:

> I went to three schools in three blocks, right around the corner . . . I never caught the bus to school, elementary, junior high, and senior high . . . However, during this span, I was incarcerated as a juvenile . . . I guess 14 or so and I didn't come back home until I was around 16. Then I was incarcerated again at 17 and didn't come back home again until I was about 22. Then I was incarcerated and came back home at 30 . . . [in] total I did 23 years.

Drug addiction made the cycle hard to escape. Forty-nine-year-old Colin graduated high school and did one year of college, but he nonetheless followed in his father's footsteps at age 20, becoming addicted to drugs and spending more than half his life incarcerated for drug dealing and related crimes:

> COLIN: Fucked my whole life up—28, 29 years of bein' incarcerated. Damn shame. I ain't nothing but 49 years, and you act like I killed somebody. And it was just forgery . . . unauthorized use of a vehicle, drugs, drugs, drugs . . . it seems like, wow, my life just took a turn . . . I have given my life to the federal, DCDC, Department of Corrections . . . I did 11 years straight, from '87 to '98, and from there I did two years, three years, two years, 18 months here, nine months here, six months here. Every year . . . these are the first two years that I have been home straight, undisturbed time since 1987 . . . I did all my life incarcerated . . .
>
> SANYU: Was there any point during that early period when you stopped to reflect or were you just in a cycle?
>
> COLIN: Yeah, a vicious cycle, going back and forth, going, going, going, like the Energizer Bunny.

Legislation and policy worked together with his drug addiction to create an individual and structural pull into a back-and-forth cycle through parole violations. And this was a national pattern. Alexander described the "extraordinary increase in prison admissions due to parole and probation violations," rising from 1% of prison admissions in 1980 to 35% of prison admissions in 2000.[116] Kevin estimated that "from 1980 to '95 . . . parole violations and stuff like that totaled about 6, 7, 8 years or something, you know, in different periods." For forty-two-year-old trans woman Hannah, "from '98, I was violating until, I kept getting out, going back in, getting out, going back until 2007. It was a violation of the terms of my release, so I kept going back, it wasn't on new charges, it was just violations." Colin described the last 10 of his 28 years in prison:

> COLIN: Went back from '99 to 2001, came out in 2001, I think I stayed in the street eight months, went back. [silence] Went back for about three years, 36 months and somethin', came out in 2004, stayed in the street from 2004 for one month, and caught a brand-new charge December 10th. They gave me 27 months. Come out 2008, go back again . . . Come out 2009 . . .
>
> SANYU: What were you going in for all those times?
>
> COLIN: Violations, dirty urine. Then I caught two new charges by bein' on parole, which is a violation. Most times I was goin' back for dirty urine.

SANYU: The three years, the two years. It was basically the habit that took you back in?

COLIN: Yes, ma'am. Drugs.

The tragic consequence of dropping out of school early and decades-long incarceration cycles during their prime working years was that respondents did not have an opportunity to get a proper foothold on life outside of prison. As forty-three-year-old trans woman Maggie put it, "I've never had my name on a lease. I've never had my own place. I always been either on mom's couch or with someone, or in jail or in some type of drug treatment." For many, reentry to prison was more stable than reentry to the community. Incarceration was not an interruption of their regular lives; prison was the more familiar home, neighborhood, and community for a generation of Black felons.

Why Did the City Turn to Incarceration to Manage Its Troubled Youth?

Given the vast amounts of money apparently available for the War on Drugs, why did the city turn to incarceration as the solution? Perhaps to take advantage of the ongoing citywide sweep; perhaps because of frustration that parents and schools were not doing more to stop the production of dropouts at high risk of turning to crime. Joseph Webb, for example, reported "that a $395,000 drop-out prevention grant [to DCPS] was going unused," and a "shake-up of top administrators" had made no difference.[117] Perhaps because so many root-cause city agencies—such as those focusing on public housing, social work, and mental health, as well as youth and adult employment agencies and drug treatment facilities (which were especially limited for poor youth[118])—were underfunded, understaffed, and necessarily did slower work and thus produced slower results. By contrast, arrests were easy to count and report to Congress, and they produced immediate, noticeable differences in the particular neighborhood that was swept.

Meanwhile, by the end of the '90s, a class action lawsuit sought receivership for the Youth Services Administration in charge of juvenile delinquents[119] due to basic neglect, the detention centers featuring "dismal facilities," overcrowding, violence from guards, and drug sales.[120] Children had been dispersed to facilities costing $100,000 per child per year.[121] Given the competition among the city agencies for a place in the budget, this, in addition to the $1 million cost for the PAUSE school, were clear cases of money that could have been used to improve schools in poor communities or work on other root causes. Instead, these funds were draining into the criminal justice system and were being used to incarcerate away predominantly Black problem children.

THE PRISON-INDUSTRIAL AND
POLITICAL-INDUSTRIAL COMPLEXES

The War on Drugs, much like other wars, is highly profitable, and billions of dollars were funneled to crisis- and symptom-management institutions. As Glenn Frankel put it: "Call it Drug War Inc. Fifty-seven federal departments and agencies now have a piece of what has become America's longest war,"[122] and entire industries were incentivized toward and dependent on the constant production of prisoners. As noted in the Part overview, managing millions of people in the criminal justice system is an expensive business. Of the estimated $305-billion annual cost for system expenditures across federal, state, and local levels, the Bureau of Justice estimated that $149 billion went to police functions, $66 billion to judicial and legal functions, and $89 billion to corrections functions.[123] In a separate study, Peter Wagner and Bernadette Rabuy estimated that about $3.9 billion went to private corrections.[124] State spending on prisoners varies widely (e.g., $59 per day in Mississippi but $315 per day in New York).[125] Prisons and the many external services they procured[126] "turned [prisoners] into commodities" who were "valued for their bodily ability to generate per diem payments to their prison keepers."[127] As routine imprisonment became mass incarceration,[128] the commoditization of prisoners made keeping bodies in prisons for as long as possible the most profitable outcome. Schwartz and Nurge observed that prisoners were

> producers of income to be fought over and welcomed. States with excess prison capacity aggressively bid to accept the overflow of prisoners from other states, and private prisons lobby hard and long to increase the number of prisoners and increase the amount of time they serve. Of course, private prisons also lobby to increase the percentage of prisoners sent to private facilities.[129]

They went on to note that the Corrections Corporation of America (CCA), a major private provider of prisons and prison services, financed and cochaired committees, such as the Criminal Justice Task Force. The task force "wrote model legislation pushing for longer sentences" and recommended "harsh sentencing laws," which would both result in more prisoners for the business.[130]

In DC, the combination of a dramatic increase in arrests, convictions, and recidivism (especially with drug addiction), led to prison overcrowding that exceeded federal regulations.[131] By 1987, Lorton, the city's main prison, was so overcrowded that prisoners went to federal prisons following court orders.[132] A prison emergency was declared in July 1987, with early releases to accommodate new offenders.[133] New drug sweeps were postponed when "corrections officials went back to court . . . and asserted that they could no longer house the increasing number of prisoners and still meet federal population caps and ensure the department wasn't violating prisoners' constitutional rights."[134] The city was in a bind, however, as residents were resistant to new prison buildings,[135] the federal government refused to accept DC prisoners,[136] and they were committed to the popular Clean Sweep as a response to the drug epidemic.[137] By 1993, Katya Lezin observed, "The District of Columbia has the highest rate of incarceration in the United States, locking up 1,651 citizens per every 100,000. The most recent statistics indicate that approximately one of every eight Washingtonians—more than 70,000 residents—is incarcerated, on probation, on parole, or under arrest."[138]

Despite prison capacity and budgetary limits, the prison-industrial complex chugged on, working to increase the number of bodies in beds. As Peter Slevin reported in 1998:

> The appeals court ruling that forced the recalculations for D.C. inmates . . . decided that time spent on parole, called "street time," would not count toward a prisoner's overall sentence if the parolee was rearrested for violating the terms of his or her release. Under the old method of calculating parole time, for example, a drug dealer sentenced to prison for nine years, paroled after four and rearrested two years later would have gotten credit for his blemish free time on parole and would have faced no more than three additional years in prison. But with the court's new interpretation, the two years on parole would not be counted toward the nine year sentence, so the prisoner could be required to serve as much as five more years . . . The ruling affects 18 percent of the 8,794 prisoners under the District's jurisdiction.[139]

For parolees addicted to drugs, this transformed staying out of prison into a Sisyphean task.

In DC and nationally, there were clear opportunity costs to massive expenditures on prisons. Increasing proportions of state and city budgets were diverted to funding jails and prisons instead of improving urban inner-city schools, which were pipelining minority youth into prison.[140] Yet reflecting the symbiotic nature of the prison- and political-industrial complexes, poor, rural community leaders solicited prison contracts to provide solid jobs for their residents, as John Eason documented.[141] Rural America is disproportionately represented in the US Congress, ensuring that rural interests can take precedence over those of populous urban districts disproportionately affected by mass incarceration.[142] Politicians also benefited. Being "tough on crime" was popular with national voters, prison contracts were popular in rural communities, and lobbyists for private prisons funneled money into political campaigns. In sum, by locking in incentives for mass incarceration, it was now in the economic interests of many Americans and their elected political representatives to manage the symptoms of the drug crisis through mass incarceration rather than to deal with the root causes.

The culmination of the city's growing budget deficit and the inability to manage the overproduction of prisoners led to pressure to shut down DC prisons and transfer jurisdiction of their prisoners to the federal system. In the Clinton Plan, accepted in 1997 as part of the DC Revitalization Act, the federal government would take charge of DC prisoners, giving huge financial relief to the city. However, as federal prisoners, they would now be subject to "longer prison terms," less discretion in sentencing, "fewer alternatives to prison time," and serve at least 85% of their sentences before eligibility for release.[143] This shift was consequential. As reporters observed, for a typical crack case, someone caught with one or two grams "under D.C. law [was] eligible for probation. But under federal standards, the same person would face 12 to 24 months in prison."[144] The plan would be phased in over five years. Lorton, the city's main prison, was closed in 2001.[145]

DC prisoners were scattered across federal, state, and private prisons around the country. Lorton prisoners were distributed to 77 federal prisons, 82% of whom were in a 500-mile radius.[146] My respondents did time in Massachusetts, Alabama, Florida, Ohio, and North Carolina, among other states. This meant a wrenching separation from kids, partners, friends, and lawyers, the former of whom now needed a lot more money and time off work to visit. In this way, imprisonment compounded the already heavy intergenerational toll on Black families.[147]

Nationally, DC prisoners were in high commercial demand even before Lorton shut down. When prisoners were transferred to Washington state, Hockstader reported: "The District is under court orders to ease crowding and Spokane officials needed the $1.1 million a year that the District will pay for the 'rent a cell' program."[148] While the prison was "a physical improvement over Lorton," there was "no chance for rehabilitation . . . and, particularly, no educational programs to pursue. Instead, the plan is to put them all to work in the jail's kitchen and cleanup details, at a wage of a dollar a day."[149] As Lorton was phased out, 1,700 prisoners were shipped to the Northeast Ohio Correctional Center, a private prison run by the CCA in 1997.[150] The Washington Lawyers' Committee for Civil Rights and Affairs noted the influence of the CCA in both national and local DC politics, as the CCA had spent several million dollars in "lobbying [efforts] at federal, state, and local levels . . . to prevent private prisons from being subjected to the same public disclosure requirements [FOIA] as public prisons."[151] The CAA also made political contributions to candidates running for the DC City Council and mayor.[152] As Martin Schwartz and Dana Nurge described,

> Youngstown, Ohio, an economically devastated area anxious for jobs, gave away valuable land and offered major tax breaks so that the Corrections Corporation of America (CCA) could build a 2,106-bed "spec prison" (Northeast Ohio Correctional Center (NOCC)) with little to no state or local monitoring. When the prison opened, it had no inmates and therefore no form of income . . . Conspiring with Washington D.C. officials to bypass the competitive bidding process, the NOCC was awarded a contract at inflated prices, with few compliance mechanisms, to immediately take 1,700 medium security inmates. However, Washington needed to close down Lorton Penitentiary quickly, so the high-risk inmates imprisoned there were sent to Ohio anyway, where they were reclassified as "high medium."[153]

Prisoners were subjected to brutal and degrading treatment by prison guards following management guidance.[154] As Santana reported, "Two inmates were fatally stabbed; 40 assaults were reported; six prisoners escaped in 1998; and in 1999, inmates won $1.65 million in a class action suit accusing guards of excessive force."[155] Meanwhile, "the American Correctional Association gave 'near perfect' ratings to the prison despite all the stabbings and deaths."[156] DC eventually removed its prisoners from the prison.

In sum, multiple institutions—the DCPS, the police, Congress, the judicial system, and the political-industrial and prison-industrial complexes—

worked together to (re)produce racial containment. Many Black youth were disproportionately pushed out of school, arrested, sentenced, and locked into decades-long entanglements with the prison system. As I illustrate in the next chapter, incarceration, ostensibly a solution to the city's syndemic, instead worked to amplify it.

ELEVEN

The DC Prison Syndemic and Community Amplification

IT IS REASONABLE TO IMAGINE that prisons ameliorated the city's drug–HIV/AIDS syndemic. Prisoners had a constitutional right to health care; thus, for poor and uninsured Americans, transitioning to prison came with not just "three hots and a cot" but also health care. Prisons were not just morally but also legally compelled to manage people with drug addiction and care for people living with HIV/AIDS. In theory, prisons should be dry, with no access to drugs, enabling people, especially those with long sentences, to become and stay clean. Similarly, sex is illegal in prison, which should eliminate sexual HIV transmission, and prisons have captive audiences for checkup appointments and routines to enable adherence to infectivity-reducing ART medication once it became available in the mid-1990s. However, as I will illustrate in the case of DC, the city syndemic was amplified in the correctional system and reverberated back to the community. This chapter examines the US and DC prison syndemic, focusing on prison policies around harm reduction (e.g., providing condoms and bleach to clean needles), HIV testing, and segregation. I then describe the drug and sexual economies and their health consequences for prisoners and the community syndemic once prisoners were released. Reflecting my interviews, I primarily focus on experiences of men and trans women placed in men's prisons.

THE DRUG–HIV/AIDS SYNDEMIC IN US PRISONS

US prisons were dominated by people who used drugs. Nationally, while most were incarcerated for violence and crimes not related to drugs,[1] as Freudenberg observed, "more than 70% of federal inmates and 80% of state

Mortality rate per 100,000 state prisoners, 1991–2004

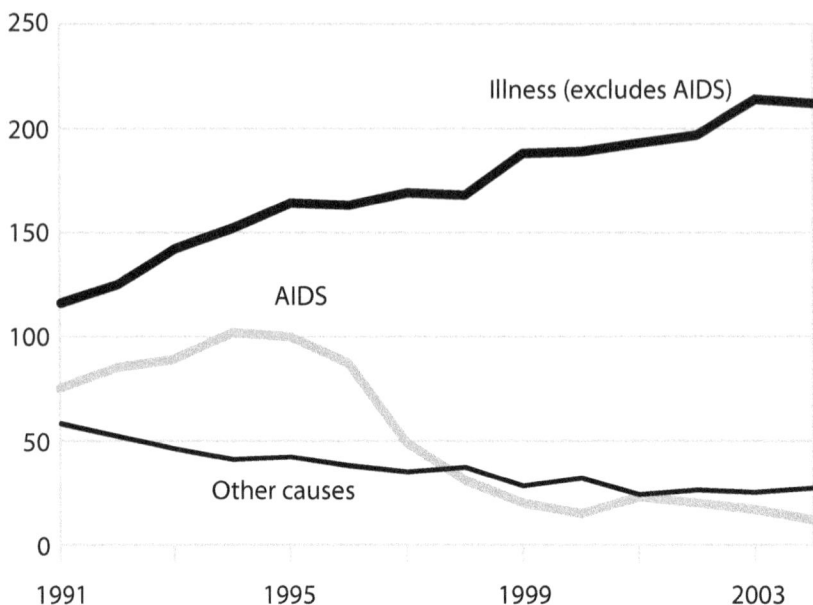

FIGURE 41. Mortality in US state prisons, 1991–2004. Data source: Christopher Mumola, *Medical Causes of Death in State Prisons, 2001–2004* (Bureau of Justice Statistics, US Department of Justice, 2007).

and local jail inmates reported a history of drug use."[2] Just over half of addicted prisoners relapsed within a month of release,[3] putting themselves at risk of overdose death[4] or reincarceration, since parole required clean drug tests. US prisons also had many people with HIV/AIDS. This was a matter of policy, as a report on HIV in correctional facilities by the National Commission on AIDS observed, "Presently, the United States maintains a de facto policy of incarcerating more and more HIV infected individuals by choosing mass imprisonment as the federal and state government's response to the use of drugs."[5]

By 1995, 2.3% of state and federal prisoners were living with HIV, with wide variation across systems; in New York, 13.6% had HIV.[6] Spaulding and colleagues noted that in 1997, an estimated "20%–26% of all people living with HIV infection in the US passed through a correctional facility."[7] Prior to ART, as the HIV epidemic escalated, AIDS became a major crisis in US prisons,[8] and the AIDS rate was "at least 5 times the rate in the general population."[9] Figure 41 illustrates mortality trends between 1991 and 2004. The impact of ART is evident in the subsequent dramatic drop in AIDS deaths. However, Laura Maruschak estimated that in 1997, "even with a sharp decline, AIDS-related illnesses were still the second leading cause of death in state prisons behind natural causes."[10] AIDS death rates in prisons were also still "five times higher than in the [general] population" in 1999.[11] AIDS deaths in prison became increasingly rare in the ensuing decade.[12]

In contrast to the national picture, in the mid-1990s in DC, Stephanie Mencimer reported that most Lorton prisoners (89%) were serving drug-related sentences and AIDS was a leading cause of death.[13] Estimated HIV prevalence was exceptionally high. Amy Goldstein reported: "A 1989 study of blood samples from 500 randomly selected inmates entering the D.C. Jail found that 16 percent were infected with the HIV virus, which causes AIDS. Prison officials estimate [in 1992] the rate may now approach 25 percent."[14] The Bureau of Justice reported DC's HIV prevalence rate as 7.8% of the total custody population in 1999, and in 2000 it was 3.3%.[15]

HARM REDUCTION IN PRISON?

Generally, prisons did not pursue harm reduction approaches because multiple laws on the books proscribed them. It was not until 2003 in *Lawrence v. Texas* that sodomy laws were declared unconstitutional. Further, because sex was illegal in prisons most did not officially provide condoms in the '80s and '90s.[16] In DC, prisoners had been denied condoms because, as Mary Campbell, the DC prisons health services educator, said to a reporter, "Under District government [law], sodomy is considered illegal. If we were to pass out condoms, then we would be going contrary to our own governing body."[17] Nonetheless, in 1992, Mayor Kelly "signed a mandate requiring the Department of Corrections to distribute condoms in all correctional institutions."[18] However, the prison

> requires that a condom-seeking prisoner first make an appointment with a case manager—which requires a wait of anywhere from several hours to several days. If an inmate is lucky enough to score an appointment, the case worker will give him a how-to-wear-a-condom "safe sex" lecture before handing him his rubber.[19]

My respondents were exposed to a wide range of condom policies around the country. In Benton's experience, for example, "some camps would allow you to have condoms and some people were gettin' 'em snuck in. Um, then we were usin' cellophane and the rubber gloves from when we clean up, we'd be usin' those. And sometimes we didn't use 'em. We just didn't use 'em ..." Trans woman Hannah, who had been placed in a men's prison, had similar experiences, noting, "Well, in a federal institution, they don't have condoms. Only at the state," because as Wynton noted, "There shouldn't be no sex going on in the penitentiary." However, like Benton, Hannah observed that even when they were available, "a lot of times people, we didn't use protection." In this respect, prisoners were no different from nonprisoners (see Part 2). However, given the necessarily dense prison sexual and drug networks, they felt that "it [HIV] was traveling a lot in the penitentiary. A whole lot, you know, because, people having unprotected sex." Similarly, correctional systems did not provide needle exchange programs, and most systems (80%) did not provide bleach (which could be subverted to use for cleaning needles and syringes) for any reason (including laundry).[20]

TESTING AND SEGREGATION

Overall, given these limited harm reduction approaches, sorting (through HIV testing) and separating (through segregation) prisoners based on their HIV/AIDS status and/or whether they had symptoms became the primary management strategies in many prisons prior to ART.[21] Their persistence after it was widely known that HIV was not spread through casual contact can only be read as a frank acknowledgement of both sex and injecting drug use within prison.

There was wide variation in HIV testing policies. Table 2, reproduced from a Bureau of Justice Statistics report, illustrates the testing policies across US prison systems in 1993, prior to ART.[22] Fifteen state systems had mandatory testing of prisoners on entry. In the DC prison system, HIV prevalence was tracked through random sampling. Otherwise, DC prisoners were tested if they had clinically indicated AIDS symptoms or by request (which in practice involved "obtain[ing] a court order requiring corrections officials to administer the blood test").[23] Jails and prisons were a common place my respondents found out they had HIV/AIDS.

In the early epidemic years, most prison systems segregated prisoners with positive tests or AIDS symptoms. Hammett and colleagues reported that "in 1985, 38 (75 percent) of the prison systems reported segregating inmates with

TABLE 2 Testing policies for the antibody to the human immunodeficiency virus that causes AIDS, by jurisdiction, 1993

| All Inmates | | Upon Release | Random Sample | High-Risk Groups | Upon Inmate Request | Upon Clinical Indication of Need | Upon Involvement in Incident |
Entering	Currently in Custody						
Alabama	Rhode Island	Alabama	Dist. of Columbia	Arkansas	Alaska	Arizona	Arizona
Colorado	Wyoming	Federal	Federal	Connecticut	Arkansas	Arkansas	Arkansas
Georgia		Missouri	New Jersey	Florida	California	California	California
Idaho		Nevada	New York	Illinois	Colorado	Colorado	Colorado
Iowa				Indiana	Connecticut	Connecticut	Florida
Michigan				Kansas	Delaware	Delaware	Hawaii
Mississippi				Kentucky	Dist. of Columbia	Dist. of Columbia	Illinois
Missouri				Minnesota	Federal	Federal	Kentucky
Nebraska				Missouri	Florida	Florida	Maryland
Nevada				Montana	Georgia	Georgia	Michigan
North Dakota				New York	Hawaii	Hawaii	Minnesota
Oklahoma				North Carolina	Illinois	Illinois	Missouri
Rhode Island				Ohio	Indiana	Indiana	New Hampshire
Utah				Pennsylvania	Kansas	Kansas	New York
Wyoming				South Carolina	Kentucky	Kentucky	North Carolina
				South Dakota	Louisiana	Louisiana	Ohio
				Tennessee	Maine	Maryland	Oklahoma
				Texas	Maryland	Michigan	Oregon
				Virginia	Massachusetts	Minnesota	Pennsylvania
				West Virginia	Michigan	Mississippi	Rhode Island
					Minnesota	Missouri	South Carolina

(continued)

TABLE 2 (continued)

	All Inmates						
Entering	Currently in Custody	Upon Release	Random Sample	High-Risk Groups	Upon Inmate Request	Upon Clinical Indication of Need	Upon Involvement in Incident
					Missouri	Montana	Tennessee
					Montana	New Hampshire	Virginia
					New Jersey	New Jersey	
					New Mexico	New Mexico	
					New York	New York	
					North Carolina	North Carolina	
					Ohio	Ohio	
					Oregon	Oklahoma	
					Pennsylvania	Oregon	
					Rhode Island	Pennsylvania	
					South Carolina	Rhode Island	
					South Dakota	South Carolina	
					Tennessee	Tennessee	
					Texas	Texas	
					Vermont	Vermont	
					Virginia	Virginia	
					Washington	Washington	
					West Virginia	West Virginia	

NOTE: Some jurisdictions reported more than one policy. Five states reported policies additional to those presented above. Alaska requires testing of those ordered by the court because of a conviction for a sexual offense. Colorado's tested inmates include those scheduled for routine physicals. In Florida all admissions to reception centers are encouraged to be tested. In North Carolina inmates are tested as a result of a court order. In Wisconsin inmates who have clinical indication of need and who agree to be tested are tested.

SOURCE: Originally published as Table 4 in Peter M. Brien and Caroline Wolf Harlow, 1995, *HIV in Prisons and Jails, 1993*, Bureau of Justice Statistics Bulletin (Aug), NCJ 152765, US Department of Justice, p. 5.

AIDS and 8 systems (16 percent) reported segregating inmates with asymptomatic HIV."[24] In some cases, male prisoners with AIDS were sent to Springfield, Missouri, while female prisoners with AIDS went to Lexington, Kentucky; both facilities had advanced medical capabilities. (Two of my respondents were sent there.) Segregation (or quarantining) had limitations from a prevention point of view. HIV's long incubation period of potentially 6–10 years meant that people were infectious several years prior to developing symptomatic HIV/AIDS. Further, since the HIV test is a test of antibodies, prisoners could be negative on entry into prison and then seroconvert afterwards. This was especially true for injecting drug users and those regularly arrested for selling sex.

By 1994, only six systems were still segregating prisoners,[25] and the last three stopped in the 2010s—Mississippi (2010), Alabama (2012), and South Carolina (2013)—following investigative reports and ACLU lawsuits.[26] Indeed, in practice, segregation was inhumane. Segregated prisoners were isolated, medically neglected, had a worse standard of living compared to others, were denied access to prison programming, and experienced discrimination, ostracism and heightened stigma.[27] For example, in Alabama's Limestone Prison, Benjamin Fleury-Steiner documented how many with HIV were in "a zone of lethal abandonment"[28] where they were "routinely denied access to treatment"[29] and subject to privatized prison health care, which prioritized cost cutting.

Officially, DC prisoners with AIDS were not segregated.[30] In practice, in the early years, prison officials dealt variably with prisoners with AIDS—some were isolated, some were not, and others served out their sentences on parole or in halfway houses.[31] Theo, incarcerated on and off between 1973 and 2003, observed that "in Lorton . . . when you were in medium [security], everybody that had HIV lived in four units. There was a cell house for 400, and over half the people there had HIV or AIDS . . ." His description of the unit suggests it was for those with symptomatic HIV or AIDS:

> I seen so many people die from this disease. Before they closed up Lorton . . . you'd see people can't get out of the bed, gettin' smaller and smaller around you, and some guys give up, just lay down in that bed and don't go to eat till they die, or they eventually come and scoop 'em up and take 'em off somewhere, and then you hear about they died a month or two later. That was somethin' to live through.

The treatment of prisoners with AIDS in DC was recognized as woefully inadequate, with documented extreme medical neglect and indifference.[32] In one case, a prisoner serving time for drug offenses "was transferred from DC General Hospital to the [DC] Jail where he" spent 10 days without care from staff.[33] His death led to protests and a judge sending the DC Jail into receivership.[34] The report that led to receivership found that the "death was one of several examples of indifferent treatment of inmates."[35] From the prison's point of view, Lezin observed, "the administrative response to Lorton's health care crisis is that inmates have a far better deal than the general public . . . The problem, according to the Lorton administration, is that inmates traditionally have received minimal health care prior to incarceration so they arrive at Lorton with 'very high needs.'"[36] The underfunded and understaffed prison system thus felt ill-equipped to make up for community lack. (The US lacks universal health care; however, DC began to shift to universal health care in 1999).[37] ART transformed the experience of living with HIV and AIDS in prison by turning it into a chronic illness managed by medication to which prisoners had access once it became available. The Bureau of Justice Statistics reported only one AIDS-related death in the DC prison system in 2001.[38]

While many do not acquire HIV in prison, it is nonetheless a site where people engaging in unprotected sex and injecting drug use can act as bridges of disease acquisition and transmission to partners in and out of prison on their release.[39] Overall, a combination of no medication (only two respondents were on ART during their entire incarceration), limited and hard-to-access HIV testing, a scarcity of condoms and bleach, and continued access to illegal drugs meant that jails and prison carried the risks of continued addiction as well as HIV acquisition and transmission.

THE DC-PRISON DRUG ECONOMY

Jails and prisons had their own drug economies within a larger citywide drug economy. The city policy, by definition, was to cleanly and efficiently sweep up DC's drug users, abusers, and dealers into penitentiaries. Using this metric, the policy was highly successful. By 1987, "more than 70% of the city's prisoners [had] tested positive for drug use."[40] Many of my respondents were incarcerated because of drugs or drug-motivated crime; in other words, they were in for carrying drug paraphernalia, selling drugs, getting caught in possession of drugs, or engaging in crime such as robbery/armed robbery, check fraud, or sex work to get money to buy drugs. However, even after entering prison, drug use continued. Lorton's prisoner drug testing in the 1980s revealed that 10% were using illegal drugs.[41] Not much had changed by the late 1990s, when "nine percent of D.C. Department of Corrections prisoners tested positive for illegal drugs during random checks in the last six months, a percentage almost four times the most recent national average for state prison systems."[42] The national average was 2.6%. "It may be the case that no correctional institution is drug free," a *Washington Post* editorial commented, but these statistics "put the District in a class by itself." It had revealed itself to be "a jail without walls."[43] Indeed, about a third of my incarcerated respondents described the continuous flow of drugs into jail and prison. In forty-nine-year-old Victor's words, "It was more drugs in jail than the streets sometimes, girl. Hell, yeah." He noted that while he was incarcerated, "I was introduced to rocks, crack cocaine in 1988. That's when I was introduced." When I asked how drugs were smuggled in, he responded: "In their anus. Stickin' it up their butt . . . Or sometimes they'll swallow it." These approaches allowed visitors and prisoners to evade strip-search detection. When I asked forty-eight-year-old Kayla whether she was clean (from cocaine and heroin) while incarcerated, she said no, elaborating, "I used to get narcotics uh every Wednesday and Saturday."

The availability of drugs in prison made it hard to quit. Those in recovery are often asked to avoid "people, places, and things" associated with their former drug use,[44] but this would be hard to do in long-term incarceration with nowhere to go. Forty-year-old Benton, who had been in and out of prison between 1991 and 2004, was unable to stay clean while incarcerated despite drug rehabilitation programs.

SANYU: So you weren't clean in prison?

BENTON: No. Well, in the beginning—no. *[laughs]* I was not for some years. I think on the end of it, when I started to get close to my release date . . . because I kept giving dirty urine, so I stopped.

He had gone to prison rehab programs; however, he found "all the drug dealers getting in the drug programs to act like they were gettin' treatment, but they were actually still continuing their business. It was wild."

Besides avoiding prolonged release, drug side effects were another motivation for staying drug free. Forty-six-year-old James, addicted to crack cocaine, explained:

SANYU: So even in jail were you able to get . . .

JAMES: Okay even in jail you're able to get it [drugs], but I don't do it in jail because I don't want to go through the paranoia, I don't want to go through the thing of I need to get up out of here. I don't want to go through that and make my situation even worse than what it is, plus due to the fact I might be caught, even though I'm already locked up.

The porosity of the prison system was well known to prison officials,[45] and the extent of drug trafficking led a judge to refuse to send a prisoner convicted of heroin possession back to the same prison, noting "that it is immoral, futile and meaningless to send a prisoner with a drug problem to the District's prison in southern Fairfax county because narcotics are as available there as they are on the streets of the city."[46] The lax supervision at the prison also reflected a chronic staff shortage. As a result, "the inmates can get anything they want at [Lorton] Central. They can get drugs. They can get wine. They can get sex."[47]

Corrections officers also participated in the drug economy. In an investigative series by reporter Leon Dash, the DC Jail director estimated that 5% or less, "a very, very small percentage" of his 600 officers, used and/or were addicted to drugs; a union official put the estimate at 25% "abusing drugs or alcohol or both."[48] Officers and prisoners who were addicted were highly motivated to acquire drugs and/or money to pay for drugs. Trafficking was also facilitated by the familiarity of prisoners and prison guards. As Warden David Roach at Lorton acknowledged to Robert Blecker:

> These men and my staff have interacted in the formative years, the embryonic years ... They grew up in the same environment, went to the same school, traveled in the same social circle. This cuts both ways: It allows the prison to operate in a more harmonious environment, yet it is not totally professional.[49]

In other words, prisoners and corrections officers were friends, neighbors, and relatives. It was thus not surprising to Blecker that the environment that produced the city's young Black men would "engulf officers no less than inmates."[50]

Investigations revealed both "heads of drug gangs [who] often continue[d] running their businesses from Lorton"[51] and prison guards involved in drug trafficking in Lorton and the DC Jail.[52] By 1992, "more than 30 guards and other employees ha[d] been charged with bribery or drug violations during the three-year undercover investigation by the FBI and the D.C. Department of Corrections."[53] By 1993, this had risen to almost 50 current or former employees, as another 17 were charged with "taking bribes and helping to supply a long-flourishing drug trade inside the sprawling Lorton Correctional

Complex in Northern Virginia ... It was the sixth time in four years that Corrections Department employees have been arrested during undercover investigations ... at Lorton and the D.C. jail."[54] Many were independent operators in crack and powder cocaine, heroin, as well as marijuana,[55] with "payments for smuggling rang[ing] from $100 to $500 depending on the amount of drugs brought inside the jail."[56] However, some were part of a ring. An investigation uncovered a large heroin ring run by Keith Gaffney-Bey out of his cell in Lorton between 1990 and 1994, earning him "$250,000 to $750,000 per year." Gaffney-Bey had already been "serving a 39-year sentence."[57] As Miller reported, he was indicted for

> bribing guards, enticing visitors to bring in drugs, smuggling heroin into the prison by mail, and arranging at least three assaults on inmates who had crossed him ... [He and other prisoners] packaged drugs they got from visitors and guards or through the mail, then made sales by using "drug runners" who went into cells. They stored money, drugs, weapons and other contraband in hiding places throughout the prison complex...[58]

Hall reported that they "smuggled more than 10 kilograms of heroin into the prison, averaging two to three ounces a week" and "carr[ied] money in and out of prison."[59] The ring had enforcers within the prison, beating and starving prisoners into compliance.[60] Gaffney-Bey was sentenced to life without parole.[61]

Fifty-year-old Wynton (in and out of prison between 1977 and 1999) described how prisoners acquired and shared needles to shoot up drugs.

> SANYU: ... were people shooting in jail, shooting drugs in jail?
>
> WYNTON: Yeah ... diabetics and stuff like that, would go to infirmary there, would get needles, they use the needles to, to take they insulin and stuff like that ... they sell them to the people ... Once they got the needles it was like, people didn't move them around but, you know, if you got friends there and they using needles and you want to use their needles, they gonna use them behind. So you never know if they can catch it [HIV] or not.

It is striking how injecting drug use and the needle economy depended on the high prevalence of other diseases in prison—in this case diabetes. Wynton observed how when people came "out of the visiting hall ... they will be waiting for you ... they'll go wait till you got to the dorm, to get, to get it ready, and bag it up and sell it." In this context, it was challenging to stay clean when drugs were regularly coming in and needles were readily available. Overall, the drug economy in the streets did not stop after incarceration but rather continued in a more concentrated fashion within DC jails and prisons, extending the city's drug epidemic and HIV vulnerability.

PRISON SEXUAL ECONOMY AND HIV RISK

There was also a vibrant prison sexual economy that carried HIV risk. Of my 21 respondents with incarceration experience, 17 had HIV during their jail/ prison years, and only two were on ART the entire time they were incarcerated. This was in part because once available, ART recommendations changed over time. At first, medication went to people with AIDS, then universal test-and-treat programs placed people testing positive for HIV on medication right away. Respondents were also on and off medication by their own decision or following doctor recommendations. This is important because the shift to universal test-and-treat programs was partly due to research showing that ART adherence significantly reduced infectivity.[62] (See also Part 2 overview.)

Prison Gendered Sexuality

While prisons were intended as sex-segregated institutions, variation in gendered sexuality at the individual level (gendered and sexual identities, presentations, practices, and bodies) and at the partner level (couple dynamics)[63] worked together to produce a queer sexual economy in this new "neighborhood," where the rules and norms around gender and sexuality were destabilized.[64] With respect to gender, in contrast to the sometimes intense transphobia on the outside, transgender respondents often found themselves in a context where their gender was validated and affirmed, and they were considered highly desirable.[65] Indeed, for some, this, along with the familiarity and longevity of incarceration, led them to begin to transition gender identities, presentations, and bodies while incarcerated. (Those I interviewed were placed in men's prisons at the time of their incarceration as they had not had official gender reassignment).

Forty-two-year-old Hannah began her transition to womanhood at age 30 "when I was in prison. I made a decision that I was gonna live my life as a woman." She felt that she "was always geared that way . . . Now I feel like I'm all that I can be. You know, it's who I am." She began hormone treatment to align her body with her identity and sense of self after she left prison. Forty-year-old Mary described:

> I was just . . . a feminine man who would dress in ladies' clothes . . . I've always lived my life that way, but I didn't begin to do anything towards the transition until my late 20's, early 30's. And that was when I was in jail . . . my first time hormone I ever took I was incarcerated. And I was incarcerated for maybe two years [that time] so I went to jail and I didn't have any breasts, and I came home from jail and I had breasts . . . so um that was the beginning of my transition . . . Another transgender woman . . . began to give me her pills . . . I went to jail with a flat chest and when I came out I was boom.

Now she felt she could "present as who I am inside, ya know, what you see is what you get, um yeah." Fifty-two-year-old Dorothy described how despite being placed in a men's prison, she was able to continue to present as a woman:

> In prison you wear the same jump suits and stuff that the men wear, yeah. But we tend to, um, change our appearance by taking lye soap and dyeing our hair, those kind of things, takin' magic markers and makin' eyebrows . . . the weekends was when we really dressed up, and the guards were like, "What the hell? Where did they get makeup from?" We took crayons and stuff and made colors, very creative.

She had to deal with the sexual harassment that often comes with womanhood, but as she aged, she transitioned from being seen solely as a sexual object, describing, "I had what I call sons, they called me Big Mama. I was their mother."

As described in Chapter 5, Dorothy was first incarcerated at age 14 for stealing women's underwear. She described a supportive atmosphere in juvenile detention:

> DOROTHY: When I left, I cried. I cried 'cause I felt like I was leavin' a sense of home, because I was more accepted there than I was at home.
>
> SANYU: Why do you think that was?
>
> DOROTHY: I think that because there's no judgment . . . we know that people still do have stigma. But I happened to go through a system, where let me just say, it wasn't all perfect, but it wasn't all bad. It was enough that I actually came out affirmed, "This is who I am." So at 16, 17, I knew affirmatively, "I am a woman. This is who I am, I'm transgender." And I wasn't gonna be changing.

Trans woman Grace was in and out of prison between 1973 and 1994, incarcerated on a variety of drug-related charges including drug distribution, possession with intent to distribute, and assault with a deadly weapon. Having spent more than half her life incarcerated, prison felt like home, and

> the final time I cried. I cried because again I left an environment where I became institutionalized, that I was used to, that I felt was like, this was my family. I was accepted. The guards loved me. The administrators loved me. "You're goin' home today. Seven years. We're gonna miss you." And I cried. My friends, actually, that came and got me, said, "You're crying? Why?" I said, "It's my family." You develop that kinship, you know.

In addition to destabilizing normative gender, this "neighborhood" also destabilized heteronormative sexuality.[66] Sex was a key medium through which masculinity was expressed or negated, and femininity was prized or degraded. Further, sex was engaged in not just by gay men or transgender women but also by straight men. As Regina Kunzel noted in an award-winning history of US prison sexuality, "Prison is but one locus from which modern sexuality has been confounded and destabilized by sexual acts, desires and identities that failed (and fail) to map neatly onto categories of 'gay' or 'straight.'"[67]

Thus, despite attempts by prison researchers and administrators to contain this instability to the prison setting, calling it for example "situational homosexuality,"[68] prison sex "challeng[es] . . . the edifice of the sexual binary," and "the homo/heterosexual binary could not capture the complexity of human sexual desire, identification and practice."[69] Indeed, sexual fluidity in the general population is common. Analyzing a nationally representative longitudinal sample, Joel Mittleman found that within a five-year period, "24% of all respondents changed sexual attractions . . . [and] 1 in 11 changed sexual identity," with most moves between bisexual and straight categories.[70] Sexual opportunity structures[71] in prison and the prominence of incarceration in many Black men's lives[72] meant that prison may have played a special role in further destabilizing the gay/straight binary among Black men. Indeed Emma Mishel and colleagues found significant increases in proportions of Black men born between 1956 and 1975 who had had male and female sexual partners, and they also found a significant association between having been incarcerated and having sex with men and women.[73] The implications of this finding for DC, where half the young men spent a sometimes significant portion of their lives incarcerated, is that they were relatively more exposed to an environment where sexuality was unanchored from heteronormative sexuality, with potential reverberations back to the community. As I will describe, based on my respondents' experiences and observations, many men they had relationships with resumed public heterosexual lives with cisgender women, with a rigidly enforced code of silence about their prison sexual practices.

Navigating the Prison Sexual Economy

My respondents described the same full range of sexual relationships that could be found in the community, including long, short-term, and casual consensual relationships; coercive and forced sex/sexual slavery; rape; and commercial sex with and without pimps. Prison reproduced and sometimes exacerbated the violent, coercive, and traumatic experiences they had had in the community, with little hope of escape before release. However, it also created conditions for long, intense, and loving relationships, reinforced by proximity in a closed environment for long periods of time. Limited medication and condom use meant all these relationships carried HIV risk.

Sexual Violence Overall, my respondents described different kinds of violent sex: sexual bondage or slavery involving "ownership" and the sale of sex, repeated forced sex, individual acts of rape, and forced sex meted out as punishment. For those subjected to these relationships, the only way out was through violence, solitary confinement, or prison release. The most extreme kind of violent sex was what appeared to be sexual bondage or slavery, which included forced sex. Forty-three-year-old Langston, incarcerated for three years, described how prisoners "belonged" to other men:

> They'd tell other inmates . . . "You know he belong to him" . . . and then if a guy liked you he would go to him and give him two or three cigarettes, and he could have you for them two or three cigarettes. So yeah . . . they sell you, you know, you wash their clothes, wash their underwear, their socks, their T-shirts. You know they sell you for a candy bar or for cookies and stuff like that, and then they knew these guys couldn't do nothing about that because they belong to him . . .

This ownership was reinforced by violence. If a person resisted,

> he'll beat you up, you, you gonna take that whupping or you fight back . . . that's how prison is. You know the, the strong prey on the weak . . . So either you did what they want you to do, or you stood up and you fought, and, and that's what it is.

Hannah spiraled down from life as a college-educated professional to selling sex and robbing stores to acquire money for her crack addiction. She was eventually arrested and began her in-and-out prison career, which lasted from 1992 to 2007. While Hannah could have acquired HIV in the context of selling sex, in her interview she attributed it to rape in prison. She went on to describe imprisonment within prison:

> HANNAH: [I] went to prison, and that's where I think I contracted the disease from . . . Because the very first time I went to prison and I got tested I was negative . . . And then I got raped in prison. It was ok. *[silence]* But you know, when somebody takes something from you, it kinda messes with your mind. So um, I'm not really sure where I contracted it . . . but I believe that it was in prison . . . after that ordeal I became hard and bitter and you know, um, it took years for me to get out of that frame of mind . . . [Prison] was mean sometimes. The COs [correctional officers] treated you bad. Sometimes the guys would be too attracted to you and make your life [a] living hell, you know, keep you in bondage, and don't want you to go out.
>
> SANYU: How? How is that possible?
>
> HANNAH: Tell you not to come out the door or they'll kill you.
>
> SANYU: *[sighs]*
>
> HANNAH: They didn't want anybody else to have you . . . we were like women on the compound.

Forty-three-year-old Sidney also attributed HIV acquisition to prison rape, though he was also exposed in multiple ways. It occurred after a condensed life of pain. He was molested as a child at 8, 11, and 14 years old. His drug use to "take away the pain I was feeling" began at the age of 11, and it escalated as he transitioned to adulthood and endured abuse from his alcoholic father and buried his mother. Drug use and armed robbery led to his first incarceration, and his incarceration cycle spanned 12 years. Two years into his first consensual relationship, which started at 17, he was incarcerated. He found out he had HIV "when I was 19 . . . I had gotten incarcerated and got raped again while I was incarcerated, and I think one of [the] guys was HIV positive that raped me when I was in jail with. So I think that's where I got HIV from."

Forty-year-old trans woman Liza's incarceration spanned from 1986 to 2007. She was diagnosed in 1990 during a jail stint and was raped multiple times.

Jail was really traumatic for me because of who I am, you know. I was feminine, I looked very feminine, and I was raped, um *[long pause]* ya know, I mean was raped on several, numerous occasions, assaulted um *[long pause]*. It was hard, ya know, um until I became seasoned and had some experience with coming to jail and stuff, you know. I could navigate around the, you know, bullshit more easily um, and then I began to inflict my pain on other people, you know what I'm saying … having unprotected sex with people *[pause]* and they don't know my HIV status, um *[pause]* you know, so. And the guilt involved with that, that's just enough you know.

Prison rape was also used by men to exert power and dominance over people who "showed a form of weakness" and to exact revenge for actions conducted on the street. Besides fighting to defend themselves or prove their masculinity so that they could be left alone, prisoners would also form "protective pairings"[74] to protect themselves from violence. This could either involve having a partner "because they were afraid that people might beat them up or take advantage of them, so they would get a boy, they would get somebody to, you know, protect them." Others would form protective groupings with older prisoners who "took me under their wing, so I was protected."

Short- and Long-Term Consensual Relationships. Respondents, including those who also had experiences of forced sex, reported a variety of casual consensual sexual encounters while incarcerated, some concurrent and some monogamous. As trans woman Carol described,

> Actually, the girls don't mind going to jail, 'cause the guys like you there. It's not a good situation because you're not free. You're not able to go to 7-Eleven, you're not able to go to McDonald's. You're not able to do things the way you want to, dress the way you want to, wear makeup and stuff. But while you're there, you have guys interested in you all the time. Like I said, they just want a hole to fuck, they want to just come, and then you get your pleasure too.

Forty-three-year-old Maggie, who transitioned from being a gay man to being a trans woman while incarcerated, described her first incarceration experience as "exciting, it was interesting … I was like, hey, candy land"; however, "[I] scattered myself around with the guys like a piece of trash and that's exactly what they treated me like, was a piece of trash, um." She described learning the hard way that "even in jail you have to respect yourself." For those wanting to find a more serious partner, in contrast to community experiences where men were scarce (see Part 2), and where those who pursued transgender women for noncasual relationships were even more scarce, in prison finding a boyfriend was easy. Hannah explained, "They were men and they were horny and they needed . . . attention and affection, so the guys would come up to you and you just pick one." Here, there was no competition with cisgender women, and there was no partner shortage problem.

Respondents also discussed long-term relationships, especially if they had longer prison sentences. Forty-nine-year-old Victor, who was gay, described short- and long-term "husband" relationships during his three-decade incarceration career. He discovered he had HIV in 1998, five months after leaving one of his stints, and started ART in 2008. As he described prison when he first arrived:

> Oh my God. The first time around was like paradise. 'Cause I was young, and it seemed like I was in popular demand. All the boys, oh, my God! [affected accent] Men, men, men, men! It's a faggy's paradise when you first started out. Oh! I'm young, the boys are young, they love me, honey! Whooh! You could just—boom! I had that. Oh! I want some of that one. And they were usin' it. They were coming! They was comin', 'cause we the closest thing to a woman anyway, and I've always been a fem queen. Girl! . . .

However, "after a while, baby, anything start gettin' old. They started gettin' on my nerves." So he decided to change strategies, describing how he "always kept a husband, you know, because once you got a husband, you just dealin' with one person. So I tried to find that one man." While his family "always made sure I had money on the books so I never had to do all that trickin' [selling sex] and all that shit like that unless I wanted to," a husband who provided was always helpful. Victor described the qualities he looked for in a husband:

> I was lookin' for, first of all, he has to be a roughneck. He has to know how to treat me. He has to know all my wants, 'cause then you know, I'm very high-maintenance. I can't stand no broke n*****, so first when they come in, first thing I'm doin' is lookin' at their shoes. "OK, he's got some shoes." I'm seein' if he goin' to the truck, which is canteen, uh, seein' if he got, you know, his swag, make sure that n***** can fight, 'cause I know I can throw 'em. So he will have to be past me, 'cause I know I knock a n*****out. So he want to keep me order, 'cause I can't stand no bitch-ass n*****. Excuse the expression! . . . They gonna be bringin' in drugs. Yeah. They're gonna be steppin' it up. They gon' be taking care of my habit, 'cause I snort dope in jail."

On occasions, Victor also "kept me a sugar daddy. He'd be paying my bills and he'll make sure that I'm all right, and he'll buy me anything off the canteen that I want and I give him a little sex." Throughout Victor's account, it was clear that his ability to successfully negotiate violence was critical to preserving his ability to choose his partners and only have consensual casual, transactional, or "husband" sex while incarcerated.

For Hannah, prison was both a place of extreme trauma as well as profound love. For her, "all the loves of my life were in prison." Describing one loving relationship, she said:

> I started doing his hair and we started getting closer. He lived in one unit, I lived in another unit, and we were just talking, and when we talking we found out we had a lot in common. And I fell in love with him and he fell in love with me.

She elaborated on how couples navigated the prison rules in order to be together:

> You get your man, you moved in the cell with him, you live together . . . you just make arrangements to move in the cell with him . . . You know you can buy a cell with stamps or a canteen, it's ways. You want somebody to move out of their cell that you're in, you just be like, "I give you fifty bucks of stamps," that was the money in jail. You know the gambling stuff. "Give me fifty bucks of stamps, you get him."

She also discussed why it was important to pick partners wisely:

> HANNAH: If you got a boyfriend that can't really take care of you, then you mess around with the other guy, so you can take care of you and your boyfriend. I've never had that happen to me, but it has happened. You go to prison and you, you choose a broke motherfucker, then you take care of both of them, you know, you trip with this one, you trip with that one to bring food in the house.
>
> SANYU: Wow. Ok. So, so part of the choosing, you, you also have to choose someone who is, who has enough money or has enough currency so that you won't have to . . .
>
> HANNAH: Be out there like that.

After Lorton closed and Hannah started doing time in federal prisons, she found they preferred—and indeed enforced—long-term partnerships because "it keeps the drama down":

The administration would tell you, you know, "Yes you, you're attractive, and you woo woo woo, but if you get caught having sex, you're going to be locked down forever. Get you a boyfriend and don't, you know, don't make my compound a havoc." You know they wanted us to get one person and be with them and, you know. *[Sanyu: Oh the prison was saying that?]* Yes. He said you got a week to get a boyfriend. *[silence]* Don't have people running in and out your dorm. I don't know who you know. Don't put my compound in an uproar or I'm gonna lock your ass on down. And when, what I mean locking down, that means solitary confinement.

Thus, rather than the prisoners pursuing her being locked down, she was held responsible for controlling men's desire for her. And as is historical for women,[75] she would be severely sanctioned if she failed.

COMMUNITY SYNDEMIC AMPLIFICATION

Correctional facilities did not just host drug and sexual economies or collect people who used and sold drugs, sold sex, or lived with HIV. They also amplified the spread of HIV within Black communities.[76] Scholars have found significant positive associations between prison release and HIV/AIDS infections in the community, even at the zip code level.[77] In the post-ART era, this can occur if prisoners are not linked to care in the community and engage in unprotected sexual or drug-use practices on release.[78] Rucker Johnson and Steven Raphael concluded that their "estimates suggest that the lion's share of the racial differentials in AIDS infections rates for both men and women are attributable to racial differences in incarceration trends."[79] In DC, with prison HIV prevalence rates as high as 16% in the '80s[80] and 7.8% in the '90s,[81] people living in prison zip codes, sending and receiving disproportionate numbers of prisoners, were especially vulnerable to HIV acquisition and transmission. My interviews shed light on how this might happen.

Prisoners were not always monogamous—some had ongoing relationships outside of prison. However, a code of silence was maintained because disclosure would mean not only disclosure of nonmonogamy but also of queer sexual practice. Trans woman Melissa elaborated:

You'll get killed telling somebody's business like that. That's considered being hot ... you'll get killed, honey, they don't play that. Your wife comes ... and then the gay person plays their position. Ok, he's like, "I'm going to visit to see my kids and my baby's momma. I'll see you when I get back, ok baby." You play your position, you play your role, you stay in your lane.

Melissa was diagnosed with HIV in 1994, two years into her incarceration cycle. She only disclosed this to one serious partner. She was on medication for part of that time, but her condom use was inconsistent. Even when relationships were very close in prison, once outside, in Melissa's view, relationships on the street took precedence:

> When you get on the street it's a whole 'nother, of course their intentions are good. We're gonna be together on the street, you know, selling you the dream. It's only a dream. That's all it is. Because when they get on the street it's gonna be something completely different, and, if you're lucky, you'll see 'em, and even if you see them on the street, you know, they don't acknowledge you, you don't acknowledge them. *[silence]*

Victor drew on his personal experience and observations in his explanation of "the way it [HIV] got into y'all world, the heterosexual world":

> Because ... [prisoners] in Lorton and in incarceration are fuckin' these boys and comin' home ... gettin' fucked by these boys with HIV, they come home to their women and kids and children, and now they're havin' unprotected sex with their wives. And they're not tellin' them what they done did in the past, in the dark ... 'cause like I say, there's a lot of kinky men that once in a while like to get plunged. And that's how it is to me, and I *know* that's how it got into the heterosexual world ... they beatin' us to the Vaseline ...

(Receptive anal sex is the highest risk sex for HIV acquisition.)[82] I asked Victor, diagnosed with HIV and not on ART for 10 years during his prison career, whether he disclosed his HIV status to prison partners and used a condom.

> You know, they give 'em out in jail. Yes, they do, hmm. And then, like I said, I always kept a husband, so I wasn't—just because I was subject to HIV, I'm not gonna pass it on like that. But no, to answer the question, I never disclosed that to any of my partners, because by lookin' at me, I don't look like it. I never had thrush, never no weight loss ... [I] didn't have no HIV signs.

Forty-year-old Benton, who identified as gay, became addicted to crack, and he started shoplifting and then engaging in burglary, selling the procured goods to buy drugs. He was in and out of prison between 1991 and 2004, and he was diagnosed with HIV in 1988. He had been on and off medication based on doctor's orders.

They had put me on a pill when I went to prison, but I went to another doctor in there and they took me off because, he said, "Your numbers are too high for you to be takin' medicine, and if you happen to get sick, you'll probably be immune, and we don't want you to be immune to the medication." So they took me off because I stayed healthy.

As noted earlier, he sometimes used condoms and sometimes did not. He described two "long, strong relationships" with bisexual men. In the first relationship, they were "just together for a long time." It was serious enough that he was "introduced to his mother, his family." The relationship ended when "I actually got busted for bringing in drugs and then they sent me somewhere else." His other relationship lasted two years. They separated when his partner was sent to another prison, but "eventually I got into a fight and I ended up getting sent right to the camp where he was, so we resumed the relationship." However, his partner was released from prison first, and he "was more of a bisexual person . . . I think he's married now." Benton disclosed his HIV status to both partners "because of the seriousness of the relationship and how we had become so connected." In both cases "they were still like, 'Man, we can just use condoms now, I'll go get checked, make sure I'm alright.'"

Transgender respondents struggled with disclosure in prison because, on the one hand, "being transgender in jail and [having] HIV was a no-no" and was therefore "like hide and seek"—hiding status and hiding medication; on the other hand, if a partner "find out you're HIV and you didn't say, you're in for it." Trans women noted that they had to be very careful whom they disclosed to, even in serious relationships. Prison provided them a unique space, affording many options to find long-term relationships, but disclosing their HIV status to the wrong person—who could be violent or spread their news and expose them to intense stigma—had the potential to negatively transform that experience, as once out in the "real world," they experienced the same community constraints they had before (see Chapter 5). Describing one such relationship, for example, Melissa noted that after a partner was released, "he came to visit me and he sent me money and stuff," but he later "told me he got married to a real woman, so I already know who that is."

Respondents on the outside also thought that prison played a role in the community's HIV epidemic, and for some it was personal. Fifty-four-year-old trans woman Della, who had never been incarcerated, described a relationship with an incarcerated partner who she believed gave her HIV. She met him when she was 22 and "went with him off and on" for the next 11 years (1977–88). What severely strained and eventually broke the relationship was that

I just couldn't keep going back and forth to jail. I went to every jail . . . in the DC, Maryland, Virginia surrounding area just to see him and stuff. I couldn't do it anymore. I was tired of it. So we kind of parted ways. I still talk to him today though. He's married and got a wife, um *[silence]*.

I asked her why she thought that he had given her HIV, and she responded, "Well because for one thing, I know that he's HIV positive. He's been since 19 . . . 85, and I found out in 1990 that I was *[silence]*." She had reason to believe he was nonmonogamous because he had twice given her an STI, syphilis the first time and gonorrhea the second.

An important dimension of Della's account is her partner's circular migration, back and forth from jail. Indeed, globally, migration has been an important vehicle for HIV spread. Circular labor migrants establishing relationships at work and at home bridged sexual networks through which HIV spread.[83] US prisoners were essentially circular migrants,[84] with parole violations for failing drug tests exerting a strong structural pull back to prison for addicted people. Some of the most frequent circular migrants among my respondents were sex workers with addiction who had especially high HIV risk (see Chapter 8). Sex workers were regularly arrested in sweeps and incarcerated for short periods of time before being released.

For many of my respondents, their circular community-prison migration spanned one or two decades during not just the prison boom but also the rapid rise of the HIV/AIDS epidemic prior to universal ART medication, which kept viral loads—and thus infectivity—consistently low. Unprotected sex was facilitated by limited condom availability and use in correctional facilities. In combination, this created feedback loops for prison and community HIV spread in prison zip codes. Regular circulation and repartnering meant that relatively few transmission events were needed to amplify racially contained neighborhood epidemics. Importantly, women in the community also had concurrent relationships while their partners were incarcerated.[85] Della believed she got HIV from her incarcerated partner; however, it was apparent in her interview that HIV may have come from other avenues because while he was locked up, "other people were interested, right?" Overall, these accounts illustrate pathways through which HIV could spread in prison, in subsequent relationships with partners after leaving prison, and through community members' concurrent relationships while their incarcerated partners were away, putting returning prisoners at risk of acquiring HIV.

This Part has illustrated how policies designed to end the city syndemic led to mass incarceration, another form of racial containment. Yet in a similar fashion to previous attempts to contain social ills in specific spaces and among particular groups of people, these efforts nonetheless served to not just replicate but also amplify both physical and social deaths of African Americans. By continuing to draw on the logic of racial and class containment to select entrants into prison, Washington, DC, reproduced and exacerbated the ill effects of its sacrifice zones through policing policies, educational policies, and crime and prison policies. Parole policies in turn drew many prisoners into multiyear, back-and-forth journeys to prison, limiting their abilities to establish stable lives outside of prison and enhancing syndemic vulnerability for prisoners and the communities to which they returned.

Racial containment also served to contain the massive effects of these policy decisions to minority communities and made it easier to then blame these same communities for the outcomes of these decisions, especially as they began to have widespread intergenerational effects.[86] Poor minority children have been growing up without fathers,[87] in poor, segregated neighborhoods, attending underfunded prisonlike schools. These conditions increase their likelihood of following in their fathers' footsteps—being pre-criminalized, disproportionately arrested, dropping out of high school, becoming incarcerated, and struggling to have a foothold on life outside prison.

Importantly, these policy decisions occurred across party and racial lines. This underscores the limitations of political blame games and distracts from the larger racialized institutional logics embedded in a variety of American institutions that work redundantly to replicate disproportionate vulnerability to social and physical death among African Americans across historical eras. In the final Part, I examine more closely how the city attempted to control the HIV/AIDS epidemic.

Racial Containment and the City's HIV/AIDS Epidemic Response

Them are the things that I think that need to be talked about in DC mainly. 'Cause to say DC has—HIV has a higher percentage than some third-world countries, that sounds like sayin', Where are we livin'? . . . This is supposed to be the capital of the world, but we can't even control somethin' like that.

THEO

THIS PART EXAMINES THE PARADOX of Washington, DC, hosting one of the nation's worst HIV/AIDS epidemics[1] even while it was the capital city, partially governed by the nation's lawmakers with access to the nation's full resources, surrounded by the nation's leading HIV-related institutions (e.g., the National Institutes of Health, the Department of Health and Human Services, and the Food and Drug Administration), and having local Black leaders whose fellow Black people were disproportionately affected. I draw on archival newspaper research, academic and other literature reviews, longitudinal city HIV/AIDS surveillance data, life history interviews with Black people living with HIV in DC in 2011 when the epidemic was near its peak, and key informant interviews with city officials, community organization leaders, and health workers (2011–23). I use these data to examine the city's successes and failures in responding to the epidemic and to understand why and how racial inequality in AIDS mortality dramatically widened *after* antiretroviral therapy (ART) became widely available. Overall, I show how the enduring role of racial containment, working through intersectional (racial, gay, and class) city politics, Congress's paternalistic relationship with the city, the city's financial bureaucratic system, and the HIV/AIDS agency, placed limits on the ability of technocratic expertise to eliminate racial health inequality.

. . .

PART 5 PLAYLIST

Louis Armstrong	When the Saints Go Marching In (1938)
Mariah Carey and Boyz II Men	One Sweet Day (1995)
Al Green	Precious Lord (1982)
Public Enemy	Meet the G That Killed Me (1990)
Disposable Heroes of Hiphopcrisy	Positive (1992)
Salt-N-Pepa	Let's Talk About Sex (Let's Talk About AIDS) (1992)
Lil B	I Got AIDS (2011)
Bill Withers	Lean on Me (1972)
Cece Winans and Whitney Houston	Count on Me (1995)
Marvin Sapp	He Saw the Best in Me (2010)
Kirk Franklin	Lean on Me (1998)
The Clark Sisters	You Brought the Sunshine (1981)
Andra Day	Rise Up (2015)
Chuck Brown & The Soul Searchers	We Need Some Money (1998)
Backyard Band	I Can Change (2011)

TWELVE

Intersectional Politics and the AIDS Epidemic

IN THIS CHAPTER, I DESCRIBE the city's racially bifurcated AIDS epidemic and the experiences of people who lived in and through it. I then show that while the city was pioneering in its response in the pre-ART years, intersectional power politics and dynamics shaped its decisions around resource allocation in ways that resulted in worse provision for poor Black people living with HIV/AIDS.

A RACIALLY BIFURCATED AIDS EPIDEMIC

Figure 42 illustrates cumulative AIDS mortality by race/ethnicity between 1983 and 2021, drawing on longitudinal city surveillance data and the latest reports (2021 and 2023). By 2021, an estimated 11,800 Black and 2,449 White people in DC had died of AIDS. The figure shows how after the ART rollout in the mid-1990s, White deaths stabilized while technically preventable Black deaths skyrocketed.

The extent of post-ART inequality is more fully captured by contextualizing the number of AIDS deaths against the racial proportions of the population. In 1983, 50% of AIDS deaths were among White people (then 25% of the city population); by 1996, they comprised 27.3% of deaths and about 27.7% of the population. By 2021, White people comprised 16.3% of the cumulative total (1983–2021) of AIDS deaths, while comprising an increasing proportion of the city population between 1997 and 2021 (27.9% in 2000, 34.8% in 2010, 38.0% in 2020). In 1983, Black people comprised 50% of AIDS deaths and 69.7% of the city population; by 1996, they comprised 70% of deaths and 62% of the population; and by 2021, they comprised 78.6% of the

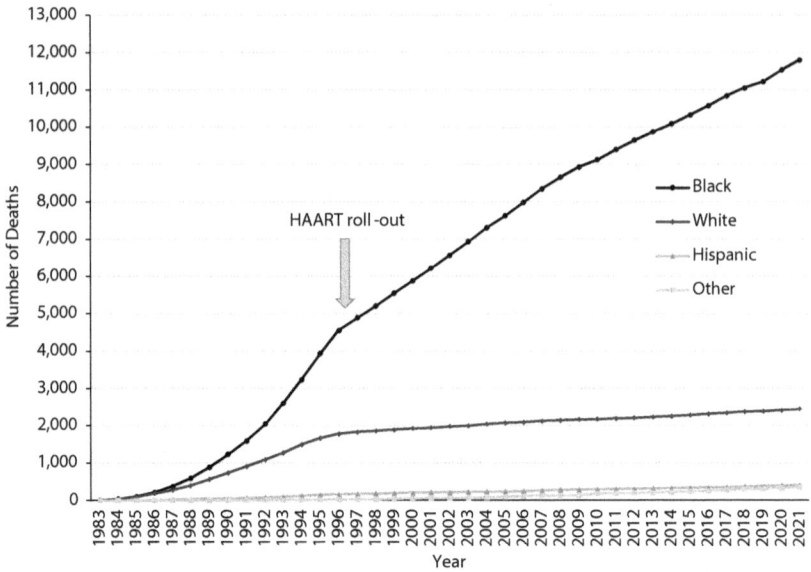

FIGURE 42. Cumulative AIDS mortality by race/ethnicity, DC, 1983–2021. Data sources: DC HAHSTA HIV/AIDS Surveillance Unit (1983–2014); DC HAHSTA, *Annual Epidemiology and Surveillance Reports*, 2021 and 2023 (2015–2021).

cumulative total of AIDS deaths, while comprising a decreasing proportion of the population (59.5% in 2000, 50% in 2010, 40.9% in 2020). To put this another way, there were an estimated 1,775 White and 4,551 Black AIDS deaths between 1983 and 1996—about 2.6 times more Black deaths; after ART, an estimated 674 White people and 7,249 Black people died of AIDS—about *11 times more* Black deaths. Thus, rather than closing the racial gap, ART greatly exacerbated it. The stabilization of White AIDS deaths illustrates what was possible once medication became available: several thousands of Black deaths could have been averted.

LIVING WITH AND THROUGH THE HIV/AIDS EPIDEMIC IN WASHINGTON, DC

Black AIDS Deaths

As HIV transformed from a silently spreading epidemic into visible mass death, racial containment meant that AIDS deaths clustered in particular neighborhoods and communities (see Figure 8). Respondents described seeing AIDS decimate their social networks of family, friends, and intimate partners. When Helen found out she had HIV, she

thought I was gonna die. I had friends around me that were dying. I mean they were dying in alleys and they was just dropping off dying 'cause I guess the epidemic back then was brand new ... so after I found out it was like a death sentence.

Describing the death of almost her entire friendship group, trans woman Priscilla pointed to a photograph on her office desk:

I took a picture at a club ... *[shows me the picture]* These are some of the girls that I grew up with when this virus first hit the city ... This is one Friday or Saturday night when we had left the club ... Every one of these girls *[each word with emphasis, pointing to each girl]*, no, well wait a minute, this one, this one, this one, this one, and this one, all of them [are] dead. These two died at the very onset of HIV when AIDS hit DC. This one I believe passed about midway into the nineties, as well as this one. This one, I think she died probably around '90, '91. This girl here and I are the only two girls out of these, this whole group, a sisterhood, just a small part of our sisterhood, we are the only two still alive. And when they died, I knew what they died from.

Ruth described losing half her network:

Nobody's around. Half of them are gone, you know. That's what happened. They wind up, you know, catching the same disease, but they, they passed, you know. I'm just one of the fortunate ones who's still here. 'Cause I know like a good maybe 30 or 40 people that I used to get high with, and they have passed from this disease ... they gone.

These descriptions are tragically typical of pre-ART mass AIDS death in White gay communities in DC and around the country. Indeed, the sexual containment of the White epidemic, and the story told by Figure 42 in the early years, meant that AIDS was particularly and proportionally devastating for White gay men.[1] However, as illustrated in the figure, over 7,000 Black people died *after* ART was widely available. Lack of or delayed ART access and use for Black people was due to both individual and structural city-level factors. At an individual level, interviews revealed the role of spillover and unaddressed mental health crises following diagnosis.

The Weight of an HIV Diagnosis

Among many of my respondents, an HIV diagnosis was emotionally devastating and received as a death sentence, with some becoming suicidal regardless of whether they were diagnosed before or after ART. When Cora was diagnosed in 1989, she "ran from it, a long time" and went on "a heroin-induced suicide mission, you know people commit suicide in different ways." Victor, diagnosed in 1998, "tried to kill myself with the drugs, and then I tried to commit suicide. Because I felt like my life was over." Fifty-one-year-old Cornelius followed "the prescription of death" after his 2004 diagnosis. He "was admitted to a psych ward because I took it so badly, and I got myself out." He "figured I was gonna die anyway ... the people I knew who had HIV were dying, so ... I didn't know what to do." So he "wouldn't take [ART] medicine, um. I had a prescription of death ... where, you don't take medicine, you don't eat, you just use drugs." Suicidality was not just a temporary state following the shock of diagnosis. For 49-year-old Theo, the experience of intense HIV stigma kept these feelings close to the surface over his 23 years living with HIV. He described how even seeing HIV stigma affected him: "[Someone] had a seizure ... and the ambulance people came, and they wouldn't even touch him, 'cause they knew he had HIV. To be livin' with this and know that's how people will treat you is hurtin' sometimes." He frequently experienced rejection in romantic relationships. Like others who felt that HIV had permanently disqualified them from love because "I'm just not good enough to love," Theo found himself fighting for his humanity and personhood, encouraging himself by saying to himself, "I'm still a person. I still have a good heart. I'm still human." He reflected that "this has not been easy ... I've felt like killin' myself. I've tried to kill myself."

The weight of an HIV diagnosis was thus compounded by a dense and multilayered community stigma—combining addiction stigma, HIV stigma, transphobia, homophobia, shame, rejection, and dehumanization—making people feel like "it's stamped on my head that I'm a tainted person" and that they were "tainted all the way around the board." Several key informants also observed this community-level stigma. A White government official observed, "The stigma was huge, the stigma in the Black community was much higher and more severe and that limited ... so much of people getting what they need on every level." Asking a Black government official whether things were better, they responded:

I wouldn't say things are better now [2011], I would say there are more resources out there. I think the biggest thing that we have is to not stigmatize the disease, and the stigma is still out there. I can remember even from the friends that I know personally who died from AIDS, they still didn't wanna let anyone know that they had the disease, and I'm talking, the most recent person died two years ago [2009]. And it's always "They're sick," ya know. You can look and figure out, 'cause if you're sick and you have cancer, people are vocal about it but when it's AIDS, it's always, "They're sick." So it's still a stigma. So no, things have not gotten better.

A transgender community leader living with HIV described the additional transphobia and having to "live such a life of stigma, demoralization, and just disenfranchised from family members."

Compounding emotional and mental health challenges, about a third of my sample also dealt with overlapping chronic diseases as they aged, reflecting how syndemics operate at both individual and community levels. HIV accelerates aging and earlier onset of chronic diseases. As Deeks and colleagues noted:

> Antiretroviral therapy does not fully restore health in all individuals; well treated HIV-infected adults have higher than expected risk of several non-AIDS disorders, including cardiovascular disease, kidney disease, liver disease, malignancy, and some neurological diseases. Although antiretroviral therapy often restores peripheral CD4+ T-cell counts, persistent immune dysfunction, inflammation, and coagulation abnormalities persist and strongly predict risk of non-AIDS morbidity and mortality.[2]

Comorbidities were a one-two punch for people who were trying to get back on their feet after an HIV diagnosis. Some had one other condition. Thirty-four-year-old Jacob had just left hospital after cancer treatment when I interviewed him. Finding out he had lymphoma "was like a blow to me, and that was like on top of my HIV status, so um. I became very depressed in the hospital." Forty-nine-year-old Hazel could only work two or three days a week now. Her chronic disease "pain is too intense." She was now on disability, and when "maybe every three or four months that I'm behind in the utility ... by the grace of God there is this company or that company that helps to support HIV folks. I can go to them and get some help. So it's eking [out] an existence." Others had multiple chronic conditions:

> I have hepatitis C now, I have chronic kidney disease that's really bad ... I have high blood pressure I didn't know about. I'm vitamin D deficient, my bones are weak. There's just a lot goin' on ... I know that I'm also bipolar ...

The complexity of comorbidities, coupled with the challenging material life circumstances of many with HIV, may have contributed to premature death. They would get "tired of taking my medicine today so I'm not taking it for another two weeks." Hazel described how

> some of my friends have passed in the middle of, ya know, you find out that you got hep C. So now you have to take the rigorous thing for hep C and your HIV meds, and something's gotta, go, so I'm not gon' take my HIV meds. Okay, so I'm beginning to get cured from the hep C and then here comes something else, and I'm dying of hep C and pneumonia complications that have nothing to do with the HIV.

The most challenging comorbidities with respect to HIV transmission were addiction and mental health challenges following diagnosis. As Ida described:

> When a person is diagnosed HIV positive, I feel that they need to get them therapy. Off the break, you need therapy . . . You know your mind is so far gone then, 'cause first of all, you already told me I'm dying . . . A lot of newly diagnosed people don't even hear the part they have HIV and you can get treated. They hear I'm dying. So now I'm going out and I, I'm gonna live recklessly . . . I was diagnosed and it was at least 10 years before I ever got on even, any, any type of medicine . . . until one day one doctor said " . . . You only have 1 T cell left in your body," and I decided to take medicine . . . I used to always say *[laughs]* if I just take another hit of crack I'd be alright *[laughs]*, but that was just the insanity of the addiction.

Cora, diagnosed in 1989, got onto treatment in 2006.

> CORA: I was always looking for *[pause]* happiness, stability, strength . . . I went in and out of the methadone clinic, in and out of the church, in and out of relationships . . . I tried the detoxes, the psychiatric wards . . . the this, the that . . . the moving, the men, the *[pause]* everything. So, nothing worked.
>
> SANYU: Oh, to try and deal with—
>
> CORA: Right. The damn mental health issues, yeah. Mm-hmm.

Indeed, over and over in interviews, the mental weight of the diagnosis with its toxic mix of stigma, denial, devastation, and suicidality led many respondents to postpone treatment and engage in high- or higher-risk practices for HIV transmission—more injecting drug use, more unprotected sex, and in the case of Tiana, "I didn't start taking medication until after [the birth], I mean, they wanted me to, I just didn't. I think I was still a little in denial. You know."

For respondents who did not start medication right away, the gap between diagnosis and treatment ranged between five and 17 years, and for at least half, it was 10 or more years. (Two respondents were long-term nonprogressors [see Part 3] living without medication for over 20 years). Limited treatment kept community viral load and transmission probabilities high. This in part reflected shifting HIV treatment policy, as noted in Part 4;[3] however, as interviews revealed, it was also about how untreated mental health crises interacted with other life challenges. (As described in Parts 2–4, for many respondents, an HIV diagnosis occurred at the tail end of a series of traumatic life events, such as child abuse, eviction from home by parents, a decades-long struggle with drug addiction, multiple family and friend deaths, persistent homelessness, intimate partner violence, and traumatic incarceration experiences). HIV pre- and post-test counseling sessions were not necessarily designed to deal with complex lifelong trauma. Steven, a community health worker, felt overwhelmed:

> At that time they had a three-day training in order to become a certified tester and counselor in DC, and that was done through the HIV/AIDS administration. It was a very, very intense training. However, when you're dealing with disadvantaged populations, people sufferin' a lot of trauma, you have to be equipped with the tools to really be able to assist them. And so I guess it was not having the counseling skills.

The brief counseling session did little to lighten the ability of an HIV diagnosis to undercut what little will some had to live, even when ART was available.[4]

Personal Safety Nets

While thousands died of AIDS, thousands more lived with HIV. I was keenly aware that I was talking to survivors, those who somehow made it through the pre- and post-ART years. Their interviews revealed the important role of personal safety nets in their survival.

Family and Friends. For many respondents, DC was where they grew up, and they had to decide whether to disclose their status to family and friends. Some, like trans woman Della, kept their status secret because "I never wanted to burden my family with my sexuality, first of all, and I definitely don't want to burden them with my health, right? So it's just something that

I deal with personally I guess." Silence, however, could be deadly. Hazel noted how not disclosing precluded life-saving, transmission-reducing support. As she reflected:

> That's part of what keeps the epidemic going is ain't nobody saying your sister sitting right [here], she HIV positive and she ain't telling you. So you can't help her to go get her meds or make her doctor's appointment 'cause she's going to get her nails done, instead of you and me are HIV positive. You ought to be saving me. "Girl you can't get your nails done, you gotta see your HIV doctor tomorrow, and I'm taking you there."

Many turned to family and friends, with varied responses. When Phyllis was diagnosed in 1995, she recalled crying out to the cab driver as she returned home, "I'm dying, I'm dying, I'm dying." When she disclosed her status to her mother on arrival, her mother refused to believe or engage with her. She then called another family member who took her to their home to process, and they were all "hugging and crying . . . it was a big old mess." The next morning, her young nephew, whose friend "watched his father die of AIDS" approached her.

> He said, "You sick aren't you?" "What?" He say, "You sick like [my friend's] dad, aren't you?" And I didn't wanna lie to him, I said, "Yeah, how'd you know?" He said, "Because of the way you all were reacting yesterday, y'all wouldn't let us come upstairs . . ." I said, "Yeah, I just didn't know how to tell you," and he said, "Yeah, I understand," and the little boy gave me a hug, and he petted me like this on my back, "It's going to be alright," and I said, "Well I guess now since you know, I gotta tell [your sister]." . . . And he said, "No, I'll tell [sister] when she's ready, I'll be able to judge." . . . He eventually told his sister. 'Cause one day she came up to me, and I think I had been sick, and I had come over to their house, and [she said] "You feeling okay? That bug ain't got you, do it? Alrighty." . . . She was an old soul too *[quiet chuckles]* . . . That was my support.

Phyllis's mother eventually believed her diagnosis after she took two more tests, and became part of her support too. But in that critical time, in the aftermath of her diagnosis, Phyllis was caught by the rich multigenerational web of her extended family and wrapped in their care, enabling her to cope.

Respondents described either themselves or their mothers telling the whole family about their status and letting the chips fall where they may. Several dealt with evolving family responses, including "the phase where everybody didn't wanna be around you . . . they didn't even want to touch you," or "the paper plate and cup thing," or taking it "one day at a time," before more education reduced stigma, and the family drew them back in. Like family, friends could also be stigmatizing, neutral, or a critical support. Caleb found varied responses among his friends. For some "I was, you know, poison towards them . . . some made jokes. And some just went along with it." When Peter was diagnosed in 1989 he was 18 years old; he said, "Initially I wanted to commit suicide because of that, but a friend of mine talked me out of it and persuaded me to live, you know, keep on living." After she disclosed to her friends, Alexandra found that "no one, none of my friends turned away from me or nothing. Um, they all, um, was supportive of me." In this way, the immediate circles around people enabled them to deal with the weight of diagnosis and move forward with their lives.

Personal Faith. Faith in God was also an important personal safety net for respondents, acting as the "third therapeutic system" (besides biomedical and alternative medicine systems).[5] It shaped how they perceived their diagnosis, provided a buffer against stigma and rejection, and gave them a reason to hope and have a sense of purpose postdiagnosis.[6] When all else failed, as Della, aged 54 years, put it, "God [was] the only entity that could possibly help." Twenty-six-year-old Moses was not alone in viewing his diagnosis through the lens of faith, as a wake-up call from God, and an opportunity to turn his life around instead of as a death sentence. As he said of God:

> He didn't want me to die, and he didn't want me to go to hell or go to jail or anything like that, and I think he woke me up. And he said, "Look, I'm gonna give you a chance that this is gonna wake you up. Here's your HIV." Stamp it. "If you really care about yourself, you will take care of yourself and you will better yourself." And I think that that's what's happenin'.

After watching so many die in the syndemic, survival left them feeling that it was God who had ultimately rescued them and had given them grace and mercy, and that God hadn't failed them. Fifty-six-year-old Elijah, whose wife died of AIDS, was "amazed every day that I'm not dead, because I put myself in situations, in those crack houses. I've seen people gettin' killed, robbed, but his mercy's been great. Harm never came to me. Harm never came to me."

Forty-six-year-old James, whose

> CD4 counts is like in the thousands, okay, and my viral load is undetectable, okay. So I'm very, very fortunate, and that's only by the grace of God. I'm very

fortunate, you know, considering all the damage that I've done to my body with the drugs and being out there on the street and soliciting and all of that, you know.

After Victor's unsuccessful suicide attempt, he felt that "hey, maybe it's not time for me to die. Maybe God's not ready for me to come home yet." This realization led him to start treatment 10 years after diagnosis.

In sum, for people who lived, friends, family, and personal faith were important personal safety nets in helping them get back on their feet and move on with their lives after HIV diagnosis. At the city level, several factors shaped the circumstances under which individual choices, lives, and deaths unfolded.

A PIONEERING AND AGGRESSIVE RESPONSE

When AIDS cases began emerging, the city was one of the nation's leaders in responding early. In 1983, the city government, led by Mayor Marion Barry, a longtime supporter of the city's gay community, allocated $25,000 from the city's budget to AIDS-related programs[7] and awarded $17,500 of it to Whitman-Walker Clinic, a predominantly White gay men's clinic for sexually transmitted diseases.[8] The clinic, under the leadership of Jim Graham, had taken an early, aggressive, and central role in the city's response and started an AIDS division that year. The city's money was to fund an AIDS information line and represented what was believed to be "the first contract in the nation to provide public money for an AIDS clinic."[9] Its AIDS Evaluation Unit was the self-described "first gay community-based medical unit in the country devoted to the evaluation and diagnosis of AIDS symptoms."[10] Along with biomedical treatment (especially for opportunistic infections that take advantage of a compromised immune system), the clinic also provided wraparound services, including counselling, anonymous testing, once available, food bank services, homes for people with AIDS, and legal services.[11] By 1986, in addition to its own fundraising, the clinic was expecting to receive $250,000 for HIV/AIDS programs and $80,000 for housing for people with AIDS from the city.[12] In 1987, as cases climbed, the city allocated $1.8 million for AIDS efforts and established "a special office to coordinate [AIDS] programs" and improve services.[13] In the 1988 fiscal year, the city's AIDS budget was set to increase to more than $3 million[14] and the Whitman-Walker Clinic received a third of that budget.[15]

As implied by these budget numbers, even before ART, HIV/AIDS was an expensive and intensive epidemic. Once established, the city's HIV/AIDS agency received both federal and city funds and then contracted with community-based organizations (CBOs), principally the Whitman-Walker Clinic, to engage in on-the-ground HIV/AIDS work. The range of required services for an effective response included HIV prevention and awareness activities, HIV testing, enrollment and continued access to ART once available, regular access to doctors for checkups, and wraparound support to enable strict adherence to ART because of HIV's tendency to mutate and become medication-resistant if one or more days are skipped. Wraparound support could include housing, food, transportation, employment and mental health services, as well as assisting eligible patients in enrolling in relevant federal government support such as Medicaid, Supplemental Security Income, and disability support.[16] These extensive services are needed because an HIV diagnosis, especially early on, often initiated a cascade of problems: multiple illnesses as HIV attacked immune systems, making it hard to reliably hold down a job; job loss because of workplace stigma; subsequent loss of employer-based health insurance; inability to secure new health insurance due to a preexisting condition (prior to the Affordable Care Act); homelessness due to stigma and lack of income; lack of food and therefore inability to tolerate medication; and so on.

Respondents described engagement with effective city programming early on. Forty-nine-year-old Ruth was tested

> on the streets of DC . . . When the epidemic first came here . . . [the] health department come around in vans, right, and they would pay you like [a] stipend to be tested. So I went on the van, and they told me that they would get back with me to let me know my results. You know at that time they had that two week thing, or a month [waiting period] . . . [when] they caught up with me, I was incarcerated. They found me . . . in the DC jail . . . someone told me that I was positive.

Ruth's experience highlights the great lengths the city's health department went to in order to inform people of their status. Fifty-eight-year-old Hiram found out at the public clinic. He had been "feeling really funny, and my energy level dropped, and I was sluggish," and he appeared to his mother to be undergoing "a whole complete change." He went to the ER for a check-up

> and what they did was they took my blood, and when they got it back . . . they told me that I needed to [go to] the um, public clinic. And when they said that, I really knew something was wrong. When I got to the clinic . . . they

ran a test on me again . . . And when I came back, I met three doctors from the CDC, and they, that's when they told me.

Hiram thus encountered multiple public institutions in his care.

The city also took on insurance companies, passing the Prohibition of Discrimination in the Provision of Insurance Act of 1986, a law that prohibited insurers from predicating decisions on AIDS tests.[17] The law was to protect people such as Alyssa, who found out she had HIV when her application for life insurance was rejected, and she was directed to see a doctor because of "abnormalities in my blood." While insurance companies were successful in overturning that law (by refusing to write insurance plans for all District residents and then lobbying Congress to veto the city's law altogether, which Congress eventually did),[18] it was nonetheless a sign that the city had put considerable weight behind fighting AIDS discrimination. The city had the first shelter in the nation for women with AIDS, sponsored by a local CBO, which opened in 1987.[19] The city also had earlier and more comprehensive sex education (including AIDS education) than its suburban counterparts[20] and controversially introduced a condom intervention program for DC high schools in 1992.[21] These bold actions, for which the city expended significant political capital and took significant congressional, national, and commercial heat, clearly show that the high number of AIDS deaths was not because its leaders did not care about the epidemic and people's suffering. A major stumbling block, however, was how intersectional power politics shaped resource allocation.[22]

RACIALLY UNEQUAL FUNDS FOR HIV/AIDS PREVENTION AND CARE SERVICES

"A Gay White Man's Disease"

When the first official reports of what is now called AIDS began to be published in *The New England Journal of Medicine* in 1981 and the CDC's *Morbidity and Mortality Weekly Report* in 1982, there was early evidence that while AIDS (at least among hospital and clinic attendees) appeared to be disproportionately affecting White gay men, it was also affecting other groups.[23] In 1982, describing their sample in the *Morbidity and Mortality Weekly Report*, Mildvan and colleagues stated: "81% were white, 15% black, and 4% Hispanic."[24] However, the racial/ethnic diversity of people with

HIV/AIDS was not immediately apparent to the public, especially in Washington, DC, which was the national center of political activism.

As many documented, in the face of government abandonment, indifference, and stigma, there was a concerted nationwide and local community-wide deployment of social capital among White gay men and allies; as a relatively wealthy community, they had resources to pour into taking care of the sick and dying, raising public awareness about the disease and about condom use, and, controversially, shutting down popular community institutions such as bath houses, especially before ART.[25] Nationally and within DC, the consequence of sexually contained gayborhoods and community institutions was that deaths were devastatingly concentrated, and within DC, hundreds and hundreds of White gay men died before ART. This mass death drove an extraordinary and strategic deployment of political capital at both local and national levels—using influential government positions and connections to the levers of power to pressure the administration to direct federal funds to research on AIDS, lobbying for access to medication during clinical trials, and working to earn seats at key decision-making tables, among other activities.[26] Activist groups led by White gay men, such as ACT UP, also applied pressure: flying in from around the country to protest in front of the White House, and the NIH and FDA in Washington's suburbs; laying quilts on the lawns of the National Mall to draw attention to mass AIDS deaths; and marching along the city streets, fighting for their lives.[27] Their heroic efforts resulted in many landmark policies, such as the Ryan White Act, which created a ground-breaking safety net for people with HIV/AIDS that lasted long after the emergency ended for White gay men.[28]

White gay activism in DC was reflected in media coverage that gave the impression to the city's majority Black population that AIDS was a sexually and racially contained disease, despite the more diverse demographic reality.[29] There were thus lags in understanding HIV/AIDS as an emergency requiring communitywide Black engagement in order to save lives.[30] Even Black health care workers in DC experienced this lag initially. Jane, a community health care worker, described how

> it started out as a "gay White man's disease" because those were the patients coming in more often. It doesn't necessarily mean that at that time Blacks were not becoming infected. But we have to think about who accesses care more often than somebody else. So clearly it's gonna show up in communities where they access care, like it's just—it's easy, right? . . .

Della worked as a caregiver for people dying of AIDS in the early years. She had seen a *Washington Blade* ad seeking home health care workers "for people who are HIV positive because didn't anybody wanna go into these people's homes." She noted that it was an

> agency that sent people out to people in their private homes to take care of . . . it was the type of thing, like, mostly White people because they had insurance . . . [but] a lot of African Americans didn't have health insurance. Most of my patients were White gay men . . .

Black Public Health Commissioner Reed Tuckson released a 58-page report in 1987 sounding the alarm that Black people comprised half (49%) of the city's AIDS cases. He publicly stated:

> The members of the black community in particular think that . . . this is not a problem for the black community . . . we strongly, strongly encourage any persons who have high risk behavior to seek voluntary, free, anonymous and easy to obtain counseling and testing.[31]

But if people did not consider themselves as engaging in high risk behavior they could exempt themselves. Many Black men who had sex with men (MSM) around the country and in DC did not identify as gay and did not see themselves as at risk. As a key informant observed, "There's no community for MSM" to inform them otherwise.[32] The city's early, primary, and longitudinal allocation of AIDS funds to the Whitman-Walker Clinic, even when the epidemic became disproportionately Black (by 1988), may have been both a result and reinforcer of the perception that this was a White gay man's disease,[33] notwithstanding mounting evidence from the coroner's office or the health commissioner's report.

However, among the city's Black gay men who were losing members by the hundreds and then by the thousands, there was indigenous organizing that was less visible to the media but no less vigorous. As a community leader observed, they

> saw the death and the dying, but no one was really reacting to it, so we began to develop our own organizations . . . a lot of organizations began to start . . . I mean there still isn't much of a reaction coming from the Black community around Black gay men [2011] . . . I think the community's concern . . . is because heterosexuals, particularly women, are becoming infected. They're not really concerned about Black gay men.

"Informal system[s] of community care" emerged, including fundraising, to take care of sick members, and support groups and CBOs were formed.[34] The first Black Pride march in the nation, organized by Welmore Cook, Theodore Kirkland, and Ernest Hopkins, was held in DC in 1991 as a community fundraising effort to support local Black HIV/AIDS CBOs.[35] As the epidemic worsened, AIDS deaths of wealthy community members, as well as the closing of clubs that had been venues of community gathering and support, such as the Club House, greatly impacted their ability to support their own prevention efforts.[36] However, many organizations survived, and as awareness grew and the epidemic became prominent among heterosexuals, a rising network of Black and non-Black community-based organizations, later supported by federal and city funding, worked alongside the Whitman-Walker Clinic to try to stem the Black epidemic.

Community Based Organizations and the Racial Allocation of Funds

Community Based Organizations. DC CBOs engaged in much of the on-the-ground work of providing care for people living with HIV/AIDS. Respondents described benefiting from a wide range of CBOs, supported by philanthropists as well as federal and city funding, including church-related organizations, drug treatment programs, the Whitman-Walker Clinic, and indigenous Black-led CBOs, among others.

The Church, a key intermediary in many people's relationship with God, was an especially important institution in the Black community. It not only served as a religious institution but also as a civil rights organization, a social and health services organization, a mediating organization, a therapeutic community, an entertainment center, and a community gathering space, among many other functions.[37] However, its role in the lives of people with HIV and AIDS was complicated, as they experienced both its compassion and its judgment. Some DC Black and non-Black ministries and leaders were pioneers in providing outreach services. Damien Ministries, initiated by Louis Tesconi and other Catholic laymen, sponsored the first shelter for women with AIDS. Nuns from Mother Teresa's order provided hospice care to people dying of AIDS. Groups of churches and interfaith groups organized gatherings to talk and raise awareness about HIV/AIDS.[38] A prominent Black-led CBO, Us Helping Us, was founded by Bishop Rainey Cheeks

(Inner Light Ministries, Unity Fellowship Church movement), along with Prem Deben, Aundrea Scott, and Howard Morris. Us Helping Us, established in 1985 and incorporated in 1988, focused on Black gay men, those who were most vulnerable to HIV/AIDS. It started in the Club House, a prominent Black LGBTQ gathering space, and transitioned to Cheeks's apartment after the Club House closed. The organization eventually expanded into a three-story building. In addition to providing core services, such as HIV testing, they also provided holistic support, such as nutrition education, stress management support, including exercise and meditation, and HIV disclosure education. It also built a rich and supportive community of Black gay men living with HIV. As Michael, a member, described:

> We were very Afrocentric, we didn't shake hands, we would hug each other. So what would happen is that, um, it got to the point where if you went into one of the Black gay clubs . . . [you would] see these guys, and there was just so much friendship, and they would all be hugging each other, hanging out . . .[39]

Another organization, Luther Place Memorial Church, merged with Miriam's House as part of its ministry.[40] The House provided a longer-term refuge for women, and especially mothers, with HIV while they tried to stabilize their lives. This support helped Ruth get back on her feet:

> I was pretty much, just wandering, you know wandering around 'cause I . . . was still homeless at the time, 'cause I had lost my, my mother, like in '85, '86. And um . . . I was taken to a shelter with health care for the homeless . . . they had a, a house up here . . . that was just for individuals who was HIV positive and had nowhere to go, who was homeless . . . And then after, there I went to a place called uh, Miriam's House. And they were just opening. So they were taking um, HIV women and kids, children . . . I stayed there another 20 months. Then my [public] housing came through and I left, you know.

These experiences notwithstanding, respondents and key informants also described experiencing the church's institutional silence, inaction, and stigmatizing practice, especially before the epidemic began affecting cisgender Black women.[41] Health worker Steven reflected:

> When HIV first came out, the African American churches were in a great position to really be at the forefront . . . But because it was associated with a particular lifestyle, they chose not to do that . . . For a long time there were churches who wouldn't bury people who died of AIDS in DC, prominent churches.

The "don't-ask-don't-tell" attitude towards gay men who richly contributed to the church did always not translate into an open embrace and care when AIDS began to decimate them.[42] From Black CBO leader Chris's cynical observations,

> [The] church only started doing it [HIV prevention] once the congregation began to get infected. They weren't doing it when the men in the choir were dying. It was again when the women began, you know, and also when the money became available suddenly, you know, then it became different. But no. *[Sanyu: Money available from—]* Government funding for the churches to do AIDS prevention programs and things like that.

(The city's HIV/AIDS agency started a Places of Worship Advisory Board in the late 2000s to encourage churches to get involved in the HIV/AIDS response).[43] Steven felt that "even now [2011] it's not addressed. I mean, in a few churches they have an HIV ministry. But it's still not addressed in the church." Respondents nonetheless went to church and found the emotional and spiritual strength they needed to carry on there. Trans woman Priscilla felt called back to church after 30 years following her diagnosis and her mother's death. Sharing her testimony, she described how her godmother reached out to her:

> And she said, "I haven't heard from you, I haven't seen you, you need to come to church." And I said, "I don't know." She said, "No I'm serious." She said, "I was praying and God told me that you needed to come to church because you just need to come to church." So I said, "Okay, I'll be there mom." She said, "When?" and I said, "I'll be there." . . . [I] went back to church . . . they baptized me Easter Sunday . . . when I came up outta that water, the drugs were gone. I didn't care about no HIV or nothing else 'cause God said he had it and I'm not gonna die from it. Now all I know I need to do is I need to live my life differently.

There were also several other organizations that respondents encountered. As noted earlier, the Whitman-Walker Clinic was the largest city-supported HIV/AIDS CBO. Several respondents—gay, straight, women, men—went there for services. For example, Kevin described how he

> became real sick due to my insurance with Kaiser lapsing, because of the job-related insurance . . . and I was cut off. I went without insurance for a period of time, and I became sick because I wasn't able to get my medicine. And a friend of mine recommended that I go to Whitman-Walker . . . They assigned me a doctor . . . she put me on a regimen, a cocktail, and I immediately started getting better.

In addition to HIV specialist physicians there, Cora mentioned access to "legal clinics . . . they have day programs . . . psychiatrists . . . gynecologists, therapists." Their HIV support groups also helped people share their unique set of challenges. As Theo explained:

> For a person livin' with HIV, you can't start a conversation on the bus or somethin' about what you feelin', what the medication's doin', what the medication's not doin', how you're only livin' off of the 600-some dollars that Social Security gives you . . . your body's not strong enough to keep a full-time job . . . Or your housing issue, or how can you find somebody new in your life without first tellin' them about that you're HIV positive? When do you tell them you're HIV positive? What's safe sex? . . . You know, talkin' about all those different things. And those things are helpin' me, you know, um.

A prominent Black-led CBO for women living with HIV was the Women's Collective, started by Patricia Nalls. She began with a phone line in 1990, and the organization expanded into a fully-fledged prevention and care organization.[44] Forty-nine-year-old Jasmine described how having such an organization enabled women to help other women:

> I go to Women's Collective. That's for HIV women. I done brought in three clients that I met off the street that wasn't taking medicine and just uh, God touched that conversation, I ain't had nothing to do with it . . . I ran into one female . . . And we talking . . . and she was saying she HIV positive. I say, "Me too." . . . So she was like, "Uh, girl, I don't know what to do." I say, "Well, I, I, we can go by the Women's Collective." . . . They opened up a file, made a file for her. Now she got somewhere to go . . . they open at nine and close at five, they got the TV rec area, they got lunch, breakfast, dinner, coffee, it's cool in there, carpet on the floor, they give out clothes, they give out food. It's just a good reach, reach out program for HIV positive women . . . if we wasn't HIV, they wouldn't had a place.

Trans woman Cheryl, diagnosed in 1995, exemplified the role of CBOs in getting people connected to care. After diagnosis, she "got high to suppress all that, 'cause I didn't really wanna know. I didn't really want to believe it." Black-led CBO Transgender Health Empowerment reached out to her for several years to "try to get me to get my life together numerous times, and I wasn't ready, and I didn't do it." She finally started ART in 2009.

Addiction treatment programs were also critical. Forty-year-old transgender woman Mary's time at a program for people with HIV was transformative. As she explained:

I went to the program and it was no distractions. You know, me being trans wasn't a distraction. Me being HIV wasn't a distraction. Everybody in there, you had to be HIV to be there, everybody was HIV, everybody took meds. I think I was the only one to be trans in there, but there was gay men and I was just accepted, so I got a chance to focus on a lot of things.

By our interview, Mary, a former sex worker and crack-addicted prisoner, was living independently, legally employed, and on the dean's list in college. As Celeste Watkins-Hayes powerfully illustrated in her award-winning book *Remaking a Life*, the irony of the HIV safety net was that it took an HIV diagnosis to unlock resources that were much needed to not just survive but thrive, resources that were absent or out of reach for poor people.

Racial Allocation of Resources. While there was a broad-based HIV safety net, it was unequally funded. Even before ART became widely available in 1993, epidemic demographics had significantly shifted—65% of AIDS deaths were among Black people and 32% among White people.[45] However, the city's allocation of HIV/AIDS resources to CBOs did not change to reflect the new demographic reality. Figure 43 by Amy Goldstein, reporting in *The Washington Post* that year, starkly illustrates that the bulk of federal and local financing went to White CBOs.[46] This mattered because of racially different epidemic profiles and attendant organizations—with the White epidemic occurring among primarily White gay men and the Black epidemic occurring among gay men, non-gay MSM, heterosexuals, and injecting drug users (see Parts 2 and 3). Black people thus had to know about and be comfortable attending White gay organizations to access the city's best-resourced services.

The Whitman-Walker Clinic tried hard to bridge the gap and share resources across races. While serving predominantly White gay clients, the clinic also served many African Americans, who comprised 40% of their clients and 35% of their staff by 1988.[47] But despite these efforts, there was a clear disconnect between where the federal government and city disseminated funds and where the greatest AIDS epidemic burden lay—in the predominantly Black and least-serviced parts of the city. This was clear early on. In a 1988 interview, Graham admitted to a reporter:

This issue has been around since 1983 . . . but we don't have a resolution . . . The issue in 1983 was, who was going to get the $17,500 in city funds to deal with AIDS and how was the city going to properly achieve racial balance in

SUBSIDIES TO D.C. AIDS ORGANIZATIONS

Figures represent the amount of money awarded by the District's AIDS agency to a variety of community groups that provide medical care, counseling, mental health services, transportation, food and other help to people who are infected with the HIV virus or have developed AIDS.

FEDERAL AID
IN MILLIONS

■ Aid to minority organizations*   □ Total aid in millions

Year	Aid to minority organizations*	Total aid in millions
1991	$1.99	$4.88
1992	$2.30	$5.88
1993	$2.18	$6.68

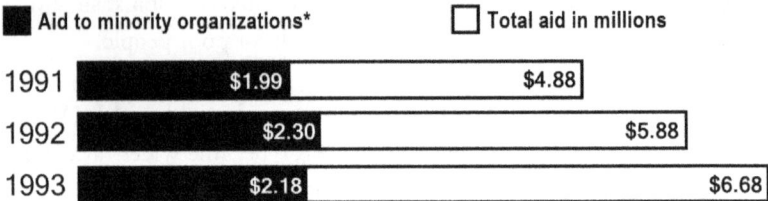

RYAN WHITE TITLE I PROGRAM
Part of the federal aid is through the Ryan White Title I program to cities that are especially hard hit by AIDS. At right are the Title I funds given to minority organizations* in the District:

IN MILLIONS

1991	$0.83
1992	$1.30
1993	$1.61

LOCAL AID
IN MILLIONS

■ Aid to minority organizations*   □ Total aid in millions

Year	Aid to minority organizations*	Total aid in millions
1991	$1.23	$4.29
1992	$1.34	$4.78
1993	$1.67	$4.89

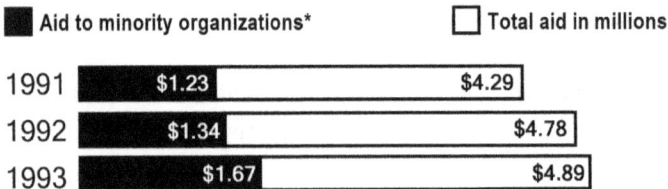

*Defined by the D.C. Public Health Commission's Agency for HIV/AIDS
SOURCE: D.C. Agency for HIV/AIDS

FIGURE 43. Racial distribution of AIDS funds. Source: Amy Goldstein, Where AIDS and Money Cross Paths, *The Washington Post*, July 11, 1993. © 1993 *The Washington Post*. All rights reserved. Used under license. https://www.washingtonpost.com/.

its AIDS efforts? I think we're providing as substantial services as anybody in town to the black community . . . But I also think we need a copartner, a vigorous, minority-oriented, minority-based AIDS effort.[48]

The clinic eventually set up a branch in the predominantly Black SE (the Max Robinson Center in Anacostia, Ward 8) a decade later, in 1993.[49] As Graham described in an interview with Genny Beemyn, archived at the Rainbow History Project, in addition to the clinic's own enthusiasm, "the city leadership wanted to see that . . . had we not been visibly committed to this [the Black epidemic], they would not have been committed to us." However, it was "a hell of a struggle. This was a hallmark of the whole black relationship . . . it's a damned if you do, damned if you don't" situation he said, describing, for example, controversy around not working with existing local organizations, and Black leaders hostility, which he felt eased over time.[50]

An important argument could be made that CBO resources were allocated unequally simply because of differential organizational capacity to provide services.[51] After all, the clinic, started in the late 1970s to treat STIs and supported by robust community fundraising, was already well set up to deal with AIDS once it appeared. It made sense that the city would give the bulk of its initial funds to a ready-to-go organization that was seen to be helping the city's most affected group and was providing outreach to other groups. However, as the epidemic unfolded, as the number of minority organizations grew and as Black AIDS deaths dramatically increased, it became clear that allocation decisions were not just about organizational capacity. Rather, as Anne Dievler and Gregory Pappas observed,[52] they were due to the intersectional politics of race, class, and sexual orientation in the city.

INTERSECTIONAL POLITICS

Racial Versus Sexual Identity Politics

Intersectional political dynamics were present during the awarding of the city's first AIDS grant, as Graham recounted to Beemyn:

> The first controversy, actually, about HIV in the District of Columbia was the summer of 1983 . . . A critical decision was who was going to get the first AIDS contract. That was hashed out in the DC AIDS Task Force, and then in the Commissioner of Public Health, and so on. The AIDS Task Force had been established in May of '83, and I was one of the first members. There were

strong feelings that this first contract should go to a Black organization in a Black city. And you had some players ... some pretty powerful players, who were saying, "This should not go to this White gay male middle class ... " But we won it. It was $17,500. It was the first remissible AIDS contract in the United States. It was. I'm sure of it.

And in the ensuing years, he said, "the proof of the matter is that the African American leadership of the city continued to place their confidence in us." Indeed, this became apparent when efforts to get the city to fund a large minority coalition failed. In summer 1993, Goldstein reported that Marion Barry, now the Ward 8 council member, "convened an AIDS summit, where 100 Black and Hispanic activists agreed to form a minority AIDS coalition. Barry said he wanted the DC Council to force the city's AIDS agency to give more money to grass roots groups."[53]

Unlike cities with significant epidemics such as New York, Philadelphia, and San Francisco, "the District lack[ed] an established, well-financed minority-based AIDS organization."[54] Twelve CBOs subsequently formed the SANKOFA Community Coalition for HIV/AIDS Services, including "the Abundant Life Center, United Response to Black America's Needs (URBAN), Impact, SALUD, HUSER, ICAN, Us Helping Us, Community Health Care, Family Planning and Counseling, Rap, Inc. and The Dwayne S. Brown Foundation."[55] As described by the Abundant Life Center's executive director, Alim Muhammad:

> The current state of AIDS funding in the District is such that White gay men, who represent the minority of new cases of HIV infection in the city, receive the lion's share of the money allocated by the D.C. government. This new coalition will work to ensure that all of the city's communities are serviced and funded at appropriate levels consistent with the proportion of AIDS cases reflective of the District's population.[56]

The power struggle between White gay and racial/ethnic-minority community organizations did not end well for the coalition, which was in competition with Whitman-Walker for city funds. Whitman-Walker won the contract.[57] Muhammad suspected "some kind of deal has been cut" because Mayor Kelly, who was up for reelection, had just been endorsed "by the Gertrude Stein Club, an influential gay political organization," a connection that "Kelly staffers have denied."[58] Nearly two decades later, the intersectional organizational tug-of-war was also reflected in a 2011 interview with Susan, a Black community health worker, who described a discussion where she gathered that gay White men feel like the disease has been stolen from them ... And I'm thinking to myself, "I'm sorry. I didn't know there was ownership placed over HIV." So I've been told, I was schooled that evening ... And funny, my partner said the same thing the other day, last night, to me. He came back from a meeting and was *so* upset and *so* drained. And I was like, "What's the problem?" "Why is it that gay White men feel we stole their disease?" "Excuse me? Disease has an ownership now?" So it came up again.

The raging Black epidemic showed the limits of existing White CBO service provision to Black people, but the continued organizational power struggle in part reflected the significant role the AIDS epidemic and its attendant infrastructures and immense resource flows had played in White gay power politics over the prior three decades. This lead to tensions in ceding ground to other minority actors when the demographic reality had clearly changed.[59]

Intraracial Black Homophobia

The early decision to allocate money to the Whitman-Walker Clinic signaled a supportive and mutually beneficial political relationship between city leadership and the White gay community even before Kelly. As Graham was quoted as saying of Barry, her predecessor, "He is a good friend of the gay community and we're a good friend of his."[60] It was not clear, however, that the leadership was a good friend of the *Black* gay community. Indeed, the battle for visibility by the city's Black sexual minorities preceded the AIDS crisis. As Darius Bost described, early DC Black gay activists "were tasked with both challenging the category of gay as 'white' and making Black bodies intelligible to the state as sexual minorities."[61] Barry was apparently "surprised to hear [from the DC Coalition for Black Gays] about discrimination by White Gay establishments,"[62] even though a law had to be passed in 1984 to end their discriminatory practices.[63] Compared to White sexual minorities, their Black counterparts appeared to have differential access to the levers of the federal government and differential "connectedness to DC's resources."[64] Black sexual minorities experienced a double standard and "hostility from the Black political establishment,"[65] which accepted, supported, and openly assisted White gay men.

DC's Black leaders' homophobic treatment of Black sexual minorities was part of a national pattern. As Cathy Cohen described in her award-winning *Boundaries of Blackness*, this was a product of the perception of HIV/AIDS as a "lifestyle-based disease" combined with the fact that stigmatized constituencies—people who used drugs and sexual minorities—were presumed to be most affected by AIDS. It was also due to the nation's first Black mayors' being concerned with maintaining racial respectability once they were finally able to govern (see Part 1).[66] This was matched by contrasting community responses, as Steven recounted:

> STEVEN: When [AIDS] came out, Caucasians united. The gay community went into the bars, they went into the bath houses, they were advocating condom use, they didn't wait on the government. They had an organization called ACT UP that was down in front of the White House that was saying, "We're not going to take this lyin' down." There has not been the same outrage among the African American community, you know. We just, "Oh, you know, we got a whole lot of HIV runnin' around here!" That's it.
>
> SANYU: Even though they're losing brothers, sisters, relatives, friends to HIV, there still hasn't been outrage?
>
> STEVEN: There hasn't been any outrage. And the outrage hasn't come from people who can be heard, people who are in the know.

Chris concurred, explaining:

> Because those were gay men. And you know about the homophobia in the community. So they didn't care. In fact, they were saying, "It serves you right," that it was God's punishment. No one was upset about that. The only ones who, uh, who saw it really were those of us who were in the Black gay community, you know. I mean, how many men were not even out to their families? For so many men, they found out their son was gay the same time— when they visited them at the hospital and he was dying, is when they would find out he was gay. So there was no outcry.

There was a sense in these and other interviews that underlying Black inertia was a certain deadly resignation. As Steven put it: "There's a saying here in certain circles, 'Charge it to the game.' What that means is, understand that there's gonna be a segment of the population that is lost."

Intraracial Class Indifference

Social class also played a role as limited funding for the city's poorest, predominantly Black wards continued on into the 2000s, even though many Black leaders held oversight and controlled levers of power over HIV spending. In January 2007, Raymond Blanks, who served on DC's Community HIV Planning Group, wrote in *The Washington Post*:

> Last year, the D.C. Council appropriated a half-million dollars to establish HIV services in Ward 7, where no services had been provided, although it had the city's second-highest rate of infection. Today, Ward 7 is still without services, although a local consulting firm was hired to assist in developing services. Even more distressing, an oversight hearing of the council's Committee on Health revealed that nearly 25 percent of the council's award was spent illegally in other sectors of the city and for other purposes.[67]

In 2009, an investigative report by Debbie Cenziper noted, "Since 2004, the city has awarded just 6 percent of $100 million in AIDS funding to specialized nonprofit groups east of the river, forcing families to scramble for care in other parts of the city."[68] The health department, responding to DC City Council pressure, "earmarked $3.5 million to bolster neighborhood groups focused on AIDS housing, counseling and case management. But the city spent more than $1 million from the fund on grants to nonprofit groups in other neighborhoods."[69] What was left was spent on " a high-end study instead of services, a neighborhood AIDS office in Ward 7 that closed within months and grants to nonprofit groups tainted by financial and operational problems."[70] Vincent Gray, DC council chairman and later mayor, followed the AIDS money into

> his home base of Ward 7. He was stunned by what he found. "There was not one grant that had been awarded to an organization indigenous to Ward 7 ... It was almost as if no one had thought about fighting this at the neighborhood and community level."[71]

Thus, even when earmarked, money for HIV/AIDS was not going to poorer Black areas.[72]

In sum, an early and aggressive epidemic response by the city ultimately failed to stem the Black AIDS epidemic. While personal safety nets and CBOs helped those who lived cope with HIV diagnoses, many died in part due to how racial and class containment worked through intersectional politics. They created blind spots and institutional lags in perceptions of who was most affected and led to unequal resource allocation, leaving deadly institutional absences in the lives of people with HIV/AIDS living in some of the worst hit and most poorly serviced Black communities.

THIRTEEN

Controlling an Epidemic

THE SUCCESSES AND LIMITS OF
TECHNOCRATIC EXPERTISE

IN ADDITION TO INTERSECTIONAL POLITICS, the city's HIV/AIDS response was greatly affected by its budget crises, which came to a head in the late '80s and early 1990s. The crises unfolded during a particularly critical period of the epidemic. HIV cases and AIDS deaths were ramping up dramatically, escalating demand for prevention and care services, and then ART became widely available in the mid-'90s, creating a large demand for treatment services. However, in the first part of this chapter, I illustrate how congressional and city measures to control the budget crises in the mid- to late 1990s instead led to service reductions across a number of agencies, including its HIV/AIDS Administration (HAA), which exacerbated the city's epidemic, especially among its poor Black residents. In the second part of the chapter, I examine the HAA, describing its troubled history and challenges, as well as how it eventually controlled the city's epidemic. I show how its spectacular success also underscores the limits of technocratic expertise in eliminating racial health inequality.[1]

THE CITY'S BUDGET CRISES

As discussed in Chapter 3, while many majority Black cities around the country experienced major financial crises, DC's was distinctive in a number of ways. Common to other settings was a loss of tax revenue as first White and then middle-class and affluent Black people departed for the suburbs. However, in contrast to other cities, Congress denied DC the right to tax commuters, forcing the city to forgo billions of dollars in revenue. Additionally, the federal government's considerable District properties were tax exempt, and the city handled institutions and programs such as courts, prisons, half of nonfederal Medicaid expenses, and growing pension liabilities that in other cities were typically handled by states.[2] Declining tax revenue and congressionally imposed restrictions on revenue generation were compounded by state-sized debt obligations and the exploding expenses from the city's SAVA syndemic and its war on drugs to combat it (see Parts 3 and 4), which brought the financial burden to a head.

For example, gun violence was expensive, costing the city an estimated $7,000 per homicide and $21,000 per shooting survivor.[3] Further, as Steve Twomey reported:

> Because most of the wounded have no health insurance, hospitals say they have dispensed millions of dollars of free medical care to the wounded, costs they seek to recover through higher charges to the paying public ... the amount of uncompensated care has become so great the Hospital Center said last month it was considering closing its trauma unit, MedStar.[4]

He followed one victim, "shot four times," for whom unpaid care cost $190,000.

Mass incarceration, the city's primary solution to its syndemic, was even more expensive. As described in Part 3, 43,000 residents were arrested in 1988 alone, and overall about 70,000 (1 in 8 DC residents) were under criminal justice supervision (parole, probation, prison, jail, etc.) by the mid-1990s, one of the nation's highest incarceration rates.[5] Setting aside the taxpayer costs for police, courts, and arrestee processing, the estimated annual cost of incarcerating an individual was $17,000 in 1990[6] and $22,000 in 1994.[7] Prison overcrowding resulted in court-ordered fines of "more than $5,000 a day," adding up to "more than $800,000" in 1987,[8] as the Corrections Department unsuccessfully struggled to accommodate mass arrests.[9] And prisons were short-staffed, with more than 300 correctional officer vacancies. However, Margaret Moore, the director, did not have budgetary authority to hire more, resulting in $21 million spent on officer overtime pay in 1994.[10] Further, as Stephanie Mencimer reported in 1993:

> Add to that the cost of acute medical care required by people with AIDS ... more than $60,000 a year. Now multiply that cost by [the number of] HIV positive prisoners, all of whom will probably develop AIDS in the next decade, and you've got a looming cost ...[11]

(As noted in Part 4, a 1989 random sample of prisoners yielded a 16% HIV prevalence.)[12] These costs were reflected in escalating annual corrections budgets, from $52.9 million in 1979 to $215 million in 1989 to $380 million in 1990 and $292 million by 1995.[13] Commenting on the 1970s to 1980s escalation, Lee Hockstader reported, "The budget increase . . . is the most rapid of any agency in the city, corrections officials have said."[14] This meant that money to deal with other city challenges was draining into the prison-industrial complex.

During the 1980s, the city had balanced budgets (with the exception of 1988, when it had a $14 million deficit); however, by 1990, DC was faced with a $93 million budget deficit.[15] The true deficit was determined to be $722 million in 1995, after an "honest accounting" arrived at after a comprehensive audit, which included previously undocumented "overspending by numerous city agencies."[16] Several attempts at austerity and budget-cutting in the late 1980s and early 1990s failed, and the alarming prospect of the nation's capital going bankrupt led to the suspension of home rule between 1995 and 2001, which included a government takeover of the city's finances, the imposition of a financial control board, and the suspension of many aspects of self-governance, as agencies that were not already under court-ordered receivership became so. The city regained control in 2001 when it had returned to fiscal health.[17]

IMPACT ON THE CITY'S HIV/AIDS SERVICES AND EPIDEMIC OUTCOMES

An early casualty of the fiscal crisis was health department programming, and after a 1989 budget cut, Commissioner Tuckson was forced to reassess how to balance existing priorities with new initiatives, and it was clear who was going to suffer most. He "complained openly . . . that city health programs for the poor and indigent are being gutted by budget cuts and staffing shortages," including a reduction of about one-third of workers in public drug and alcohol programs, one-tenth of workers in neighborhood health clinics, and $3 million worth of drug treatment and AIDS care programs.[18] Abramowitz reported that budget documents showed that money allocated for AIDS programming, such as "public education initiatives, financing for the drug AZT and money for an intermediate care facility for AIDS patients," was being cut to accommodate existing programs. Tuckson reasoned, "If I spent all the money on AIDS, I would have had to close down the ambulatory health clinics in the city and stop infant mortality [prevention efforts]."[19] It was clear to

Roger Doughty, a Gay and Lesbian Activists Alliance activist, that "AIDS programs ... are being raided to pay for other programs."[20]

The city was unable to spend even federal funds specifically earmarked for AIDS. By 1991, the HAA had not had a permanent director for two years because of a hiring freeze, which meant Commissioner Georges Benjamin could not hire a new director.[21] The hiring freeze resulted in 15 federally funded positions at HAA being left vacant.[22] Millions in federal AIDS funds went unspent for four years and some were returned.[23] This became a major catalyst for AIDS activist protests both by groups, like Oppression Under Target,[24] and by individuals, like Hank Cadre, who in 1991 went on a three-day hunger strike outside the health department to protest the failure to spend federal AIDS funds.[25] When a new HAA director, Caitlin Ryan, was finally hired in 1991 in response to the protests, she found

> no secretary. No contracts officer. No budget officer. No epidemiologist. No fax line. No computer ... What the office did have was an infusion of federal money, courtesy of the Ryan White Comprehensive AIDS Resources Emergency Act. But there was no process in place for dispersing its grants. Often, some money would go unspent.[26]

Even after Caitlin Ryan left in 1993 and a new director, Frank Oldham Jr., took over in January 1994, he was confronted with the same problem, unable to hire employees or spend money to provide "help for dozens of shoestring community groups working to slow the epidemic or assist people who already are sick." He noted: "'Without a doubt, other bureaucracies have been more responsive.' He said the city will not become truly effective in fighting AIDS unless his agency reports directly to the mayor, circumventing the usual rules for hiring workers and awarding contracts."[27] He left after only six months.

In 1996, John Cloud, writing for the *Washington City Paper*, noted that

> according to city figures, from 1991 to 1995 the city delayed spending $11.1 million in federal grants from the Ryan White CARE Act. That amounts to more than a third of all money given to the city under the act, Congress' main HIV/AIDS annual funding bill. The city carried over more than $3 million in unspent Ryan White funds last year alone.[28]

The inability to spend funds was due to the city's financial bureaucratic process. Cloud described the problem:

Unlike 23 states (including Virginia), the city doesn't require that federal grants be in city bank accounts before a check can be written, according to Valerie Holt, the city's acting treasurer. Instead, the city has long paid contractors out of its own pocket and then received reimbursements from the feds. That system works fine as long as the District has the cash to pay contractors. When it doesn't, all hell—for lack of a bureaucratic term— breaks loose.[29]

This problem was compounded when Congress passed the Cash Management Improvement Act, which "took effect" in 1994 and "required that the city be specific about when it would draw down federal money, and in precisely what amounts. 'In the past, you could just estimate the disbursements,' [Holt] says. The city's antique computers couldn't handle the required precision."[30]

Lack of cash and new federal requirements meant the city was unable to pay its community-based organization (CBO) contractors, even though millions were available, contributing to deadly service delays. As reported by Alvin Peabody in *The Washington Informer*, Anthony Williams, the city's chief financial officer (CFO) and future mayor, noted in 1996:

"I think we've reached the conclusion that the process of paying vendors who do services for the District, is completely flawed." . . . The CFO went on to single out the more than 10 HIV/AIDS vendors in the District, most of whom haven't been paid by the city for 30 to 60 days. "In a normal fashion, that would seem fine. But when it comes to a life-threatening illness such as HIV or AIDS, I think it's disgraceful that we have to wait that long to pay these people," Williams said. "Payment to these vendors is also a violation of an agreement we made last year that said that the city would pay them promptly."[31]

Among the affected vendors in the early to mid-'90s was Whitman-Walker Clinic, which, along with other nonprofit CBOs, relied on timely city payment. Jim Graham, its director, observed, "Last year on any given day, Whitman-Walker Clinic carried overdue payments of a million dollars. I was at wit's end." In response, it began to limit patient services. Other CBOs, unable to survive for months without payment for work rendered, reduced services or simply closed.[32] This meant reduced citywide provision of HIV/AIDS prevention, care, and treatment.[33]

Because Ryan White funds were the "payer of last resort," the people most affected by spending delays were the poorest and most vulnerable people with AIDS, which in DC meant predominantly Black people living in Wards 7 and 8. Not spending available federal funds—to the tune of $11 million— also extended to Department of Housing and Urban Development funding for the Housing Opportunities for Persons with AIDS program.[34] As noted earlier, housing was a much needed service for people with AIDS. Eventually, the federal government took over and started making direct payments of Ryan White funds to local AIDS service providers, entirely circumventing the city.[35]

The budget crises also meant that between 1994 and 1996, the DC Bureau of Laboratories, which conducted HIV testing, was periodically (for months at a time) unable to buy the necessary chemical reagents.[36] Funds were available, as testing was CDC financed, but because the city did not have cash in hand, blood samples sat untested.[37] DC General's AIDS response also suffered. Both *The Washington Informer* and *The Washington Post* reported in 1995 that the city's only public hospital was apparently left with one AIDS physician caring for 800 patients (the other two resigned because of budget crisis–induced job insecurity) and just one public STI clinic, which provided free screening and treatment after the other one closed.[38] These services are critical, as STIs increase the likelihood of HIV acquisition and transmission.[39]

Perhaps the deadliest impact of the budget crisis was cutting off access to ART once it became available. In February and April of 1996, the city's AIDS Drug Assistance Program (ADAP) stopped operating because the city was months behind on payments to the pharmacies which provided the drugs.[40] (ADAP, part of the federally funded Ryan White program, covers medication for uninsured/underinsured people[41] because the annual out-of-pocket cost for AIDS drugs was and is thousands of dollars). Later that year, Peabody reported that HAA "released a statement declaring a temporary suspension of services to new clients involved in DC's ADAP" because

> increases in client enrollment, coupled with the addition of new, but costly medication treatments, have caused monthly programs expenditures to rise dramatically. "We are excited about the new drug protocols for people with HIV/AIDS, but we have to make very difficult decisions in order to continue to responsibly provide services to our existing clients," Wilson said. "We will eventually get on track to assist new ADAP clients." In the meantime, [they] will be placed on a waiting list, which will be prioritized according to client's medical and financial needs.[42]

As noted earlier, ART prolonged lives and reduced infectivity. Those most affected by ADAP suspension were likely the city's poorest, who were predominantly Black.

Intermittent or interrupted ART access can be deadly, as HIV mutates and can become medication resistant. The impact of starting and stopping medication was captured in retrospective phylogenetic studies examining the city's HIV transmission chains.[43] Between 1994 and 2013, Kassaye and colleagues found "persistently high and longstanding TDR [transmitted drug resistance]," representing 28.9% (1994–1996), 24.7% (1997–2006), and 19.7% (2007–2013) of the sample.[44] They observed that "to our knowledge, this is the highest prevalence of TDR mutations reported within the United States or in any region within Europe or Australia where ART therapy use has been long-standing."[45] Their findings reflected "delays in treatment initiation, suboptimal treatment adherence, and interruptions in care."[46] Even while they "observed a downward trend in the overall prevalence of TDR compared with the early period . . . continued high levels of drug resistance are evidence of fragmented care."[47]

Fragmented care happened in part because needed wraparound services (see Chapter 12) also suffered from budget cuts. Between 1990 and 2004, Lazere and Nickelson found that city "funding has fallen dramatically for several services targeted on low-income and other vulnerable populations in the areas of housing, human services, and employment services." They calculated an 80% reduction in employment services, a more than 50% reduction in affordable housing programs, a 33% reduction in Department of Human Services programs (which "reflects cuts in . . . child care, homeless services, emergency assistance and welfare"), a 15% reduction in non-Medicaid health services (including addiction services), and a 21% cut in mental health funding.[48] As described in Chapter 12, without a stable place to live and without addiction and mental health services, it was hard to regularly adhere to a treatment regimen, increasing HIV transmission risk.

In sum, the budget crisis contributed to limited and delayed HIV testing and access to ART, limited numbers of available HIV/AIDS specialists, reduced funding for CBOs that helped link people to care, and reduced wraparound services, such as housing, addiction treatment, and mental health care, which could prevent HIV transmission. Both racial and class containment were reflected in the outcomes. Congressional rescue for the city ultimately resulted in widening racial health inequality; it exacerbated the epidemic among the poor—those least able to purchase private help—

and among Black organizations and Black people located in poor neighborhoods in particular, who, as described in Chapter 12, were already experiencing the effects of disproportionately low city spending.

THE HIV/AIDS ADMINISTRATION (HAA): 2001–2022

A central actor in the city's HIV/AIDS response was the HAA.[49] It was both "the biggest liability of the whole response," as a key informant noted, as well as an unprecedented success in turning the city's epidemic around and bringing it under control. However, as I illustrate at the end of this chapter, little changed with respect to racial inequality in HIV/AIDS.

A Troubled HAA

The HAA was beset with problems in the 2000s, including agency corruption, contributing to misspending of funds; very high leadership turnover in what was a highly politicized job; limited long-term strategic thinking about and planning for the epidemic; poor and/or nonexistent epidemic surveillance, resulting in an outdated and inadequate response; and subsequent poor prevention, testing, and counselling services, contributing to late diagnoses and AIDS deaths.

Agency Scandals. Even after the city became fiscally sound, the HAA's financial problems did not end. The Gay and Lesbian Activists Alliance and DC Council members such as Jim Graham (1999–2015) and David Catania (1997–2015) played an important role in holding the HAA's feet to the fire and demanding accountability. Throughout the 2000s, several scandals compounded the lack of spending of available federal funds. For several years, the Alliance complained about a lack of transparency in and oversight over how HAA was spending AIDS funds, pointing to a five-year gap between oversight hearings (July 18, 1998 to May 15, 2003).[50] There were city and FBI investigations in 2006 into accusations of corruption and "widespread fraud and theft" in the HAA office,[51] and in 2009, an investigative *Washington Post* report by Debbie Cenziper estimated that the HAA "awarded more than $25 million from 2004 to 2008 to nonprofit agencies marked by questionable spending, a lack of clients, or lapses in record-keeping and care ... Many of the groups have since closed or are no longer providing AIDS services."[52] At that point, the Department of Housing and Urban Development also "threaten[ed] to cut off $12.2 million" worth of AIDS housing program funds because of lack of transparency in spending.[53] Key informant interviewees discussed ghost employees in the HAA who "hadn't shown up to work for two and a half years," and the federal government placed the whole Department of Health on manual drawdown because of "mismanagement of HRSA and CDC dollars." This meant that the department was now required to get "permission in advance for every single expenditure on every line on every grant" instead of filing quarterly or annually. As a departmentwide mandate, this also impacted the HAA.

High Leadership Turnover. The HAA, as well as the whole health department, also had very high leadership turnover. The jobs of health commissioner and HIV/AIDS chief were especially challenging. They involved managing multiple local and sometimes competing constituencies; navigating intersectional power politics; navigating city, federal agency, and congressional laws, policies, and preferences; and managing the full national and local media glare—all while managing several overlapping worst-in-the-nation epidemics. A 1987 interview of Commissioner Tuckson was telling. He raised the epidemic alarm early on and subsequently tried hard but struggled to mount an effective response. He told *The Washington Post* that he was fully aware of the challenges, predicted very high HIV/AIDS cases in the next five years, and was aware of the urgency inherent in his position, observing that administrators didn't last long. He noted of himself, "I know I probably only have two years."[54] This was apparent looking at both the length of his eventual tenure and those of others that followed.

Table 3 illustrates the very high turnover in the health department and the HAA in particular.[55] (The HAA was later put in charge of hepatitis, STIs, and TB, and became the HIV/AIDS, Hepatitis, STD, and TB Administration or HAHSTA.) There have been at least[56] 17 public health directors/commissioners between 1984 and 2015 (just under two years per director on average over the 31-year period) and at least 16 HIV/AIDS chiefs between 1986 and 2013 (just under two years per director over a 27-year period). Only in the last decade did administrators have long tenures: Commissioner LaQuandra Nesbitt (2015–22) and Chief Michael Kharfen (2013–21) were the longest serving in their respective positions, staying seven or more years each.

HAA chiefs left for a variety of reasons.[57] The official notices for departures described chiefs as being fired or mentioned that they left abruptly.

TABLE 3 DC public health leadership turnover, 1984–present

DC PUBLIC HEALTH DIRECTORS/COMMISSIONERS	
Ayanna Bennett	2023–present
Sharon Lewis (Acting Director)	2022–2023
LaQuandra S. Nesbitt	2015–2022
Joxel García	2013–2015
Saul Levin (Interim Director)	2012–2013
Mohammed N. Akhter	2011–2012
Pierre Vigilance	2008–2011
Carlos Cano (Interim Director)	2007–2008
Gregg A. Pane	2004–2007
James Buford	2002–2004
Ivan Walks	1999–2002
Marlene Kelly (Acting Director)	1998–1999
Allan S. Noonan	1997–1998
Marlene Kelly (Transitional Director)	1997
Harvey I. Sloane (Acting Commissioner)	1995–1997
Mohammed N. Akhter	1991–1995
Georges Benjamin (Acting Commissioner)	1990–1991
Reed V. Tuckson (Acting Commissioner from 1986–1987)	1987–1990
Andrew McBride	1984–1986

DC HIV/AIDS CHIEFS (HAHSTA SENIOR DEPUTY DIRECTORS)	
Clover Barnes	2021–present
Anjali Talwalker (Acting Director)	2021
Michael Kharfen	2013–2021
Gregory Pappas	2011–2013
Nnemdi Kamanu Elias (Interim Director)	2010–2011
Shannon Hader	2007–2010
Gregg Pane (Interim Director)	2007
Marsha Martin	2005–2007
Lydia Watts	2004–2005
Ronald Lewis	1998–2003
Chukwudi Saunders (Acting Director)	1997
Melvin H. Wilson	1995–1997
Frank Oldham Jr. (Director, HIV/AIDS Agency)	1994
Caitlin Ryan (Director, Office of AIDS Activities)	1991–1993
Iris Lee (Acting Director, Office of AIDS Activities)	1990
Jane Silver (Director of AIDS office, created in 1987)	1987–1989
Jean Tapscott (AIDS Coordinator for the District)	1986–1987
Selma DeLeon (AIDS Coordinator for the District)	1986

Underneath these explanations, interviewees and reports noted that while some left on their own accord, others left because of perceived or real incompetence, that is, because they were scapegoated or because they were actually responsible for service delivery failures. Some left because they were unable to manage the city's tedious bureaucracy and budget crises, which made it hard to hire staff to engage in prevention or to disburse funds, hard to carry out new initiatives, especially around prevention, and hard to fund small CBOs, especially as contracting was seen as particularly prone to corruption. Several were caught up in entanglements with the city's intersectional politics, and in particular, they did not build a broad enough coalition among the city's many constituencies; this meant they did not have enough political capital to survive when they inevitably ran up against city bureaucracy. Importantly, the job was highly politicized—new mayors and commissioners often wanted their own person in the job. This latter reason may partly account for the longevity of Kharfen and Nesbitt, as Muriel Bowser has been mayor since 2015. Regardless of the reason, the high turnover pattern clearly undermined efforts to establish long-term strategies to control the epidemic.

"The True Extent of the Epidemic Is Unknown": Poor Epidemic Surveillance. In August 2005, the DC Appleseed Center released a report following its investigation of the HAA. They were following up on Mayor Anthony Williams's puzzlement over why so much money had been spent on the epidemic over the years while so many were still dying from it.[58] Further, life-saving medication had been available for almost a decade and was free for the uninsured. A telling comment in the report was the statement, "The true extent of the HIV/AIDS epidemic in the District is unknown."[59] They attributed this to the HAA's poor or lacking disease surveillance system. The city was "not systematically collecting and analyzing data about the epidemic in a way that would allow it to plan prevention and care effectively."[60] In a continuation of the situation from 1991, they found a 50% staff vacancy in the surveillance unit (representing 13 federally funded positions) occurring because of "bureaucracy at HAA, DOH and the Office of Personnel."[61] This likely explained their so-called passive surveillance system, with staff waiting for reports to come in as opposed to being proactive, and with staff also not checking on errant reporters (e.g., doctors not reporting cases).[62] An additional problem in the surveillance office was neglect, as Chief Marsha Martin, who took over in September 2005, noted.[63] Three months before her arrival,

as Jose Vargas reported for *The Washington Post*, an office evacuation to deal with contamination uncovered misplaced boxes containing "HIV and AIDS cases . . . 2,000 to 3,000 [of them] that had yet to be entered into the city's database."[64] Under Chief Shannon Hader, who took over in 2007, the city reviewed death certificates with the CDC, uncovering underreporting of AIDS deaths, and had to begin an intervention with the city's doctors and labs to improve it.[65]

Poor epidemic surveillance meant that the true number of AIDS deaths may be much higher than illustrated in Figure 42 simply because of inadequate reporting. The Appleseed report also criticized the department for only conducting AIDS surveillance instead of HIV surveillance. Indeed, prior to 2007, the city was out of compliance with CDC mandates for reporting core HIV/AIDS metrics. It had apparently never submitted an HIV report and had not submitted an AIDS report in five years. Knowing AIDS rates was relevant for helping the very sick and dying, but less so for HIV prevention. Pre-ART, given the average six-to-ten-year gap between acquiring HIV and developing AIDS,[66] AIDS rates were a lagged indicator of where the HIV epidemic was six to ten years ago. As a result, as a city health official observed, "the response never evolved." This was particularly problematic for "long-standing AIDS service organizations [which] had not updated their response for the epidemic that we're seeing now." Thus, the public perception of the epidemic, especially among cisgender Black women, was also lagged. Forty-eight-year-old Kayla did not believe her 1999 diagnosis, observing, "When it first came and they said it's a White man's gay disease, so I, I, it excluded me. Right? And I was like 'I don't believe it.'" With no change in the message, as a Black woman city politician explained:

> Everyone is eliminating themselves, you try to eliminate yourself as much as possible. Ok, gay White men, then, okay um, gay lifestyle period . . . then drug use, okay, so you don't use IV drugs or drugs in general so you eliminate that way. Then jail, you don't talk to anyone who's ever been incarcerated, so then you knock that out, okay.

This resulted in a false sense of safety—and shock when diagnosis came.

Indeed, it became and were made clear to me in interviews and reports about missing data above, that the full longitudinal data underlying Figures 23 (HIV) and 42 (AIDS) were unavailable in real time to HAA until the first surveillance report in 2007. In addition, they did not know the extent to which it had shifted from an epidemic among gay men and injecting drug users to a generalized epidemic (across the whole population), and so they were unable to communicate the change in time. Further AIDS deaths in the poorest wards of the city blinded them to the widespread nature of new HIV infections occurring throughout the city, even among nonpoor straight Black people. Because of the latter's financial ability to manage their illness through health insurance and purchase necessary wraparound support, they could better keep AIDS and AIDS death at bay, making them invisible to the city's AIDS-based surveillance system. It also meant that people who were not in traditional "risk groups" did not know they were vulnerable and needed to protect themselves until it was too late. In sum, without knowing the true extent of the HIV epidemic, prevention efforts could not be directed to people or areas where resources were most needed, and the alarm could not be fully sounded. As such, the initial understanding developed in the pioneering years continued to serve as a template for the HAA as it disseminated funds to groups based on the historic perceptions of the epidemic as opposed to focusing on currently and newly vulnerable groups. The Appleseed report's findings galvanized the city's mayors, the HAA, and the city at large, and slowly but surely things began to change.[67]

Controlling the Epidemic

"Know Your Epidemic": Fixing the Surveillance System. A key turning point was a 2006 HIV testing campaign aimed at getting all DC residents to know their status (akin to UNAIDS guidelines to know your epidemic).[68] It was started under Chief Marsha Martin, who took over in 2005 after the Appleseed report was released, and continued under Interim Chief Gregg Pane (January through September 2007). As described by George Washington University professors Amanda Castel, Alan Greenberg, and colleagues, who were key actors, the HAA partnered with George Washington University, the CDC, OraSure Technologies, and local CBOs, among other actors, to run an intervention campaign to routinize HIV testing called "Come Together DC—Get Screened for HIV" so that people could know their HIV status earlier.[69] This involved creating an opt-out rather than opt-in testing policy throughout the health care system. In addition, free testing sites became widespread, not just in the city's emergency rooms but also places like the Department of Motor Vehicles.

The campaign yielded results used in the city's first HIV surveillance report, produced by the HAA's surveillance unit led by Tiffany West-Ojo in partnership with a George Washington University team led by Amanda Castel and Alan Greenberg.[70] It was released in November 2007 when newly appointed Chief Shannon Hader (under Mayor Fenty) was in her first few months. (Reports have been released annually since then). The 2007 and 2008 reports made clear how the epidemic had evolved. They revealed just how high the city's HIV prevalence was—3%, which was likely an underestimate—and the disproportionate impact on Black people, among whom 4.3% had HIV, compared to 1.4% of White people. They revealed that Black women's HIV prevalence was equivalent to White men's (2.6%) and that Black men had the highest prevalence—6.5%.[71] It also illustrated a citywide epidemic; while between 2003 and 2007, Ward 8 had the highest rate of newly reported HIV/AIDS cases, Wards 5, 1, 7, and 6 were also greatly impacted,[72] necessitating a citywide strategy, not just one focused on the poorest wards. In other words, HIV/AIDS had crossed the class containment barrier. The reports also revealed that the epidemic had become generalized across the population (above 1% prevalence), escaping the sexual containment barrier and reflecting the crossover from an epidemic predominantly among men who had sex with men (MSM) and injecting drug users to one that fully included heterosexual men and women. Shockingly, it found, 9% of the entire nation's mother-to-child HIV transmission cases in 2005 were in Washington, DC.[73] Also alarming was that "between 1997 and 2006, almost 70% of all AIDS cases progressed from HIV to AIDS in less than 12 months after the initial HIV diagnosis, primarily due to late testing."[74]

Developing Data-Driven, Evidence-Based Interventions. Armed with this data, Hader kicked off what would be over a decade of data-driven, evidence-based interventions carried out under her and subsequent HAA chiefs Elias, Pappas, Kharfen, and Barnes to tackle key epidemic drivers. They continued to emphasize routinized HIV testing, which sometimes required fighting with insurance companies to get them to cover proactive testing that was not clinically indicated, as well as getting private providers to test their patients. Indeed, the city launched a social media campaign for a direct-to-consumer "Ask for the Test" campaign[75] in order to encourage privately insured patients to ask doctors for an HIV test. The HAA ironically found it easier to effect change at scale in the public health care system, which poorer patients were more likely to access, than in the private system. As a result, as an official observed, outcomes may have been more successfully and quickly achieved in the city's poorest neighborhoods once interventions began.

The HAA also ran "Rubber Revolution," a public sector condom distribution campaign, ramping up from 115,000 condoms distributed in 2006 to 1.5 million by 2008.[76] Cross-departmental openness to the campaigns was in stark contrast to that experienced by Commissioner Tuckson when he tried to run mass awareness campaigns in 1988 and 1989, and Metro refused to put up condom posters in public transport vehicles.[77] The HAA also worked with CBOs to update their responses and approaches, including linkages to care, which before meant testing in one place and getting care in another. This would mean shorter gaps between diagnosis and treatment, which in turn would reduce AIDS deaths and transmission. Another important intervention, "It's Free to Treat Your HIV," combatted what was found to be a lack of awareness of free ART, thus providing motivation for testing and ART uptake. Given the urgency to get people with HIV onto ART, pre-exposure prophylaxis (PrEP)—preventive use of ART for HIV-negative people—was understandably not a major component of the city's intervention strategy.[78] (As described in Part 3, Congress lifted its ban on needle exchange programs in 2007, allowing the city to partner with CBOs to bring the HIV epidemic among injecting drug users under control, with dramatic effect—see Figure 34).

The HAA's interventions had an astounding effect on the epidemic, as evidenced by dramatic declines in newly diagnosed HIV cases and AIDS deaths, indicating very high linkage to ART. By 2016, an estimated 76.2% of people with HIV were in care and 62.7% were virally suppressed (i.e., had undetectable levels of the HIV virus).[79] And by 2022, 80.5% were retained in care and 68.6% were virally suppressed,[80] indicating a lower community viral load[81] that conferred a sort of "herd immunity" on the population as a whole. The city's HIV epidemic was well on its way to being under control (UNAIDS goals aim for 90% in care and 90% suppressed). The HAA's spectacular success was accomplished through utilizing comprehensive real-time data to develop data-driven, evidence-based analyses to identify where the biggest challenges lay; its liberally drawing upon university-based expertise, private media marketing know-how, and CBO's on-the-ground knowledge to design and implement interventions; and its ability to depend on mayoral and broad multisectoral government support to accomplish its goals.

While the HAA's efforts led to a controlled epidemic, they reduced but did not eliminate racial health inequality. Figure 44 reveals a tale of two epidemics. The top panel illustrates the White HIV and AIDS epidemic and the middle panel illustrates the Black epidemic. The bars show a disproportionately high overall burden of HIV among Black people compared to White people, and the trend lines show that for both groups AIDS deaths rose before and fell following ART. However, Black deaths rose dramatically higher and faster pre-ART, and while they also fell dramatically, they stabilized at a high level, and gains were reversed during COVID. (As noted in Chapter 12, the post-ART era was also an era of declining proportions of Black residents and increasing proportions of White residents—see Figure 10). The bottom panel illustrates new HIV diagnoses, with the initial rise likely reflecting the citywide 2005–7 testing campaign. While new Black diagnoses then fell dramatically, they stabilized at a level 9.6 times higher than White people by 2022.

Spatially, even though gentrification has shifted the city's racial residential patterns, Figure 45 illustrates a clear relationship between where Black people lived and new HIV diagnoses (top map) and living cases (bottom map). Overall, wards with higher proportions of Black people had higher numbers of new diagnoses and people living with HIV.

Finally, data from the 2023 HAHSTA report makes racial health inequality in the epidemic even more apparent. As Table 4 illustrates, while Black people comprised an estimated 43.4% of the city's population, they comprised almost three-quarters of living (70.6%) and newly diagnosed (73.3%) HIV cases and almost 80% of AIDS deaths. By contrast, White people comprised an estimated 37.5% of the city population, 14.7% of living HIV cases, 7.6% of new cases, and 10.4% of AIDS deaths.[82] Among new diagnoses in 2022, while Black MSM comprised a third (37%) of cases, Black heterosexual women comprised a higher proportion of new cases (16%) than White MSM (8%) or Black heterosexual men (9%).[83]

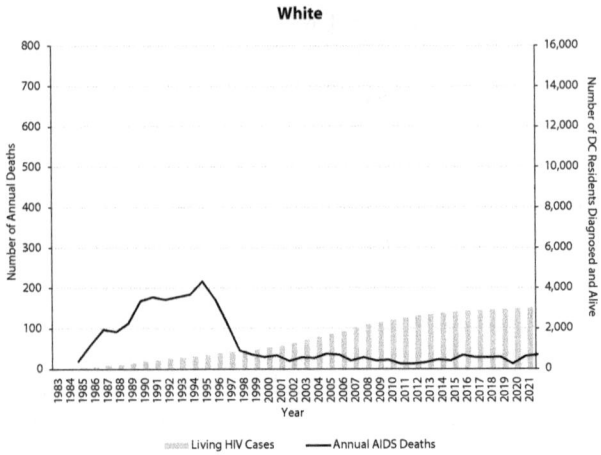

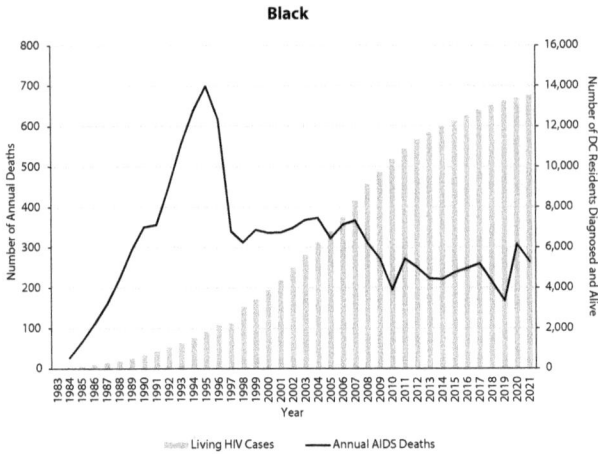

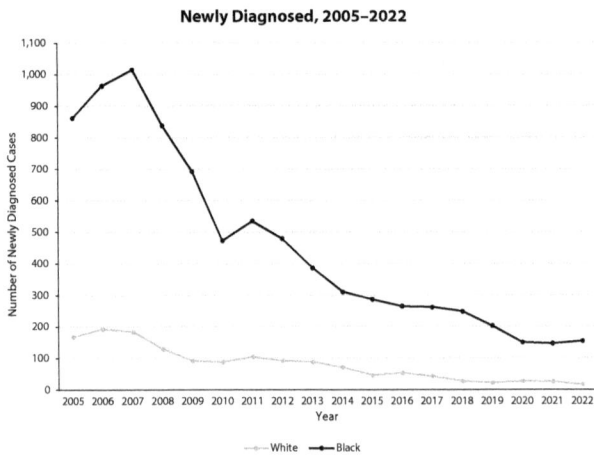

FIGURE 44. The DC HIV/AIDS epidemic, 1983–2022, by race. Data sources: DC HAHSTA HIV/AIDS Surveillance Unit and *Annual Epidemiology and Surveillance Reports* (1983–2022).

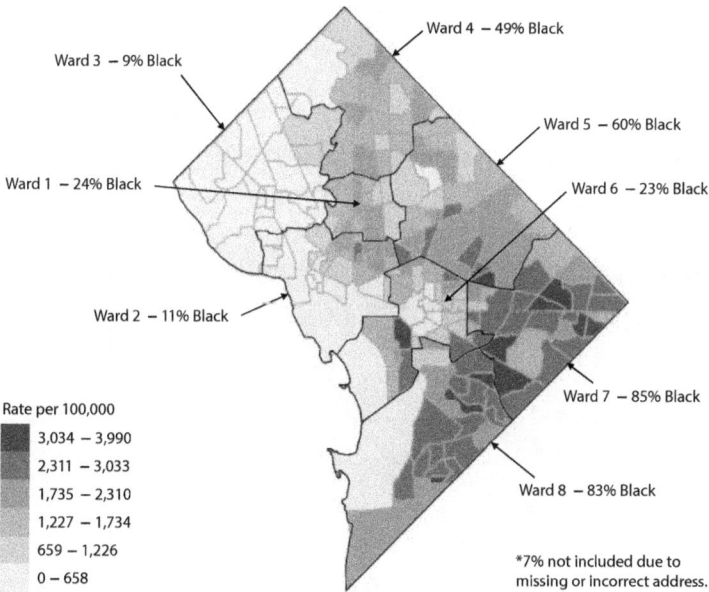

Rate of Newly Diagnosed HIV Cases in the District by Ward and Census Tract, District of Columbia, 2022 (N = 210*)

Ward 4 — 49% Black
Ward 3 — 9% Black
Ward 5 — 60% Black
Ward 1 — 24% Black
Ward 6 — 23% Black
Ward 2 — 11% Black
Ward 7 — 85% Black
Ward 8 — 83% Black

Rate per 100,000
121 – 172
91 – 120
61 – 90
31 – 60
1 – 30
0

*5% not included due to missing or incorrect address.

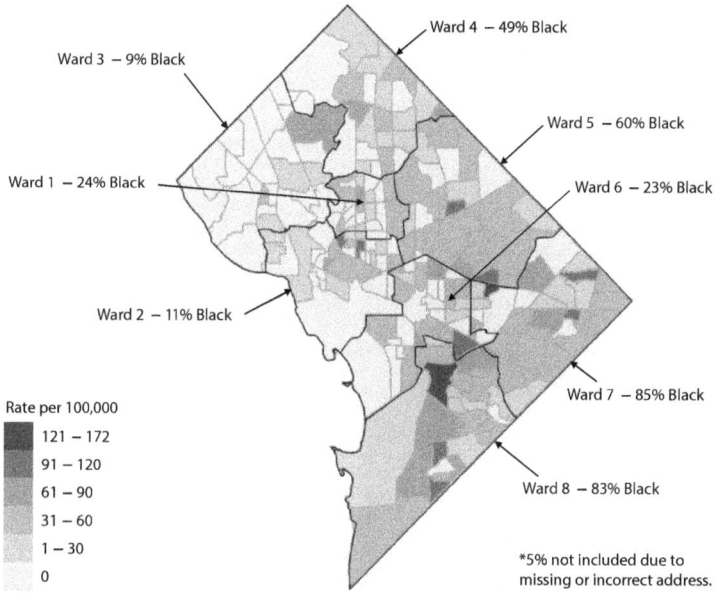

Rate of HIV Cases Living in the District by Census Tract, District of Columbia, 2022 (N = 11,747*)

Ward 4 — 49% Black
Ward 3 — 9% Black
Ward 5 — 60% Black
Ward 1 — 24% Black
Ward 6 — 23% Black
Ward 2 — 11% Black
Ward 7 — 85% Black
Ward 8 — 83% Black

Rate per 100,000
3,034 – 3,990
2,311 – 3,033
1,735 – 2,310
1,227 – 1,734
659 – 1,226
0 – 658

*7% not included due to missing or incorrect address.

FIGURE 45. Rates of newly diagnosed HIV cases and people living with HIV by race, ward, and census tract, DC, 2022. Data sources: DC HAHSTA, *Annual Epidemiology and Surveillance Report*, 2023; American Community Survey.

TABLE 4 Racial/ethnic distribution of HIV/AIDS cases in DC, 2021–22

Race/ Ethnicity	% of DC Population, 2022	% of Total Living HIV Cases, 2022	% of New HIV Cases, 2022	% of AIDS Deaths, 2021
Black	43.4	70.6	73.3	78.9
White	37.5	14.7	7.6	10.4
Hispanic/Latino	11.7	8.6	13.8	3.0
Other	7.4	6.2	5.2	7.7

DATA SOURCE: DC HAHSTA, *Annual Epidemiology and Surveillance Report*, 2023.

CONCLUSION

Overall, this Part illustrates that even after ART medication became available, the city's HIV/AIDS outcomes reflect both the life-saving presence and the lethal absence of or actions by a range of institutions and actors, such as Congress, the city government, the HAA, and a wide range of local CBOs. Congress's paternalism and the city's intersectional politics and antiquated financial systems and policies, as well as HAA corruption and its insufficient surveillance system, worked together to create lagged and outdated responses, limiting services and medication access for Black, especially poor, people. Yet even when Congress and national agencies were supportive, city government was efficient, medication was universal and free, and the HAA performed spectacularly to control the epidemic, the lack of change in racial health inequality highlights the fact that technocratic expertise and universal health care were necessary but not sufficient in neutralizing the role of racial containment in producing and reproducing unequal life and death outcomes.

Conclusion

We hold these truths to be self-evident, that all men are created
equal, that they are endowed by their Creator with certain unal-
ienable Rights, that among these are *Life*, Liberty and the pursuit of Happiness.—That to secure these rights, Governments
are instituted among Men, deriving their just powers from the
consent of the governed,—That whenever any Form of Government becomes destructive of these ends, it is the Right of the
People to alter or to abolish it, and to institute new Government,
laying its foundation on such principles and organizing its powers in such form, as to them shall seem most likely to effect their
Safety and Happiness.

DECLARATION OF INDEPENDENCE, 1776
[my emphasis]

RACIAL CONTAINMENT AND RACIAL
HEALTH INEQUALITY

This book examined why Washington, DC, has one of the nation's worst
racial life-expectancy gaps. I have argued that this is not accidental but by
design. I have shown how intersecting systems of inequality worked through
racial, class, and sexual containment to recurrently produce health inequality
across generations. In particular, I have shown how the racial containment
principle with its negative cultural schema (comprised of coagulated and
automated beliefs, assumptions, and stereotypes about Black people's inferiority) shaped default institutional ways of seeing, thinking about, and acting
towards Black people, and especially poor Black people. Taking a system-
wide and historical approach lifts our gaze from the ghetto and focuses on

the social forces that create and sustain it. The book illustrates how racial containment was entrenched and embedded in interlocking and interacting laws, regulations, procedures, practices, and policies governing the operation of multiple public and private institutions over time. I show how this played out in a succession of congressional bodies, federal agencies, and local government institutions, even with changing casts of White, Black, Republican, and Democratic actors. Racial containment was deployed not just through a range of health policies but also through policies concerning city finances, banking, land valuation, housing, education, police, criminal justice, and prisons, among others. The sheer range of institutions and policies deployed in racial containment reflects redundancies in the system of racism aimed at maintaining and reproducing White and class privilege across generations, ensuring that even ostensibly race- and class-neutral policies were continually undermined. For example, policies for decent, middle-class style public housing for the poor were undercut by ignoring building codes and building on environmentally unsound land, followed by the denial of Black loans and racial covenants, which led to racial inequality in the ability to escape to the suburbs, followed by federal denial of funds to maintain and repair public housing, followed by federal government funding to improve housing stock for the wealthy, further squeezing out the Black poor.

The book also illustrated how intersectional politics, and class containment in particular, undergirded racial containment. It showed how racial containment can turn a community in on itself through presenting singular solutions to social problems that required the deployment of class containment. For example, Black mayors pursued gentrification to balance the books and avoid losing home rule, per congressional rules, but in the process they facilitated the displacement of the Black poor; the Black middle class and affluent escaped to the suburbs to pursue better city services, safety, and education for their children, taking their tax dollars with them (as Congress did not permit commuter taxation) and exacerbated city poverty and racial health inequality; and mass incarceration was targeted at Black people of lower socioeconomic status in the absence of effective drug interdiction or funding for mass addiction treatment. However, intraracial class containment was only partially successful. Racial health inequality still followed many Black people into the suburbs, albeit to a significantly lesser degree than in the city. Within the city, public housing projects were sited in middle-class Black neighborhoods, ensuring spillover effects from city syndemics. And mass incarceration rebounded on the community when it dramatically distorted marriage markets, contributing to high levels of nonmarriage, and amplified the HIV/AIDS epidemic, which escaped class containment barriers.

Racial and class containment clustered together social ills, producing syndemic zones in poor Black neighborhoods. These zones of disinvestment and political abandonment had overlapping and interacting epidemics, which worked together to amplify the occurrence of each epidemic as well as give birth to spillover epidemics. They were characterized by poor city services, such as neglectful garbage collection and poor enforcement of housing codes, as well as by poor or limited federal, business, and local government investment, poor public transportation, poor response to resident complaints, and poor schools. They were also unhealthy environments, located near garbage dumps and highways, with high pollution exposure, and on environmentally unsound land. Given this combination of factors, people living in city sacrifice zones were vulnerable to illness and premature death, starting from infant mortality through to multiple exposures to HIV, drugs, gun violence, and homicide, as well as spillover chronic disease epidemics. This was illustrated in cascading epidemics unfolding in the same places, clustering premature deaths from multiple causes and tearing through multiple generations of Black families and neighborhoods.

Ironically, the solutions to the problems racial containment created often resulted in the reproduction of racial health inequality. People were displaced from alleys and slums to eliminate syndemics through urban renewal. They moved into overcrowded and poorly maintained housing, which contributed to ill health, or into public housing buildings that deteriorated due to lack of maintenance and subsequently served as ground zero for new syndemics for subsequent generations. Mass incarceration, another form of racial containment, was the primary solution to those syndemics. But prisons hosted syndemics, which through circular migration amplified Black community syndemics. Numerous institutional redundancies undergirded each recreation of racial containment. In the case of mass incarceration, multiple institutions, such as the police, schools, and the political- and prison-industrial complexes, and multiple congressional and local laws and policies, such as sentencing laws, zero tolerance school policies, and the structural pull of parole law, contributed to the (re)production of this form of racial containment. As noted in the Introduction, racial and class containment are both spatial (segregation) and nonspatial (clustering together privileges or social ills). This was illustrated in the city's response to the AIDS epidemic, with disease framing that lagged the coroner's office reports, disproportionate resource allocation to White CBOs despite changing demographic realities, and Congress and the city resolving financial challenges by cutting programs and services to the poor, exacerbating their health challenges. The intransigence of racial health inequality is evidenced by the glacial pace and/or reversals of progress regardless of actor intentions, political affiliations, and/ or race, especially in the face of new epidemics, as evidenced by COVID-19. In combination, I have argued that racial containment amounts to death by design—a concept capturing not just the deliberate cause-effect design of social policies, processes, procedures, and laws, but also more benign policies, such as entrenching the conditions of possibility for disproportionate Black deaths in poor Black neighborhoods.

While I have focused on Washington, DC, and on Black people, this story also speaks to the intergenerational reproduction of marginality in communities across the country. For example, many Native American and poor White communities have also been subject to containment dynamics. Many live in economically disadvantaged, politically abandoned, environmentally challenging places, and are beset with multiple overlapping epidemics as well as disproportionately clustered premature deaths that have unfolded across generations.[1] This was more recently exemplified by the opioid and COVID-19 epidemics, with rising poor White mortality and worsening of the already persistently low Native life expectancy.[2] For these communities too, health outcomes are not just a function of individual choices. They are also a product of intersecting systems of inequality working through a range of institutions and policies to recurrently produce unequal health outcomes in the same places among the same populations.

ELIMINATING HEALTH INEQUALITY

Limitations of Current Approaches

This book illustrates the limits of overreliance on the criminal justice and health care systems to solve health crises. In the case of DC, mass incarceration ultimately worked to amplify Black community syndemics. And even when federal, university, and health department technocratic expertise was combined with community knowledge and universal health care, racial health inequality remained stubbornly in place. This is because health departments and the criminal justice system are last-resort institutions, managing outcomes of exposure to a lifetime of societal ills. Without placing emphasis on demand-side policies,[3] money drained into the criminal justice and health care systems and out of root-cause institutions aimed at countering these cumulative exposures and working to prevent or delay entrance into these systems. This neglect positioned the health department and criminal justice system in the role of putting out fires, at large expense, often in the same zip codes among disproportionate numbers of people from the same groups, over and over again, as epidemics came and went. Because syndemic zones give birth to multiple epidemics, without improving places and investing in America's marginalized and sickest communities through multisectoral action, health inequality will remain in place, by design.

The Need for Systemic Change

The redundancies created by systems of privilege and inequality illustrate how they work to undergird each other. Tackling these systems is necessary as they reproduce social problems more reliably than individuals who come and go can fix them. In the long run, it is much cheaper and more efficient to fix defective systems than it is to deal with the many challenges of people exposed to them. Focusing on systems also avoids the trap of what William Ryan called blaming the victim. Because, he noted,

> the ultimate effect is always to distract attention from the basic causes and to leave the primary social injustice untouched. And, most telling, the proposed remedy for the problem is, of course, to work on the victim himself. Prescriptions for cure ... are invariably conceived to revamp and revise the victim, never to change the surrounding circumstances. They want to change his attitudes, alter his values, fill up his cultural deficits, energize his apathetic soul, cure his character defects, train him and polish him and woo him from his savage ways.[4]

As evidenced by the civil rights, feminist, and LGBTQ movements, systemic changes to racism, classism, and heteropatriarchy have required a combination of (a) legal battles to change laws, policies, and regulations across multiple institutions, such as the workplace, the education system, and the health system; (b) media engagement and other activities aimed at changing negative cultural schemas about groups such as women, the poor, non-White people, nonheterosexual people, and/or gender nonconforming people; and (c) protests to exert pressure on policy makers and create ongoing public awareness of injustice.[5] Systemic multisectoral change is needed to weaken institutional redundancies that undergird unequal health outcomes.

Focus on Place-Based Interventions

In addition, the groundedness of health crises also suggests the need for a renewed focus on place-based interventions centering on America's sickest neighborhoods, communities, and counties, which are invariably poor minority and White neighborhoods.[6] The US has a long history of experimentation with place-based interventions in the country's poorest communities, with ideas proposed and tried by both Democrats and Republicans, suggesting agreement about the root problem. In the last half century, these have included the multiagency Model Cities Program in the 1960s, initiated under Lyndon Johnson, and the National Commission on Severely Distressed Public Housing, established in 1989 under George H. W. Bush, the recommendations of which led to the establishment of the public housing Hope VI program, funded with congressional appropriations in 1993 under Bill Clinton. More recently, the Obama administration initiated Promise Neighborhoods in 2010 through the Department of Education and Choice Neighborhoods through the Department of Housing and Urban Development, and the Trump administration initiated Opportunity Zones in 2017 through tax incentives.[7]

Overall, the interventions have had varying degrees of success and have been subject to criticism. Failures have often been attributed to poor program targeting—they have not always been narrowly focused on the poorest people and/or the poorest neighborhoods; place identification has been left up to gubernatorial or mayoral discretion and thus subject to patronage; interventions have been under-resourced, with funds spread too thinly to effect change; policy favor has changed from administration to administration; there has been bureaucratic infighting among the multiple agencies involved; and there have been power struggles among governors, mayors, private businesses, and community groups when large amounts of federal funding are in play.[8] As this book has illustrated, such intersectional politics often divert even earmarked resources away from the poor. Nonetheless, past failures should not lead to the abandonment of place-based initiatives. Rather, new interventions should aim to identify lessons learned and improve upon past efforts.

Bipartisan and continuous state and congressional will to reduce health inequality and extend the lives of residents in the most marginalized and sickest communities in the United States could turn the tide on their unacceptably low life expectancy. This would contribute not only to higher average life expectancy in their respective states but also to higher overall life expectancy in the United States as a whole.

Washington, DC

Enduring and extreme racial health inequality in the nation's capital undermines the main reason for government according to the US Declaration of Independence—securing life for *all* its citizens. Congress has been experimenting with different versions of federal city governance throughout its history—variously giving and taking away power, giving independence and meddling in city affairs, respecting and overriding the will of the people, financially setting the city up to fail and then dramatically coming to the rescue.[9] Regardless, it is clear that the current system of governance is not working when Black girls and boys born in the capital of the United States can expect to live 12 and 18 years less than their White counterparts, respectively. Throughout the city's history, the seesaw between congressional "racism and paternalism,"[10] indifference and micromanagement, mapped onto local intersectional politics have combined to produce disproportionate Black physical and social death. Congress and the city often engage in seemingly intractable and endless debates about the commuter tax, reparations, having no voting representation on final legislation in Congress, and statehood. This book will no doubt add fuel to those debates. However, poor Black residents in the city's poorest places, and poor Black men in particular, have been neglected and considered disposable for far too long and need immediate solutions and investment on a Marshall Plan scale. They should no longer be ignored, corralled, or gentrified away from their home city. It is my hope that this book compels congressional and city leaders to engage in concerted multisectoral action to close the racial health gap and finally end the suffering of generations of poor Black DC residents.

. . .

CONCLUSION PLAYLIST

Public Enemy	Fight the Power (1989)
Kendrick Lamar	Alright (2015)
Common & John Legend	Glory (2015)
Nas	I Can (2002)
Beyoncé	Freedom (2016)
Michael Jackson	Man in the Mirror (1988)
Roy Ayers	DC City (1983)
Janet Jackson	Rhythm Nation (1989)
Aretha Franklin	Amazing Grace (Live at New Temple) (1972)
Al Green and Deniece Williams	Lift Every Voice and Sing (1985)
Yolanda Adams	And Still I Rise (1998)
Mahalia Jackson	We Shall Overcome (1947)
Duke Ellington	New World a-Comin (1943)
Mambo Sauce	Welcome to DC (2011)

Methodological Note

STAGE ONE—"A SMALL SUMMER PROJECT"

Why Is the HIV Prevalence Rate So High Among African Americans in DC?

This study began after I read a newspaper article about DC's HIV epidemic and was bothered by the fact that its Black residents were so affected, despite living in the capital of the most powerful nation on earth. At the University of Colorado Boulder, where I began my career, junior faculty were given a small pot of use-it-or-lose-it research money. So I decided to use the award to conduct a small summer project in DC over five weeks in June and July 2011. My plan was to conduct key informant and individual interviews to try to understand why the rate of HIV was so high among African Americans. I began by looking online for DC organizations working with people living with HIV and also asked friends and colleagues for leads. While a few key informants were recruited through referrals, most were recruited through cold calling/emailing, as well as showing up to organizations to ask for interviews. Key informant interviews stretched between 2011 and 2023, but most were conducted during the summer of 2011. I conducted 10 in-depth key informant interviews with six cisgender men and four cisgender and trans women. Respondents included District public health and local government officials, African American community leaders, and heads and staff of community-based organizations, including neighborhood churches, hospitals, and HIV/AIDS prevention and service provision organizations. I asked about their biographies, how they got involved with their organizations, and what their organizations did. I also asked how they thought larger city dynamics might be impacting the HIV epidemic.

After these interviews, I gave key informants study fliers with my contact information and asked if they could share them with people who might fit the study criteria— African Americans living with HIV in DC. Interested interviewees then called me to request participation in the study. From there, recruitment occurred through snowball sampling—with participants hearing about the study from other participants or key informants. I interviewed 37 people living with HIV—18 cisgender men, 10 cisgender women, and 9 trans women. Respondents had a variety of sexual identities, some of which had changed over time, and they ranged in age from 20 to 61, with most in their 40s and 50s (all but three were aged 40 or more). (As noted in Part 3, this age distribution mirrors DC's HIV demographics.) Interviewees were paid $30 for their time, and I tried to keep interviews to about an hour, though some were longer and some were shorter. I interviewed respondents at locations of their choosing throughout the city, including in homes (permanent, transitional, or borrowed), community organizations, restaurants, and workplaces. My experiences travelling to and from interviews were instructive in helping me better understand my respondents and the city's many worlds.

I decided to follow a compressed life history format in my interview schedule. Rather than narrowly focusing on asking respondents about practices they think led to HIV acquisition, I was interested in contextualizing their acquisition, and I decided to ask them to tell me about their lives as a whole, leading up to and following diagnosis. As a result, interviews covered a wide range of topics, including respondents' parents' biographies, their own early childhood and family life growing up, residential, educational, and employment histories, friendships, current family life, sexual and romantic relationship histories leading up to their current or last relationship, condom use, HIV acquisition and transmission, HIV status disclosure, drug and sexual risk and protective behaviors, and current experiences living with and managing HIV and any comorbidities. I also asked them about their current everyday lives and their future hopes and dreams. Toward the end of each interview, after respondents had shared their life story, I asked each respondent for their own theories of why the rate of HIV was so high among African Americans in DC to gain insight into the city's epidemic through their eyes and life experiences.

My interviewees placed me in different social categories. Most often, I was simply a Black girl (girl!) interviewing her fellow Black people, and I was readily inserted into DCs distinctive Black color hierarchy (more than one respondent referred to my skin color as a reference point, e.g., "He was your complexion, I like dark men"). Other times I was an African, signaled, for example, by comments about Africa and Africans regularly sprinkled throughout the interview. I was a professional Black woman, ma'amed with formal responses to questions; and yet other times I was specifically an academic, responded to in ways that made clear that a respondent had participated in other academic studies. In these interviews, respondents would package all the information they thought I wanted to know in a neat and efficient paragraph at the beginning. I often spent the rest of the interview carefully unpacking that paragraph and drawing out respondents to underscore my interest in their life as a whole, not "just the facts." I was often shifted in and out of these categories in the course of an interview. My positionality, with respect to race, nationality, class, and gender, thus created both familiarity and distance, and I tried hard to monitor the emotional tenor of interviews, build rapport with respondents, and make them feel comfortable sharing their life stories.

My positionality was shaped by my heritage and life experiences. The United States has been my home for more than two decades, and I entered the category of African American on gaining citizenship. However, growing up, I had a certain obliviousness about race and ethnicity. Born on a continent where most people shared my race, I had a Ugandan mother from a dominant ethnic group and a Kenyan father from two different ethnic groups (one politically marginalized, one politically useful to those in power), and I spent part of my childhood in Tanzania, a country whose revolutionary first president, Julius Nyerere, worked hard to neutralize the power of ethnicity. As such, for much of my postcolonial East African childhood, the consequences of race and ethnicity were things that happened to other people. My obliviousness continued even when scholarships enabled me to regularly encounter and live alongside White people in a boarding school with missionaries' and diplomats' kids in Kenya, and with children of wealthy parents at a private boarding school in England. However, as I grew older, going on to university in England, coming to the US for graduate school in Chicago, and then moving on to various jobs, I experienced both gradual awareness and rude awakenings as I encountered racism that was expressed both overtly (e.g., racist words shouted at me on the street, being followed around in a store, etc.) and subtly (e.g., looks, silences, strange marginalizations, social invisibility, etc.).[1] However, my respondents' life stories and the many rabbit holes they led me down to write this book showed me exactly how racism could become deadly—getting under the skin, imprinting itself on psyches, bodies, neighborhoods, and a city, and how it could recurrently produce poor Black health across generations.

The combination of a short period of fieldwork and a compressed life history format made for a particularly intense five weeks. By the end, though I had more interviews lined up, I stopped interviewing because I had reached saturation (hearing repeated responses across interviews) and due to my own overwhelm after hearing so much pain and trauma. My counseling psychologist mother suspected "secondary trauma" when I struggled with emotional and analytic paralysis for many years after. While the interviews were transcribed shortly afterwards and I was able to begin thinking about the larger story, it was several years before I stopped running from the interviews and began the reading/rereading process and started to code and analyze the transcripts "objectively."

STAGE TWO—HISTORICIZING AND CONTEXTUALIZING

As I conducted my interviews, it became clear to me that there was a larger story going on beyond individual lives and choices. For example, after many respondents described prison experiences, research revealed that it was not an artifact of my snowball sample but characteristic of a generation of young Black men. I wondered about the extent of drug addiction disclosed by respondents, and research revealed that this, too, was not an artifact of the sample but a major phenomenon in the city. My interviews also quickly revealed the limits of trying to use contemporaneous data to understand current events. As respondents, largely aged 40–60, told me their life stories, I realized that to fully understand their current outcomes, I had to at least start looking at the city's history starting in the 1950s through the 1970s, when many were born. Key informant interviews also mentioned historical phenomena that underscored the importance of digging into the city's history.

The study's expansion continued when some of my initial historical research revealed that HIV was just one of many worst-in-the-nation city epidemics, suggesting there was something about the city that made it particularly prone to epidemics, and epidemics which predominantly affected African Americans. HIV/AIDS was thus the latest epidemic, the latest cause of death, and what I was really looking at was an instantiation of the reproduction of racial health inequality. Eventually I decided it would be better to just start from the city's founding in 1790 and work my way forward, examining the city's recurrent health crises up until the HIV/AIDS and then COVID-19 epidemics. The connections between HIV and drug addiction in my interviews, as well as drugs and homicide in the city, led to a deeper focus on the SAVA syndemic that unfolded between 1960 and 2022.

As the project became more historical, I oriented myself by reading classic texts on urban epidemic political histories, such as Charles Roberts's work on cholera, Keith Wailoo's work on sickle cell anemia in Memphis, Samuel Roberts's work on tuberculosis in Baltimore, and James Colgrove's work on the public health administration in New York City. My historical thinking about DC built on older histories by Constance McLaughlin Green, Letitia Woods Brown, Howard Gillette Jr., James Borchert, and Betty Plummer, among many others, as well as recent histories by Chris Myers Asch and George Derek Musgrove, Sarah Shoenfeld of Prologue DC, Genny Beemyn, Justin Shapiro, Kwame Holmes, and Rebecca Dolinsky, among many others. Collectively, these histories were helpful guides for my own archival work, especially in identifying primary sources and the types of primary sources to look for.

Key primary sources for my reconstruction of the city's early health history were Board of Health reports, which are digitized and easily accessible. I read and took notes on all the Board of Health reports from 1872 through 1890 and then picked one report from each subsequent decade (1900, 1910, 1920, 1930, 1940, 1950, 1960 reports) to read and analyze. For 1970 through 2022, I drew on a variety of hard copy reports, including the city's own Vital Statistics reports (1974, 1980, 1985), the city's Biennial report (1980), as well as digitally available National Vital Statistics and Life Table reports which included information on Washington, DC, to fill in the gaps (1970, 1990, 2000). For 2010 through 2022, I drew on digitally available academic articles, grey literature, as well as city health reports, including a 2010 community needs assessment report and its annual HIV/AIDS surveillance reports (2007–23).

To reconstruct the city's drug, homicide, mass incarceration, and Black HIV/ AIDS histories, I conducted archival research drawing on reporting in *The Washington Post*, focusing on articles published between 1960 and 2010 on cocaine, heroin, AIDS, and Lorton prison. I supplemented this research with more focused triangulating searches in other papers such as the *Washington Examiner*, the *Washington City Paper*, *The Washington Informer* and the *Washington Blade*. I read and took notes on articles chronologically to get a clear picture of how the epidemics unfolded and how they were perceived to have unfolded by various actors. I supplemented archival newspaper research with historical and contemporary reviews of academic, government, and grey literature as well as interviews (including two oral histories from the Rainbow History project) to fill in gaps, triangulate, check newspaper claims, where possible, and thicken the analysis.

Finally, I drew on longitudinal quantitative datasets to further ground, triangulate, and substantiate the study. These included data from DC's HIV/AIDS surveillance unit (1983–2015), DC's HIV/AIDS surveillance reports (2016–23), the National Center for Health Statistics/Vital Statistics (1880–2022), the Disaster Center (1960–2010), the Global Health Data Exchange (IHME, 2000–2019), the US census (1880–2020), and the American Community Survey (2010–22).[2] Overall, this historical and contextual turn added several years to this project because of its large scope, multiple methods, and the slow and laborious process of archival research.

STAGE THREE—THEORIZING, ANALYZING, AND WRITING

Theoretically and analytically, I used both a sociohistorical and socioepidemiological approach to locate my respondents and their health challenges within the larger historical, political, and social contexts of the city in which their lives unfolded. I took inspiration from C. Wright Mills's noting in *The Sociological Imagination* that "neither the life of an individual nor the history of a society can be understood without understanding both."[3] Thus, in Glen Elder's words, I sought to "join human lives with their [historical] times."[4] My interview schedule and coding strategy (both manual and NVivo coding) was explicitly geared towards exploring my respondents' life course histories. I deductively examined life stages, and domains and turning points within those stages, such as childhood (family life, friendships, neighborhood life), the transition to adulthood (educational, employment, residential, and romantic/sexual experiences), and middle and older age. I inductively examined emergent themes, such as prison experiences, drug use (personal, family, and friend use, selling drugs, etc.), religion, and friend and family deaths.

I also utilized a "whole system,"[5] "web of causes"[6] socioepidemiological approach. I examined both individual health trajectories—deductively examining HIV/AIDS (diagnosis, transmission, disclosure, and management), as well as drug addiction and other comorbidities—as well as the full range of institutions that shaped peoples' lives and health outcomes as they transitioned into and through adulthood, such as those they directly encountered (schools, health care settings, families, workplaces, prisons, clubs, etc.) and more distal institutions such as local and federal government agencies. This approach necessarily stretched the project across disciplines and sociological subfields. A system-wide approach attendant to institutions enabled me to see the many redundancies in the system of racism as they cumulated in respondents' lives as they aged. Joining interview analysis with qualitative and quantitative archival research also enabled me to see how processes unfolding long before my respondents were born shaped the circumstances of their life choices, risk factors, and health outcomes.

Guided by these approaches, data analysis and writing proceeded through triangulation among data sources. Triangulation was especially important in mitigating some of the limitations of my sample. I interviewed survivors of the SAVA syndemic, and snowball sampling meant, to some degree, that I was interviewing social networks. I was also not interviewing a random sample of people but a highly select group comprising some of the most marginalized people in the city. Thus, I was interested in both locating *these* lives in the flow of the city's history as well as understanding the extent to which respondents were unique or typical of the larger DC population. I first drew on interview coding and analysis to draft thematic chapters (on drugs, prison, sexual transmission, etc.) and then began to historize and contextualize each section, going as far back and as broadly as I thought was necessary to locate and understand respondents' lives and outcomes. Individual respondent narratives stood in for the many, illustrative of larger city trends and dynamics, and also took center stage as singular experiences of people who lived through the syndemic.

Finally, as I noted in the Introduction, this is a partial story.[7] A key challenge throughout the project was balancing breadth and depth. I often felt that each Part could be more fully fleshed out and more deeply researched in a standalone book; so much remains to be told. A story should be told of the heroic White gay activism in the city. The Hispanic story, which is complex and paradoxical, deserves a full unpacking. And even within the Black story, there is a richer and more complete story to be told. Many more actors than appear in these pages played crucial roles in the city and community responses to mitigate the various epidemics that faced DC, and their stories should also be told. Finally, a rich story should be told of the legal, political, and social grassroots resistance to racial health inequality throughout the city's history.

ACKNOWLEDGMENTS

This book has greatly benefited from a large number of people and institutions. I first thank all my interview respondents for sharing their life stories. At the University of Colorado Boulder (CU-Boulder), I thank the Council on Research and Creative Works, the Population Program at the Institute of Behavioral Science, and the Undergraduate Research Opportunity Program, which provided primary funding for the fieldwork and interview transcriptions. I have also benefited from administrative and computing support from population research centers at CU-Boulder, the University of Michigan, and Princeton's Office of Population Research (OPR). At OPR, I am grateful for the wonderful staff and especially Associate Director Nancy Grinius-Cannuli, Mary Lou Delaney (now retired), and Kristen Neri for their assistance and support.

Over the years, I have also greatly benefited from hard working and persistent assistants, including undergraduate students Rosemary Rast and Sara Watkins, graduate students Allison Scott Pruitt, Miriam Peterson, Erin Ice, Janette Norrington, Lemeng Liang, Beza Taddess, Marley Olson, and Rob Kemp, and postdoctoral associate Jolene Tan, who helped to gather data, file public records requests, source information, and conduct quantitative analyses, among other tasks. I am especially indebted to Jolene Tan for her crucial assistance in the final year of this project, in working on many of the book's figures and helping to get them press-ready.

I thank my father Aloo Mojola for giving me such a grand introduction to the full range of African American music when I was growing up, my brother Luka Mojola for helping me to curate the book's playlists, and Margo Mahan for cluing me in to DC's go-go music. I thank Julie Dombrowski for her introduction to then DC HAHSTA Director Michael Kharfen, and him as well as then Strategic Information Officer Rupali Doshi and then Chief Epidemiologist Adam Allston for access to DC HIV surveillance data. I also thank current HAHSTA Director Clover Barnes and Chief Epidemiologist Kate Drezner for access to more recent surveillance data.

Many academic staff provided crucial assistance, including Boriana Pratt, OPR's statistical programmer; GIS/cartography specialists Jeffrey Blossom (Harvard), Caitlin Dickinson (Michigan), and Gabe Moss (Moss Maps); and librarians, especially Joann Donatiello (OPR/Princeton), along with Nicholas Reynolds (Princeton), and Kirsten Graupner and Stefan Gellner (Wissenschaftskolleg zu Berlin). I am also very grateful to Mitch Duneier, Princeton Sociology's chair extraordinaire, for his encouragement and instrumental support, enabling me to keep making progress on this book amidst myriad administrative responsibilities directing OPR. I am grateful to Donna DeFrancisco in Sociology for her administrative support and kindness. I also thank my OPR predecessor Doug Massey and, at Princeton's School of Public and International Affairs, current dean Amaney Jamal and former dean Cecilia Rouse for their encouragement, support, and belief in me.

This book would have taken years longer if it were not for fellowships from Harvard University's Hutchins Center, the Wissenschaftskolleg zu Berlin, a German Institute of Advanced Study (Wiko), and the Religion and Politics Cluster of Excellence at Westfälische Wilhelms-Universität-Münster, Germany. These fellowships granted uninterrupted time away to think deeply, write, and participate in interdisciplinary scholarly communities. At the Hutchins Center, I benefited from a 2015–16 Hutchins Fellowship from the W. E. B. Du Bois Research Institute and am grateful to its director Henry Louis Gates Jr., my assigned mentor William Julius Wilson, and the staff, in particular Krishna Lewis, Velma DuPont, and Justin Sneyd. Justin's poster advertising my presentation at the Center inspired this book's cover. I also thank the Center fellows who gave early feedback. At Wiko, I benefited from a 2021–22 sabbatical fellowship and am grateful to its rector Barbara Stollberg-Rilinger, the staff, in particular Vera Pfeffer and Daniel Schönpflug, the librarians mentioned above, and the Villa Jaffe housekeeper Ellen Lehmann. I greatly benefited from the many fellows who gave feedback; in particular, Bernardo Zacka, Adrian Favell, Hannah Landecker, and Liza Lim. At the Cluster, I benefited from a 2022–24 visiting fellowship allowing for several short visits over winter, spring, and summer breaks, enabling me to briefly escape and write. I am grateful to its Speaker Michael Seewald, the staff (in particular Judith Grubel and Angela Marciniak) and the faculty for their generosity and warm hospitality. The German time zone gave me a clear morning to think and write, keeping my US administrative responsibilities at bay while prospective email writers and callers were (mostly) asleep. I also benefited from independent writing retreats at the Rondo Retreat Center in the Kakamega Rainforest of Western Kenya and the Highlights Foundation Writing Retreat Center in Boyds Mill, Pennsylvania, where I was wonderfully taken care of and left alone to think and write.

The book has been greatly enriched by many academics. From the project's beginnings, and as I entered new literatures, disciplines and sub-disciplines over the ensuing years, I benefited from orienting conversations and references.

CU-Boulder colleagues Patti Adler and Tim Wadsworth, as well as David Kirk, Andrew Papachristos, Megan Comfort, and Brian Kelly provided helpful entries into drug and criminology literatures; Derek Hyra, Michael Bader, and Liza Weinstein provided helpful entries into urban sociology literatures; Josh Pacewicz encouraged me to look at city budgets; and as the project became more historical, conversations with Andrew Abbott and Princeton colleagues Keith Wailoo and Alison Isenberg were especially helpful. I additionally benefited from opportunities to present work in progress at many institutions, receiving important questions, comments, and critiques from many audience members and in one-on-one conversations. These helped to put the book's arguments through their paces, often sent me back to the drawing board, and pushed me to fill in crucial gaps and thicken my analysis. I am very grateful for the audiences in university sociology departments at American, Arizona-Tucson, Brown, Columbia, Georgia, Massachusetts—Boston, New York, Northwestern, Princeton, and the American Sociological Association's Social Dimensions of AIDS session. I am also grateful to audiences in population research centers at Harvard, Cornell, Columbia, Penn, and CUNY; inequality centers at Cornell and Columbia; health and behavioral science centers and departments at CU-Boulder, CU-Denver, University of Washington/Fred Hutchinson Center for AIDS Research, Columbia, Michigan, Vanderbilt, and American; and Yale's History of Science and Medicine program and Ethnography Project.

In addition to hearing presentations, many colleagues also read and provided invaluable feedback and critique on various versions of papers and chapters as they developed. My first audiences at CU-Boulder included members of our Sociology Junior Faculty Workshop including Stefanie Möllborn, Christina Sue, Amy Wilkins, Isaac Reed, Jenn Bair, Hillary Potter, and Jill Harrison, as well as Jason Boardman, Fred Pampel, Rick Rogers, Patti Adler, and Tim Wadsworth. At Michigan, I am grateful to the Urban Sociology working group members Alexandra Murphy, Jeremy Levine, Jacob Lederman, and Karyn Lacy, who pushed me to revise and thicken what is now Part 1 and to do more to flesh out the city's health history. That part was also enriched by comments and critique from the Witwatersrand Institute for Social and Economic Research (WISER) in Johannesburg, South Africa, whose participants included Sarah Nuttall, Achille Mbembe, Keith Breckenridge, Hlonipha Mokoena, Pamila Gupta, Richard Rottenburg, and Isabel Hofmeyr. Brian Kelly, Andrew Papachristos, Christina Sue, Stefanie Möllborn, and Princeton colleagues Jean Grossman, Rhacel Parreñas, and Laurence Ralph provided helpful feedback on other chapters. I am especially grateful to colleagues who participated in a 2022 book manuscript workshop organized by Mitch Duneier, which included him, Keith Wailoo, Shamus Khan, Judy Auerbach, and Matthew Desmond. While I did not follow all their recommendations, their deep engagement with my work, detailed comments, trenchant critiques, and critical questions pushed me intellectually and greatly improved the book's theoretical apparatus, content, arguments, and readability. I am also grateful to the University of California Press, whose reviewers, including Andrea Leverentz and an anonymous reviewer, provided very useful comments and critiques. I am indebted to Naomi Schneider, my editor, for her incredible patience and steadfast belief in me over the many years between proposal and finished product, her advocacy on my behalf, and the many (many many!) extensions I was granted. I also thank the press staff, including Aline Dolinh and the entire production team, for their hard work and dedication getting this book to press.

Finally, I have been fortunate to have a rich community of colleagues, friends, and family who encouraged, supported, and believed in me and this project. I am grateful for my Princeton colleagues, and especially Kathy Edin, Tim Nelson, and Matt Desmond, along with Viviana Zelizer, Mitch Duneier, and Dalton Conley for their warm welcome, kindness and generous friendship, especially when I first arrived at Princeton. I am grateful to Daniel Jordan Smith for his advice and support at critical junctures of my career. I remain ever grateful for the steadfast support, wisdom, and guidance of my long-time mentors Jane Menken, Dick Jessor, Janet Jacobs, Judy Auerbach, Andy Abbott, and Patrick Heuveline whose confidence and belief in me from the very beginning gave me the courage to take scholarly risks. In DC, Zuzana Johansen generously hosted me, and her encouragement, support, and kindness were crucial in sustaining me through many low points of fieldwork. I also thank Nicole Angotti for her steadfast support and encouragement and for generously connecting me to local DC scholars. Old friends, especially Stef, Christi, Fernando, Carew, Joanne, Eric, Jayme, and Kirsten, and new friends, especially Michael, Alyx, Ilya, David, Sofía, Jess, Sean, Mark, and Juan kept my spirits up, graced me with kindness, wisdom, generosity, hospitality, and delicious food, and most of all kept me laughing. My Kenyan/Ugandan family, immediate and extended, and especially Aloo, Freda, and Luka Mojola have been my sharpest interlocutors and biggest cheerleaders. I am forever grateful for them. Soli Deo Gloria.

INTRODUCTION

1. Figure 1 estimates are drawn from Arias et al 2024. This is the most recent report from the National Vital Statistics System. (See note 2 of the Appendix for details.)

2. See also Montez et al 2020.

3. Harper et al 2014; M. Roberts et al 2020; A. Silva et al 2023; Hendi 2024.

4. Hendi 2024:418–9. Nationally, Hispanic and Asian Americans have a higher life expectancy than White Americans (Dwyer-Lindgren et al 2022). This was also the case in DC. While overall Black life expectancy was 72.7 years, White, Hispanic, and Asian American life expectancy was 88 years, 88.3 years, and 89.9 years, respectively (https://www.countyhealthrankings.org/health-data/district-of-columbia?year=2021&measure=Life+expectancy*&tab=1). To understand the Hispanic health advantage, see Markides and Eschbach 2005 and Riosmena et al 2013. To understand the Asian health advantage, see Acciai et al 2015. Since 2007, Native Americans have had the lowest life expectancy in the US (Dwyer Lindgren et al 2022).

5. D. Williams and Sternthal 2010; see also D. Williams and Jackson 2005; Rogers 1992; Schwandt et al 2021.

6. Wrigley-Field 2020.

7. See also Andrasfay and Goldman 2021.

8. Johnson et al 2022; Waidmann et al 2025.

9. Hendi 2024:419 (Table 2).

10. Xu et al 2022; M. Roberts et al 2020.

11. Case and Deaton 2015, 2020; see also Metzl 2019.

12. Kochanek et al 1994; Harper et al 2007; Harper et al 2012; Elo et al 2014a; Fuchs 2016; Sharkey and Friedson 2019; Schwandt et al 2021.

13. Fuchs 2016:1869 (Table).

14. Krieger 1994; Wilkinson 1996; Berkman and Kawachi 2000; US Department of Health and Human Services, https://health.gov/healthypeople; Centers for Disease Control and Prevention, https://www.cdc.gov/about/priorities/social-determinants-of-health-at-cdc.html?CDC_AAref_Val=https://www.cdc.gov/about/sdoh/index.html.

15. Fielding-Miller et al 2020; Karmakar et al 2021; Millett et al 2020; Feldman and Bassett 2021.

16. Link and Phelan 1995; Gutin and Hummer 2021; Kawachi and Berkman 2003; Diez Roux and Mair 2010; Williams and Collins 2001.

17. Rhodes et al 2005:1027.

18. Singer 1994; Milstein 2001; Singer and Clair 2003; Singer and the Hispanic Health Council 2000; Singer et al 2017.

19. Edlin et al 1994; Singer and Clair 2003; Kwan and Ernst 2011; J. P. Meyer et al 2011; Freudenberg et al 2006.

20. Singer and the Hispanic Health Council 2000.

21. Stall et al 2008; Egan et al 2011.

22. Stall et al 2008; J. P. Meyer et al 2011.

23. Islam et al 2021.

24. Linas et al 2021; Holland et al 2021; Piquero and Roman 2024.

25. Millett et al 2020.

26. Including Berkman and Kawachi 2000; Williams and Collins 2001; Diez Roux and Mair 2010; Sampson and Wilson 2005; Massey and Denton 1993; Sharkey 2008; Friedman et al 2009; Auerbach et al 2011; Blankenship et al 2005; Kuzawa and Sweet 2009; Singer 1994; Singer and Clair 2003; Milstein 2001.

27. For structural sexism and health, see Homan 2019. For structural heteropatriarchy and health, see Everett et al 2022. For SES and health, see Link and Phelan 1995; Gutin and Hummer 2021. For structural racism and health, see Bailey et al 2017; T. Brown and Homan 2024.

28. Umberson 2017; Umberson et al 2017; see also Abraham 1993.

29. See for example Newell 1998.

30. Goosby et al 2018; see also Kuzawa and Sweet 2009.

31. Barker 1990; De Boo and Harding 2006; Goosby et al 2018; Kuzawa and Sweet 2009.

32. Goosby et al 2018:330; see also Geronimus 1992.

33. Singer and the Hispanic Health Council 2000.

34. While space and place are distinct phenomena (Gieryn 2000), in this book, I use the terms interchangeably to capture both physical settings as well as the less tangible ways in which people are contained to social locations.

35. I first started thinking about and working with the idea of *containment* when encountering its usage in a 1948 national report on segregation that referred to the residential containment of Black people to particular parts of the city. Other usages include A. Hirsch, who in the foreword to the 1998 edition of his 1983 book on Chicago ghetto-making, noted, "What we experienced was the ferocious application of a domestic 'containment' policy—the word itself was frequently used by contemporaries in this context—that complemented American foreign policy in rhetoric and imagery" (1998:xv). Manning (1998:335), writing on Washington DC, also discussed a "racial containment strategy."

36. Wilson 1987; Massey and Denton 1993; Tilly 1998, 2000; Weber (1922) 1978; Starr 2019; Desmond 2023; Logan and Molotch 1987.

37. Chetty et al 2016.

38. Bischoff and Reardon 2014; Reardon et al 2018. Though see Leung-Gagné and Reardon 2023 for debate on estimates.

39. See also W.J. Wilson 1978; Killewald et al 2017.

40. W.J. Wilson 1987.

41. Edin et al 2023.

42. Desmond 2016, 2023.

43. Lerner 2010.

44. Bullard 1990; Bullard et al 2008; Lerner 2010; Commission for Racial Justice 1987; Singer 2011.

45. See for example Noonan 2005.

46. Sampson 2012. For literature reviews, see Kawachi and Berkman 2003; Diez Roux and Mair 2010. See also Ross and Mirowsky 2001; Fitzpatrick and LaGory 2003; Boardman et al 2005; Morenoff 2003.

47. See for example D. Williams and Collins 2001.

48. Massey and Denton 1993. See also Drake and Cayton 1945; K. Clark 1965; A. Hirsch 1983; Venkatesh 2000; Duneier 2016.

49. For histories, see Limerick 1987; Blackhawk 2023. For life expectancy, see Dwyer-Lindgren et al 2022; Goldman and Andrasfay 2022.

50. A. Morris 2015.

51. Du Bois 1899.

52. Elbers 2021.

53. D. Williams and Collins 2001.

54. Hendi 2024.

55. D. Williams and Collins 2001. See also Phelan and Link 2015; Bailey et al 2017.

56. D. Williams and Collins 2001; Bailey et al 2017; Brown and Homan 2024; R. Walker et al 2010; Crowder and Downey 2010.

57. LaVeist and Wallace 2000; J.P. Lee et al 2020.

58. Commission for Racial Justice 1987; see also Bullard 1990; Bullard et al 2008.

59. Ladner 1986; Collins 1990; Crenshaw 1991.

60. Collins 1990.

61. Braveman et al 2010:S192 (Figure 1a). See also Schoendorf et al 1992; Fishman et al 2021.

62. Massey and Denton 1993; LaVeist et al 2011.

63. Sampson and Wilson 2005:180.

64. Sharkey 2013:27–28.

65. Sharkey 2008:933.

66. Schwandt et al 2021:6.

67. Schwandt et al 2021:6.

68. Spain 2014.

69. Risman 2004; West and Zimmerman 1987; Acker 1990; Schilt and Westbrook 2009; Westbrook and Schilt 2014; Courtenay 2000; Connell 2012; Dovel et al 2015.

70. Connell 2005; Connell 2012; Rubin 1993 [1984]; Everett et al 2022.

71. Moen 2001; see also Mojola et al 2021, 2022.

72. Verbrugge 1985, 1989; Case and Paxson 2005; Courtenay 2000; Read and Gorman 2010; Moen 2001.

73. Nicolosi et al 1994.

74. J. Becker et al 2017.

75. Bird and Rieker 1999; Courtenay 2000; Connell 2012.

76. Daly and Wilson 1988; Kanazawa and Still 2000; Madfis 2014; Ashforth 1999; Courtenay 2000; D. Cohen and Nisbett 1994.

77. Krieger 2000; Miller and Grollman 2015; Schilt and Westbrook 2009; McKay et al 2023.

78. Mojola et al 2021.

79. See S. Lee 1993:78 (Table 1); see also Prewitt 2005; Cohn 2010; Parker et al 2015:19–31; Jensen et al 2021.

80. Omi and Winant 1994:55; Winant 2000; Saperstein et al 2013. For global perspectives, see Bethencourt 2014.

81. Treitler 2013. See also Bonilla-Silva 2004; J. Lee and Bean 2004. Though for rejoinder, see Alba 2009.

82. Hamilton 2019; J. Collins et al 2002; Hamilton and Hummer 2011; Elo et al 2014b; Hamilton and Green 2018; Ifatunji et al 2022.

83. Bonilla-Silva 1997:466. See also Feagin 2013; Feagin and Bennefield 2014; Bonilla-Silva 2021.

84. Bonilla-Silva 2006.

85. Ray 2019.

86. Reskin 2012.

87. Friedland and Alford 1991; DiMaggio 1997; J. C. Scott 1998; Boutyline and Soter 2021; Ray 2019; Ridgeway and Correll 2004; Acker 1990; Starr 2019.

88. Ray 2019; Reskin 2012.

89. Reskin 2012; see also Bailey et al 2017; Mojola et al 2021; Fernández-Kelly 2015.

90. Pedulla and Thébaud 2015; England et al 2020.

91. Starr 2019.

92. Monk 2021:40.

93. Krieger 2021:xi, 24. Krieger extends Pierre Bourdieu's discussion of "embodied history" with respect to bodily habitus to examining how health is embodied (2021:44–46), and how "literal 'pathways of embodiment' connect … this lived experience to population distributions of health outcomes" (45).

94. Krieger 2021; Goosby et al 2018; Chowkwanyun 2011; Hammonds and Reverby 2019; McBride 1991; Edin et al 2023.

95. Krieger 2021:43, 67.

96. C. Rosenberg 1962; Wailoo 2001; S. Roberts 2009; Colgrove 2011.

97. Mbembe 2019:66.

98. *Washington Informer*—Nov 16, 2022—Barnes; *Washington Examiner*—Aug 30, 2010—Jaffe (see print newspaper sources at the end of the bibliography). See also Waters 1997; Dula 1994.

99. Washington 2006; D. Roberts 2017.

100. National Advisory Commission on Civil Disorders 1967:1.

101. Duneier 2016:11.

102. Ruble 2010; Jaffe and Sherwood 2014; Gillette 1995; Manning 1998; Asch and Musgrove 2017.

103. *Post*—Jan 23, 2015—Brown; *Post*—Jun 29, 2022—Van Dam; Perry et al 2022:6 (Table 2).

104. *Washington Times*—May 23, 1994—Eberstadt; Jaffe and Sherwood 2014; Asch and Musgrove 2017.

105. *The New Republic*—May 5 2015—Vinik.

106. *NBC Washington*—Feb 8, 2018—Jacob; *Post*—Mar 14, 2018—Nirappil.

107. Jaffe and Sherwood 2014:254; *Post*—Nov 24, 1990—Escobar.

108. For DC, see Edwards et al 2009; *Post*—Mar 17, 2016—Shaver and Hedgpeth. For Flint, see Hanna-Attisha et al 2016.

109. Magnus et al 2009; *Healio Infectious Disease News*—Jan 1, 2008—Ellis.

110. The phrase was popularized by George Clinton and Parliament Funkadelic.

111. Hyra 2017.

112. I was inspired to do this after a question from Australian composer Liza Lim about whether there was a soundtrack or an underlying music to the book as I wrote. See also Wailoo 2001.

113. Wendland 2022.

PART I

Overview

1. Georgetown University 2016. See also C. King et al 2022.

2. DC estimates for 2022 from censusreporter.org.

3. https://coronavirus.dc.gov/page/2021–2022-coronavirus-data.

4. Hendi 2024.

5. District of Columbia Department of Health 2014, 2019; King et al 2022.

6. Link and Phelan 1995; D. Williams and Collins 2001.

7. Naveed 2017. See also J. Bernstein et al 2006.

8. Naveed 2017:1.

9. Naveed 2017:2.

10. DC Policy Center 2021.

11. https://planning.dc.gov/page/census-and-demographic-data-ward-3; https://planning.dc.gov/node/1180945 (estimates drawn from the American Community Survey 2010–14).

12. https://planning.dc.gov/page/census-and-demographic-data-ward-8; https://planning.dc.gov/node/1181226 (estimates drawn from the American Community Survey 2010–14).

13. https://planning.dc.gov/sites/default/files/dc/sites/op/publication/attachments/Key%20Indicators%202017-2021_1.pdf.

14. Reproduced from District of Columbia Department of Health 2014:19, 32, 33 (Figures 16, 41, and 42).

15. Reproduced from District of Columbia Department of Health 2019:9.

16. See also King et al 2022.

1. The First Era: 1790–1890

1. Gillette 1995:27; Asch and Musgrove 2017.

2. L. W. Brown 1972:130–131.

3. L. W. Brown 1972.

4. Gillette 1995:28–29.

5. Gilette 1995; L. W. Brown 1972; C. Green 1962.

6. Asch and Musgrove 2017:17.

7. Gillette 1995:37.

8. Hodder 1936:525.

9. Hodder 1936.

10. See https://www.senate.gov/artandhistory/history/common/image/DCEmancipationAct.htm. See also Asch and Musgrove 2017.

11. Manning, 1998:332.

12. National Committee on Segregation in the Nation's Capital 1948:18 (hereafter National Segregation Report 1948). See original 1872 city code at https://code.dccouncil.gov/us/dc/council/code/sections/47-2907.

13. National Segregation Report 1948:22.

14. District of Columbia Black Homeownership Strike Force Final Report 2022:7, https://dmped.dc.gov/sites/default/files/dc/sites/dmped/page_content/attachments/BHSF%20Report%20FINAL%20FINAL%20.pdf.

15. C. Green 1967; Gatewood 1990; Moore 1999; Byrand 1999; E. Taylor 2017; Asch and Musgrove 2017.

16. Gatewood 1990:38.

17. Asch and Musgrove 2017:171.

18. C. Green 1962:91 (see also Table 2 on p. 92).

19. C. Green 1962:91.

20. Grigoryeva and Ruef 2015; Groves and Muller 1975:173–4.

21. Asch and Musgrove 2017:189; Groves 1974.

22. Fletcher 2008.

23. Borchert 1980.

24. Groves 1974:270–271.

25. Borchert 1980:39.

26. Borchert 1980.

27. Borchert 1980:12.

28. Borchert 1971/1972; Plummer 1984; Groves 1974.

29. Borchert 1980; Groves 1973:264.

30. Byrand 1999.

31. Asch and Musgrove 2017:137; see also Downs 2012.

32. Asch and Musgrove 2017:138; see also C. Green 1967.

33. Asch and Musgrove 2017. See also Shoenfeld 2019a.

34. Gatewood 1988; Gatewood 1990.

35. Gatewood 1990:65–66.

36. R. M. Johnson 1984; Ruble 2010; Asch and Musgrove 2017:185–88.

37. Asch and Musgrove 2017:185–88.

38. Asch and Musgrove 2017; Borchert 1973/1974.

39. Groves 1974:271.

40. Groves 1974; see also Borchert 1971/1972.

41. C. Green 1962; C. Green 1967; Borchert 1971/1972; Groves and Muller 1975; Borchert 1980; Gilette 1995; Asch and Musgrove 2017.

42. C. Green 1962; C. Green 1967; Borchert 1971/1972; Groves and Muller 1975; Borchert 1980; Gilette 1995; Asch and Musgrove 2017.

43. Board of Health 1872:42.

44. Board of Health 1872 (supplemental report):135.

45. Plummer 1985:220.

46. Board of Health 1875:68.

47. Borchert 1973/1974.

48. Board of Health 1877:46.

49. Board of Health 1875:68–69.

50. Borchert 1980.

51. Board of Health 1890:640. The apparent rounding up of population sizes between 1883 and 1890 suggests that these were estimates. Indeed, in the 1890 report, while the death counts appear to be specific, the health officer, Smith Townshend, MD, discussed why he was assuming a population size of 250,000. (The 1890 Census listed the city's total population at 230,392, with 75,572 Black and 154,695 White people. He was thus overestimating by about 20,000 people—15,305 White and 4,428 Black). His reasons included potential census undercounting (it was conducted in June when the city had significant summer out-migration), the city's transient visitors, and an unusually high death rate of members of Congress (Board of Health 1890:660–661). He concluded by stating: "In fact I am satisfied that a reenumeration of a few of the districts made today would demonstrate that upon the whole 20,000 additional is a very small margin upon which to proceed" (661). If we recalculate the 1890 death rates based on the mortality table death counts and the 1890 census population sizes, we get 34.80 for "Coloreds" and 18.97 for "Whites." So the overestimates do not change the basic conclusion concerning racial death inequality.

52. Board of Health 1890:668.

53. Plummer 1985:218.

54. Board of Health 1876:249.

55. Board of Health 1875:92–93.

56. Groves 1974:274.

57. Groves 1974:274.

58. Clark-Lewis 1994; C. Green 1962; Asch and Musgrove 2017.

59. Borchert 1980:174–176. I present DC racial trends in widowhood (1880–2020) in Part 2, Figure 28. See also C. Green 1962; C. Green 1967; Borchert 1971/72; Groves and Muller 1975; Asch and Musgrove 2017.

60. Board of Health 1875:91.

61. C. Green 1962; National Capital Housing Authority Report 1944:136.

62. Board of Health 1877. See also C. Green 1962.

63. Board of Health 1877:26.

2. The Second Era: 1890–1950

1. National Committee on Segregation in the Nation's Capital. Hereafter National Segregation Report 1948.

2. Manning 1998:333; see also Massey and Denton 1993.

3. A. Hirsch 1998 (1983).

4. S. Roberts 2009.

5. C. Green 1962:147–154; Borchert 1971/72; Gillette 1995.

6. De Graffenried 1896:14.

7. National Capital Housing Authority Report 1944 (henceforth NCHA 1944).

8. NCHA 1944:139.

9. https://millercenter.org/the-presidency/presidential-speeches/december-6-1904-fourth-annual-message.

10. See S. Roberts 2009 for the case of Baltimore.

11. NCHA 1944:42; Groves 1974:271; Gillette 1995.

12. 63rd Congress. Session II. Chs 310. Pg 716–717, H.R.13219 (1914) (enacted). https://uscode.house.gov/statviewer.htm?volume=38&page=716.

13. Gillette 1995; NCHA 1944.

14. Borchert 1980:34–35.

15. NCHA 1944.

16. https://www.fdrlibrary.org/housing; NCHA 1944:112.

17. Brabner-Smith 1936:631.

18. Brabner-Smith 1936:631.

19. Brabner-Smith 1936, 1937.

20. NCHA 1944:81.

21. NCHA 1944:13, 11, 42.

22. NCHA 1944:13, 11, 42.

23. Meier and Rudwick 1967; National Segregation Report 1948.

24. The research committee of the National Segregation Report was Louis Wirth (chair), Will W. Alexander, Charles H. Houston, Joseph D. Lohman, Donald Young, Robert C. Weaver, Charles Dollard and E. Franklin Frazier. For reaction to the report, see Woodson 1949; Green 1967; Pritchett 2005.

25. National Segregation Report 1948:62–63. See also Meier and Rudwick 1967.

26. Cited in Jaffe and Sherwood 2014:10.

27. National Segregation Report 1948:55.

28. National Segregation Report 1948:57.

29. C. Green 1967; Manning 1998; Asch and Musgrove 2017.

30. NCHA 1944; Gillette 1995.

31. NCHA 1944:55–58, 60–64.

32. See S. Roberts 2009 for the "infected house" approach in the case of Baltimore.

33. NCHA 1944:8.

34. Swope 2018:709.

35. Swope 2018:710.

36. NCHA 1944:143.

37. NCHA 1944:145.

38. National Segregation Report 1948:91.

39. Jaffe and Sherwood 2014:10.

40. Jaffe and Sherwood 2014:10.

41. S. Roberts 2009.

42. NCHA 1944:17.

43. National Segregation Report 1948:32–33.

44. *Post*—Feb 6, 1944—Meyer (see print newspaper sources at the end of the bibliography).

45. Gillette 1995.

46. Lavine 2010:447.

47. Swope 2018; Lavine 2010.

48. Lavine 2010:443.

49. Lavine 2010:444, 448.

50. Asch and Musgrove 2017:321.

51. https://www.cdc.gov/std/treatment-guidelines/timeline.htm#:~:text=1943%20%E2%80%93%20Penicillin%20used%20for%20the,government%20focus%20on%20gonorrhea%20control; https://www.cdc.gov/world-tb-day/history/?CDC_AAref_Val=https://www.cdc.gov/tb/worldtbday/history.htm.

52. Lavine 2010:458.

53. *Pittsburgh-Washington Courier* in 1949, cited in Gillette 1995:163.

54. Gillette 1995; Lavine 2010.

55. Ammon 2009:188.

56. NCHA 1944.

57. NCHA 1944.

58. The National Association of Real Estate Exchanges became the National Association of Real Estate Boards (NAREB). This later became the National Association of Realtors. https://www.nar.realtor/about-nar/history.

59. Barnes 1980:474.

60. Barnes 1980:456.

61. NCHA 1944:58–59.

62. NCHA 1944:59.

63. NCHA 1944:59.

64. *Post*—Dec 19, 1965.

65. Gillette 1995:164; Jaffe and Sherwood 2014:13. See also Kofie 1999.

66. Manning 1998:335.

67. *Post*—Dec 19, 1965.

68. See also Oliver and Shapiro 2006 (1995); K. Taylor 2019; Golash-Boza 2023.

69. NCHA 1944:98.

70. Barnes 1980:454.

71. A. Hirsch 1983.

72. Bullard 1990; Bullard et al 2008; Lerner 2010.

73. https://www.nar.realtor/about-nar/history/1924-code-of-ethics.

74. Winling and Michney 2021:51, 48, 53–54.

75. Winling and Michney 2021:57.

76. Michney and Winling, 2020:156.

77. National Segregation Report 1948:88; on Bilbo, see https://www.senate.gov /about/origins-foundations/electing-appointing-senators/contested-senate-elections /126Theodore_Bilbo.htm.

78. Gillette 1995; Manning 1998; National Segregation Report 1948.

79. National Segregation Report 1948:32.

80. National Segregation Report 1948:30 (quote); Shoenfeld and Cherkasky 2017 for 1921.

81. Manning 1988:335.

82. See Shoenfeld 2019b.

83. Winling and Michney 2021:60; Jackson 1987.

84. Shoenfeld 2019b; https://mappingsegregationdc.org/resident-sub-areas .html.

85. Golash-Boza 2023.

86. This racialized spatial coding exercise was a nationwide process, as Jackson (1987) and Rothstein (2017) have comprehensively documented.

87. See Grigoryeva and Ruef 2015 for primary and tertiary segregation.

88. National Segregation Report 1948:25.

89. Fullilove 2004.

90. National Segregation Report 1948:33.

91. National Segregation Report 1948:26.

92. In this section I draw on Board of Health (BOH) reports from 1900, 1910, 1920, 1930, 1940, and 1950 (see BOH 1910:10, 247 for Figure 19).

93. The 1900 BOH report did not record overall death rates by race (see 1900:6) nor did it provide population sizes by race. However, it did provide death counts by race (3,325 White deaths and 2,628 "Colored" deaths). I used population sizes from the 1900 census (White population = 191,532; Black population = 86,702) to calculate the crude death rates reported in the main text ((Death count/Population size)*1000).

94. BOH 1900:6.

95. BOH 1910:12–13.

96. BOH 1910:12, 252.

97. BOH 1910:253.

98. BOH 1920:82.

99. BOH 1920:82. It is important to note that the average age of death differs from life expectancy in that the latter is a prospective estimate of how long someone can expect to live.

100. BOH 1920:84.

101. National Segregation Report 1948:48.

102. National Segregation Report 1948:49.

103. National Segregation Report 1948:48.

104. According to the 1950 census, DC was 64.6% White (517,865/802,178) and 35% Black (280,803/802,178), totaling 99.6%. As such, in DC the non-White category still functionally meant Black.

105. BOH 1950:155.

106. BOH 1950:154, 157 (table).

107. BOH 1950:157.

108. BOH 1950:156. See also BOH 1940:139.

109. BOH 1950:153.

110. National Segregation Report 1948:49–50.

111. National Segregation Report 1948:52.

112. National Segregation Report 1948:49.

113. National Segregation Report 1948:50.

114. Baker et al 2008.

115. National Segregation Report 1948:53.

3. The Third Era: 1950–Present

1. Hyra 2017.

2. Figure 10. See also Hyra 2017; Asch and Musgrove 2017; Sturtevant 2014.

3. See Chapter 2; see also Manning 1998; Lacy 2007; Jackson 1987.

4. Jaffe and Sherwood 2014; Asch and Musgrove 2017; Golash-Boza 2023.

5. US Census. Estimates were calculated from the underlying data used to construct Figure 10. US Census data for the District of Columbia was downloaded from IPUMS: https://usa.ipums.org/usa/index.shtml. Ruggles et al 2025.

6. US Census. Estimates were calculated from the underlying data used to construct Figure 10. US Census data for the District of Columbia downloaded from IPUMS: https://usa.ipums.org/usa/index.shtml. Ruggles et al 2025.

7. Gillette 1995; Golash-Boza 2023.

8. Gilbert 1968; J. S. Walker 2018.

9. Jackson 1987.

10. Lacy 2007.

11. Lacy 2007.

12. Gillette 1995; Jaffe and Sherwood 2014.

13. For 1947 and 1960, see Manning 1998:337. For 1970–2000, see Lacy 2007:45. See also Sturtevant 2014; Hyra and Prince 2016; Hyra 2017.

14. Sawyer and Tatian 2003:9 (Table 1).

15. Sturtevant 2014; Hyra and Prince 2016; Hyra 2017.

16. Gillette 1995.

17. Jaffe and Sherwood 2014:361.

18. Sawyer and Tatian 2003:9 (Table 1); B. Williams 1988; Kofie 1999; DC Fiscal Policy Institute 2011.

19. See also Sturtevant 2014; DC Fiscal Policy Institute 2011.

20. Squires et al 2002; Lacy 2007.

21. See also Lacy 2007.

22. Jaffe and Sherwood 2014:12. See also Lacy 2007 for suburban intra-racial inequality.

23. Dawson 1995.

24. Gillette 1995; Asch and Musgrove 2017.

25. US Census. Estimates were calculated from the underlying data used to construct Figure 10. US Census data for the District of Columbia downloaded from IPUMS: https://usa.ipums.org/usa/index.shtml. Ruggles et al 2025.

26. https://statehood.dc.gov/page/faq.

27. Meyers 1996:47 quoted in Prince 2014:50; See also Jaffe and Sherwood 2014.

28. Bouker 2016:85.

29. *Post*—Feb 17, 1997—Williams (see print newspaper sources at the end of the bibliography).

30. Goldfield 1980:462.

31. Gillette 1995:196.

32. Gillette 1995; Prince 2014.

33. Friesema 1969 drawing on Stokely Carmichael and Charles V. Hamilton's arguments in their book *Black Power*.

34. *National Intelligencer*—Dec 22, 1800—Woodward. See also Gillette 1995; https://statehood.dc.gov/page/faq.

35. Musgrove 2017; see also Asch and Musgrove 2017.

36. C. Cohen 1999; Higginbotham 1994.

37. Friesema 1969; Keller 1978; Biles 1992; Kraus and Swanstrom 2001; Hopkins and McCabe 2012.

38. W. J. Wilson 1978, 1987.

39. Biles 1992:116; Friesema 1969.

40. Biles 1997:115.

41. Biles 1992:122.

42. Friesema 1969:77–78.

43. Kraus and Swanstrom. 2001:103.

44. Sturtevant 2014. See also Asch and Musgrove 2017.

45. Kofie 1999; Jaffe and Sherwood 2014; Gillette 1995; Prince 2014; Hyra and Prince 2016; Hyra 2017; Golash-Boza 2023.

46. Goldfield 1980:457–458.

47. Jaffe and Sherwood 2014.

48. Goldfield 1980:460.

49. Goldfield 1980:459–460.

50. Goldfield 1980:460.

51. Gillette 1995:216.

52. Hyra 2017:153.

53. For the quote, Goldfield 1980:463; see also p. 462 for fuller discussion.

54. Prince 2014:134.

55. Lewis 2010:184.

56. Lewis 2010:184, 196.

57. Lewis 2010:206–207.

58. Golash-Boza 2023:199.

59. Merton 1968.

60. Golash-Boza 2023:5.

61. NCHA 1944.

62. Shapiro 2020.

63. B. Williams 2001. See also the map at https://anacostia.si.edu/barryfarm/investigate/division-and-displacement.

64. Gillette 1995:158–9.

65. Gillette 1995:155.

66. Gillette 1995:159.

67. Gillette 1985.

68. Shapiro 2020; Currie et al 2014.

69. NCHA 1944.

70. Shapiro 2020:81.

71. *Post*—Jun 25, 1981—Sargent.

72. Shapiro 2020, 2024.

73. Shapiro 2020:174; Shapiro 2024.

74. Shapiro 2024:15.

75. Shapiro 2020:185–187. See also Shapiro 2024.

76. Engels and Dutt 1872.

77. Shapiro 2020:119.

78. *Post*—Sep 16, 1972—Scharfenberg.

79. *Post*—Sep 16, 1972—Scharfenberg.

80. Shapiro 2020:125.

81. Shapiro 2020.

82. See Shapiro 2020:214–215.

83. *Post*—Jun 25, 1981—Sargent.

84. *Post*—Jun 25, 1981—Sargent.

85. *Post*—Apr 18, 1993—Boo.

86. *Post*—Apr 18, 1993—Boo.

87. *Post*—Apr 18, 1993—Boo; Cunningham 1999.

88. Cunningham 1999.

89. *Post*—Apr 18, 1993—Boo; Cunningham 1999. See also Post—Oct 18, 1996—Boo.

90. Cunningham 1999.

91. *Post*—Aug 16, 1995—Loeb.

92. Cunningham 1999.

93. Jaffe and Sherwood 2014:141. See also *Post*—Dec 26, 1990—Melton and Abramovitz; *Post*—Feb 10, 1997—Williams for help for the Black poor.

94. *Post*—Dec 26, 1990—Melton and Abramovitz.

95. Jaffe and Sherwood 2014.

96. Jaffe and Sherwood 2014:210. See also *Post*—Jan 29, 1995—Loeb; *Post*—Mar 3, 1995—Loeb and Adams.

97. Asch and Musgrove 2017; Bouker 2016; Cunningham 1999. See also *Post*—Jan 29, 1995—Loeb; *Post*—Jul 12, 1995—Locy.

98. Bouker 2016; Asch and Musgrove 2017.

99. Jaffe and Sherwood 2014; Asch and Musgrove 2017.

100. Jaffe and Sherwood 2014; Lewis 2010; Asch and Musgrove 2017.

101. Magnus et al 2009; District of Columbia Department of Health 2014, 2019; Georgetown University 2016; King et al 2022; Hendi 2024.

102. Du Bois 1935.

103. NCHA 1944; Golash-Boza 2023.

104. BOH 1960:179.

105. National Center for Health Statistics 1966:376.

106. National Center for Health Statistics 1963:1–50: Table 1-AA.

107. National Center for Health Statistics 1963:3–8: Table 3-E.

108. See N. Turner et al 2020:2 (Table 1).

109. National Center for Health Statistics 1963:1–40 (Table 1-V).

110. BOH 1960:181.

111. National Center for Health Statistics 1975:9–4.

112. National Center for Health Statistics 1974 I-54–5 (Table 1–13).

113. DC Department of Human Services 1980:23.

114. National Center for Health Statistics 1974:I-73 (Table 1–17).

115. National Center for Health Statistics 1985:9-3.

116. DC Department of Human Services 1980:35.

117. National Center for Health Statistics 1985:9-3.

118. DC Department of Human Services 1980:35.

119. DC Department of Human Services 1980:23.

120. Ahmed et al 1991:665.

121. National Center for Health Statistics 1998:4.

122. National Center for Health Statistics 1998, White men pp. 14–15 (Table 5), Black men pp. 26–27 (Table 11).

123. Wei et al 2012:4 (Table A).

124. Miniño et al 2002:105 (Table 36).

PART 2

Overview

1. My sample comprised 12 gay and bisexual men, 6 heterosexual men, 10 cisgender women (7 heterosexual, 3 bisexual), and 9 transgender women.

2. *Healio. Infectious Disease News*—Jan 1, 2008—Ellis (see print newspaper sources at the end of the bibliography).

3. Morgan et al 2002. See also: https://www.unaids.org/en/frequently-asked-questions-about-hiv-and-aids; https://www.cdc.gov/hiv/about/index.html.

4. Patel et al 2014:5 (Table 1). See also: https://www.cdc.gov/hiv/risk/estimates /riskbehaviors.html.

5. Chan et al 2014; Chu et al 1994. But see Oster et al 2015. None of my cisgender women respondents discussed getting HIV from another cisgender woman. For oral sex, see Patel et al 2014.

6. Hollingsworth et al 2008.

7. See Galvin and Cohen 2004.

8. See for example Laumann et al 1994, 2004; Blackwell and Lichter 2004; Curington et al 2021.

9. Oster et al 2015:446.

10. See for example Elbers 2021; Hall et al 2019; United States Government Accountability Office 2022; Lipka 2014; Candipan et al 2021; Curington et al 2021.

11. Benjamin 2019; see also Curington et al 2021.

12. Mojola et al 2021:959.

13. See for example Ellingson et al 2004; Laumann et al 1994, 2004; A. Green 2008.

14. See Morris and Kretzschmar 1997; Morris 2004; Bearman et al 2004.

15. Guttmacher Institute 2019.

16. Kreisel et al 2021.

17. Chesson et al 2021.

18. Chesson et al 2021.

19. CDC 2024a.

20. https://www.hiv.gov/federal-response/ending-the-hiv-epidemic/overview.

21. https://www.hiv.gov/hiv-basics/overview/data-and-trends/statistics.

22. https://www.hiv.gov/hiv-basics/overview/data-and-trends/statistics/; Aral et al 2008.

23. Hess et al 2017.

24. CDC 2024a; CDC 2024b.

25. CDC Fact Sheet, https://www.cdc.gov/nchhstp/newsroom/docs/factsheets /cdc-hiv-aa-508.pdf.

26. Patel et al 2014. See also M. Cohen et al 2011.

27. Kaiser Foundation 2024. BRFSS 2022—Analysis by Kaiser Foundation. https://www.kff.org/hivaids/fact-sheet/hiv-testing-in-the-united-states/#:~:text= According%20to%20the%20CDC's%20Behavioral,%2Fethnicity%2C%20and%20 other%20factors.

28. Copen 2017.

29. See for example Harawa et al 2004; Millett et al 2007; Hallfors et al 2007; Magnus et al 2009; Lo et al 2018.

30. Hallfors et al 2007:125.

31. Magnus et al 2009.

32. Aral et al 2008; Adimora et al 2006; Auerbach et al 2011; Friedman et al 2009; Watkins-Hayes 2014; Blankenship et al 2005.

33. Fiscella et al 2000; Kirby et al 2006; Vyas et al 2020.

34. Kanny et al 2019; Beer et al 2016.

35. J. Hirsch and Khan. 2020.

36. Laumann and Youm 1999.

37. Laumann et al 1994, 2004; Laumann and Youm 1999; Service and Blower 1995; Bearman et al 2004; Adimora et al 2006; Carey et al 2010; Bingham et al 2003; M. Morris et al 2009; Oster et al 2015.

38. *Post*—Mar 14, 2009—Vargas and Fears.

39. Magnus et al 2009:1278.

40. District of Columbia HIV/AIDS, Hepatitis, STD, and TB Administration (HAHSTA) Annual Report 2010 (henceforth cited as DC HAHSTA Report). HAHSTA estimates are likely underestimates as they are counts of those who have tested; thus untested/undiagnosed HIV positives are not included in counts of people with HIV.

41. Over the 40-year period, the city consistently updated data as reporting standards changed such that there are year-to-year changes in estimates of the number of people living with HIV when looking at the city's reports. For Figure 23, I used 1983–2016 surveillance data given to me by the city and drew 2017 data from the city's 2022 report appendix. The overall 1983–2016 estimates for numbers of people living with HIV in this figure were consistent with the 2017 HAHSTA report. I drew 2018–2022 data from the 2023 report appendix. I also looked at earlier published studies: P. Rosenberg and Biggar 1993 estimated that in 1991, HIV prevalence among DC residents aged 20–64 was 4.9% among Black men, 2.9% among White men, 1.6% among Black women, and 0.3% among White women. See also P. Rosenberg et al 1992.

42. Analysis of raw HAHSTA HIV surveillance data. I am unable to disaggregate transgender people from the cisgender population in the overall population trends for mode of HIV acquisition, as it is unclear how sexual contact for transgender people is classified (the categories for sexual modes of transmission are for men who have sex with men, heterosexual sex, and a combination of sex and drug use). As such, I report the overall population trends, and then the specific trends for transgender people.

43. Calculated using data from DC HAHSTA Report 2023 Appendix, p. 54 (Table B3).

4. The HIV Epidemic Among Gay and Bisexual Men

1. I follow my respondents in using the terms *gay*, *homosexual*, and *bisexual*; I also use the terms *queer* and *sexual minorities* to broadly refer to people with non-heteronormative (straight) sexual identities. No respondents used other terms, such as *same-gender loving*, for example, to describe their identity.

2. National Segregation Report 1948; C. Green 1967:108–9.

3. See Beemyn 2014; Holmes 2011; Dolinksky 2010; Hersker 2002.

4. See Ellingson and Schroeder 2004 for a theory of sex markets.

5. Beemyn 2014; Hersker 2002; Lait and Lee 1951.

6. Beemyn 2014.

7. Beemyn 2014.

8. For DC, see Beemyn 2014; for national story, see Bérubé 1990; D'Emilio 1998.

9. Beemyn 2014.

10. Asch and Musgrove 2017.

11. Adkins 2016.

12. Beemyn 2014; Adkins 2016.

13. Beemyn 2014.

14. Bérubé 1990; D'Emilio 1998.

15. See oral history interview at https://www.loc.gov/item/afc2001001.05208/.

16. Beemyn 2014; Dolinsky 2010.

17. Chauncey 1994:22. See also Bérubé 1990; D'Emilio 1998.

18. Chauncey 1994. See also Kunzel 2008.

19. Levine 1979.

20. Ghaziani 2014. See also Levine 1979.

21. D'Emilio 1998; see also Orne 2017.

22. Ghaziani 2014.

23. Holmes 2011.

24. Holmes 2011:4.

25. Hersker 2002:2.

26. Holmes 2011; Dolinsky 2010.

27. *Washington Blade*—Oct 15, 2019—Chibbaro (see print newspaper sources at the end of the bibliography).

28. https://www.whitman-walker.org/our-history/.

29. Dolinsky 2010; Holmes 2011; *Post*—Jun 8, 2005—Schwartzman.

30. *Post*—Jun 8, 2005—Schwartzman.

31. Dolinsky 2010; Holmes 2011; Beemyn 2014. See also Bost 2015.

32. Dolinsky 2010; Holmes 2011; Beemyn 2014.

33. Dolinsky 2010. See also Bost 2015.

34. Nero 2005.

35. Ellingson and Schroeder 2004

36. Rosenfeld 2007.

37. For the paradigmatic example of this in Harlem, New York, see Garber 1989; Hawkeswood 1996; Chauncey 1994. See also Andriote 1999.

38. See Ward 2015; T. Silva 2017.

39. Wright 1993; E. P. Johnson 2011.

40. Holmes 2011.

41. Dolinsky 2010:207. See also Bost 2015.

42. Beemyn 2014; Bost 2015.

43. Holmes 2011:45.

44. Dolinsky 2010.

45. Holmes 2011; Dolinsky 2010; Holmes 2016.

46. https://historicsites.dcpreservation.org/items/show/1290.

47. *Washington Blade*—Sep 8, 2011—Staff reporters.

48. Holmes 2011, 2016; Dolinksky 2010. https://dchistory.org/the-clubhouse/.

49. Chauncey 1994; Hawkeswood 1996.

50. *Black Light* was started to increase coverage of Black sexual minorities, responding to perceived limited coverage in the *Washington Blade*.

51. For 2010, see https://williamsinstitute.law.ucla.edu/publications/us-census-snapshot-2010/; for 2023, see https://williamsinstitute.law.ucla.edu/publications/adult-lgbt-pop-us/. The Williams Institute estimated that 14.3% of the city is LGBT.

52. These odds are calculated based on the city's HIV prevalence in the HAHSTA 2010 report, which illustrated that 7.1% of Black men and 2.9% of White men were living with HIV.

53. An obvious and important limitation of these odds is they do not distinguish between gay and heterosexual odds; so the odds for White gay men may well have been higher due to being a numerical minority in the city, especially if in gay enclaves.

54. At the time of my interviews (2011), pre-exposure prophylaxis had not been introduced. It was first approved in the US in 2012. See https://www.niaid.nih.gov/diseases-conditions/pre-exposure-prophylaxis-prep.

55. Here *straight* is not just a sexual identity, an opposite gender partner preference, or a set of preferred sexual practices, but also a culture inscribed in a society's laws and dominant norms and sanctions. For straight culture, see for example T. Silva 2019. On gay men's nonmonogamy norms see for example van Eeden-Moorefield et al 2016; Philpot et al 2018.

56. For debate, see J. King 2004; Denizet-Lewis 2003; Boykin 1996; Ford et al 2007; Saleh and Operario 2009; Millett et al 2005; Snorton 2014; Malebranche et al 2010. See also Collins 2004.

57. For "down low" White men, see for example Ward 2015; T. Silva 2017.

58. Oster et al 2015:450 (Figure 3B).

59. Oster et al 2015:448 (Table 2).

60. Some long-term nonprogressors are able to transmit the disease, while others are "elite controllers" whose bodies also keep their HIV viral load low. See https://clinicalinfo.hiv.gov/en/glossary/long-term-nonprogressors-ltnp; https://clinicalinfo.hiv.gov/en/glossary/elite-controllers.

61. Gardner et al 2011.

62. DC HAHSTA Report 2010, 2023.

63. See Castel et al 2012a:350 (Table 2) for DC community viral load.

64. Havlir and Beyrer 2012; Auerbach 2019.

65. Ghaziani 2014.

66. Seidman et al 1999; Brekhus 2003; Orne 2017.

67. Ghaziani 2014; Orne 2017.

68. A. Green 2007, 2008.

69. Hersker 2002; Holmes 2011.

70. Hersker 2002; Ghaziani 2014.

71. Hersker 2002:3.

72. Hersker 2002.

73. Leap 2009:212.

74. Leap 2009; *Post*—Jun 8, 2005—Schwartzman.

75. Leap 2009:216.

76. *Post*—Jun 8, 2005—Schwartzman; Leap 2009.

77. Hawkeswood 1993, 1996; Dolinsky 2010; Bost 2015.

78. DC HAHSTA 2023 Report: Appendix p. 64 (Table B11). For national picture, see https://www.cdc.gov/hiv/data-research/facts-stats/gay-bisexual-men.html; https://www.cdc.gov/hiv/data-research/facts-stats/race-ethnicity.html#:~:text=Black%2FAfrican%20American%20people%20and,new%20HIV%20infections%20in%202022.

5. The HIV Epidemic Among Heterosexual Men, Women, and Trans Women

1. People whose sex assignment at birth aligns with their gender identity. See Aultman 2014. I hereafter simply use the terms *men*, *women*, and *trans women* and only use *cisgender* when explicitly distinguishing between cisgender and transgender women.

2. Magnus et al 2009:1282.

3. DC HAHSTA Report 2010:4 (Figure 3).

4. DC HAHSTA Report 2010:4 (Figure 2).

5. DC HAHSTA Report 2010:9 (Table 4)—2009 column.

6. Morgan et al 2022.

7. S. Clark 2004; J. Hirsch et al 2009.

8. DC HAHSTA Report 2010:24 (Table 9).

9. Same-sex marriage was illegal in the US until 2004 (when it was legalized in the first state) and 2015 (when it was legalized nationally). A Gallup poll found that about 3.5% of the population identified as LGBT in 2012 (https://news.gallup.com/poll/234863/estimate-lgbt-population-rises.aspx), and in the BRFSS 2020–21, 5.5% identified as LGBT (https://williamsinstitute.law.ucla.edu/publications/adult-lgbt-pop-us/). Of the LGBT population 10.7% identify as Black and 52.3% as White; this translates to national proportions of 0.59% Black and 2.9% White LGBT people. About a quarter of Black LGBT people (27%) and almost half of White LGBT people (45%) were married or cohabiting between 2012 and 2017—both lower proportions than their non-LGBT counterparts (https://williamsinstitute.law.ucla.edu/visualization/lgbt-races/#Intro-text). As such, while proportions of same-sex marriages are growing, they do not yet significantly change the overall depiction of heterosexual marriage trends in the US in the figures in this section.

10. Analysis of the ACS shows that divorce rates were slightly higher in 2019 for Black men (18.6%) and women (22.8%), and White men (15.1%) and women (17.6%), before declining in 2020 and 2021. This is likely due to the COVID-19 pandemic.

11. Fry and Parker 2021; see also Marsh 2023.

12. https://www.census.gov/library/stories/2022/07/marriage-prevalence-for-black-adults-varies-by-state.html; *Newsweek*—Oct 20, 2009—Connolly (see print newspaper sources at the end of the bibliography); McConnell and Sayin 2023.

13. By historical period effect, I mean phenomena such as the Great Depression, World War II, and the Prison Boom years, for example. I elaborate on this later. By cohort effect, I mean age groups such as those in their 20s, 30s, and so on.

14. A key assumption of this claim is different drivers of never marrying by age 50 for White and Black populations. While I assume a missed window for the Black population, and assume their disproportionate indigeneity and long-term residence in the city, for the White population, I assume disproportionate White outmigration to the suburbs for those who married, leaving a select sample of people aged 50 and over in the city. Connolly (see note 12 above) suggests that the city's large LGBT population (see note 51 of Chapter 4), may also have impacted the city's marriage rates, especially since marriage was not legal in DC until 2009.

15. Waite 1995; Kposowa 2013. Kposowa finds that nationally, for men, marriage is protective against AIDS mortality.

16. Lotke 1998.

17. Pager 2003.

18. Pager 2003; Western 2006; Pager et al 2009; Edin and Kefalas 2011; Amato and Beattie 2011.

19. Landry 2002; K. Johnson and Loscocco 2015; see also Dow 2019; Pinder-hughes 2002; W.J. Wilson and Neckerman 1987; Raley et al 2015. See Hochschild 1989 for second shift.

20. W.J. Wilson and Neckerman 1987.

21. Pinderhughes 2002; P. Cohen and Pepin 2018.

22. The census and ACS were used to identify sex, race/ethnicity, marital status, and employment status. Data from the Bureau of Justice Statistics (National Prisoner Statistics Program) yielded the number of prisoners.

23. Collins 1990:158; Collins 2004:293.

24. Collins 2004; Johnson and Loscocco 2015; Pinderhughes 2002.

25. See, for example, D. Roberts 2017.

26. See for example M. Alexander 2010; Faber 2020; Pager 2003; Curran and Abrams 2000; Western 2006; Squires et al 2002; Wakefield and Wildeman 2013; Turney 2017; Edin and Nelson 2013; Fernandez-Kelly 2015.

27. Liebow 1967; Hannerz 1969; Majors and Billson 1993; Collins 2004; Bowleg et al 2004; Whitehead 1997.

28. Liebow 1967; Edin and Kefalas 2011; Edin and Nelson 2013.

29. Morris and Kretzschmar 1997; M. Morris et al 2009.

30. Wiederman 1997.

31. Adimora et al 2002; Adimora et al 2007; Laumann et al 2004; Whitehead 1997; Bowleg et al 2004; Fullilove et al 1990; Bontempi et al 2008.

32. Dworkin 2005, 2015; Higgins et al 2010; Dauria et al 2015. See also Adimora et al 2002; Adimora et al 2007; Laumann et al 2004; Whitehead 1997; Bowleg et al 2004; Fullilove et al 1990; Bontempi et al 2008.

33. Oster et al 2015.

34. Magnus et al 2009.

35. Kuo et al 2011.

36. Whitehead 1997; Carey et al 2010; Bowleg 2004; Bowleg et al 2011.

37. Amaro 1995; Aral et al 2008; Adimora et al 2006; Sobo 1995; Wingood and DiClemente 1998; Kerrigan et al 2008; Bontempi et al 2008; Bowleg 2004.

38. Bowleg et al 2004.

39. DC HAHSTA Report 2023 Appendix, p. 55 (Table B4).

40. DC HAHSTA Report 2023 Appendix, p. 57 (Table B5) (Data for 2022).

41. DC HAHSTA Report 2023 Appendix, p. 57 (Table B5) (Data for 2022).

42. Herbst et al 2008; Becasen et al 2019; Clements-Nolle et al 2001; Operario et al 2008; Nemoto et al 2004.

43. Becasen et al 2019. See also Herbst et al 2008.

44. DC HAHSTA Report 2016:10 (Table 1).

45. Flores et al 2016b:3 (Table 1). See also Flores et al 2016a.

46. DC HAHSTA Report 2016:10 (Table 1).

47. The HAHSTA 2023 report did not provide transgender HIV prevalence rates (see note at bottom of Appendix Table A4, p. 47). For 2022, I draw the DC transgender population size from Herman et al 2022:9 (Table 4), who estimate 5,300 transgender people in DC; and race/ethnic population sizes from Herman et al 2022:11 (Table 5), who estimate 1,800 White and 2,400 Black transgender people in DC. (Estimates from 2017–2020 BRFSS data.) The HAHSTA 2023 report (Table B3, p. 54) provided 2022 transgender HIV cases by race/ethnicity. The report does not break out transgender cases by gender, so I cannot calculate rates for trans women. Notably, as for cisgender populations, these are not random samples of the transgender population but counts of those who test positive. As such, these are likely underestimates of the true number of people with HIV in the city (the untested/undiagnosed).

48. DC HAHSTA 2023:9. Since there is no cure for HIV, lower HIV prevalence in 2022 compared to 2010 meant that people with HIV had died or they had moved out of DC.

49. LaVeist and Wallace 2000; Mackenzie 2013; J. P. Lee et al 2020.

50. *Post*—Aug 6, 1977—Stevens.

51. *Post*—Apr 1, 1993—Harriston.

52. Some transgender women also sold sex to pay for hormones to aid the expensive gender transition process, especially if they didn't have medical insurance or if it did not cover transitions. See also Herbst et al 2008; Clements-Nolle et al 2001.

53. For truly disadvantaged, see W. J. Wilson 1987. For matrix of domination, see Collins 1990, 2004.

54. Badgett et al 2019:39.

55. National Center for Transgender Equality 2017:1.

56. National Center for Transgender Equality 2017:1.

57. Xavier et al 2005.

58. Bockting et al 1998; Sugano et al 2006; Nemoto et al 2004; Melendez and Pinto 2007.

PART 3

Overview

1. See the Introduction; Singer and the Hispanic Health Council 2000.

2. See Zinberg and Harding 1979; P. Adler et al 2012; Rhodes et al 2005; R. Wallace 1990; D. Wallace and Wallace 1998; Crum et al 1996; Boardman et al 2001; E. Roberts et al 2010; Dunlap and Johnson 1992; Ciccarone and Bourgois 2003; Parsons et al 2009; Bauermeister 2008; Friedman et al 1999.

6. First Comes Heroin: 1960–2016

1. Schneider 2008:5. See also Courtwright 2001; Jonnes 1996.

2. Courtwright 2001:48. See also Musto 1999; Jonnes 1996; Schneider 2008.

3. Musto 1999; Courtwright 2001; Jonnes 1996; Schneider 2008.

4. Musto 1999; Jonnes 1996.

5. Jonnes 1996:112.

6. Kosten and Gorelick 2002.

7. Musto 1973; Jonnes 1996; Courtwright 2001:147–49.

8. Jonnes 1996; Courtwright 2001.

9. M. Alexander 2010.

10. M. J. Alexander et al 2018.

11. Jones et al 2019; Barlas 2017.

12. J. Friedman and Hansen 2022 find that Black overdose mortality rates subsequently increased, were equal to White rates in 2019, and surpassed them in 2020. In DC, Kiang et al 2021 found that in 2019, Black people's opioid-related mortality "was 11.3 times higher than White [people's]. . . . This inequity was substantially higher than any other jurisdiction on both the relative and absolute scales" (589).

13. Ruttenber and Luke 1984.

14. See Jonnes 1996; *Post*—May 22, 1961—Dixon; *Post*—May 23, 1961—no author; *Post*—Dec 10, 1961—Kluttz; *Post*—Feb 28, 1964—Anderson; *Post*—Jan 2, 1966—Thompson; *Post*—Dec 18, 1970—Ungar; *Post*—May 23, 1976—Dash (see print newspaper sources at the end of the bibliography).

15. *Post*—Jul 15, 1960—Lewis; *Post*—Oct 27, 1960—no author; *Post*—Oct 22, 1966—Morgan.

16. *Post*—Oct 22, 1966—Morgan.

17. *Post*—Jan 30, 1968—Bernstein.

18. *Post*—Oct 20, 1966—Morgan.

19. *Post*—Feb 6, 1970—Kessler.

20. M. Greene 1974:3.

21. DuPont 1971:320.

22. *Post*—Jun 23, 1968—Asher.

23. *Post*—Oct 18, 1965—Lewis; DuPont 1971.

24. *Post*—Feb 6, 1970—Kessler.

25. *Post*—Feb 6, 1970—Kessler.

26. I come to this conclusion because DuPont 1971 reports that a special coroner's office study found that 21 people died of heroin overdose in 1967, and 21 died in 1969 (DuPont 1971:320). Assuming a peak heroin-usage incidence in 1969, it is unlikely that hundreds of people died of overdose between 1960 and 1966.

27. *Post*—Sep 9, 1965—Downie. For quote, see *Post*—Oct 20, 1966—Morgan.

28. M. Greene 1974:4.

29. DuPont 1971:323.

30. The Model Cities program was a place-based government intervention to commit government resources and funds to the most disadvantaged parts of cities in the US. See Hetzel and Pinsky 1969.

31. DuPont 1971:320, 323; DuPont and Greene 1973.

32. *Post*—Oct 23, 1966—Morgan.

33. *WAMU Metro*—Nov 21, 2014—Sheir.

34. *Post*—Feb 16, 1969—Carter.

35. DuPont 1971.

36. *Post*—Feb 16, 1969—Carter.

37. *Post*—Feb 16, 1969—Carter.

38. Public Law 89–793 [H.R.9167], Nov 8, 1966.

39. Dole and Nyswander 1965; *Post*—Apr 11, 1972—Claiborne; Dupont 1971.

40. M. Greene 1974.

41. *WAMU Metro*—Nov 21, 2014—Sheir.

42. *Post*—Apr 11, 1972—Clairborne.

43. DuPont 1971; *Post*—Mar 16, 1972—Woodward; *Post*—Jul 7, 1972—Valentine and Woodward; Courtwright 2001.

44. *Post*—Nov 10, 1974—Feinberg; *Post*—Nov 8, 1975—no author; *Post*—Mar 17, 1976—Auerbach; *Post*—May 24, 1976—Dash.

45. *Post*—Apr 18, 1976—Dash.

46. *Post*—Sep 6, 1976—Dash; *Post*—Nov 14, 1976—Williams and Darling.

47. Hser et al 2001.

48. See for example Robins et al 1974; Waldorf et al 1992.

49. Leshner 1997; Kosten and George 2002; Zinberg and Harding 1979.

50. Cora did not directly attribute her HIV acquisition to heroin use, but she described sharing needles in the course of her addiction.

51. Des Jarlais et al 1989; Friedman et al 1999.

52. Patel et al 2014.

53. *Post*—Apr 1, 1976—Dash; *Post*—Nov 14, 1976—Williams and Darling; *Post*—Mar 17, 1976—Auerbach.

54. *Post*—Apr 20, 1976—Valentine; *Post*—Jun 30, 1976—Dash; Dole and Nyswander 1976.

55. Craig 1978.

56. *Post*—Aug 26, 1979—Valentine.

57. *Post*—Aug 26, 1979—Valentine; Jonnes 1996.

58. Jonnes 1996; *Post*—Aug 26, 1979—Valentine; *Post*—Feb 8, 1980—Robinson and Valentine; *Post*—Jan 24, 1979—Shaffer and Meyer.

59. *Post*—Aug 26, 1979—Valentine.

60. *Post*—Aug 26, 1979—Valentine; *Post*—Feb 8, 1980—Robinson and Valentine.

61. *Post*—Jun 24, 1979—Tofani.

62. *Post*—Sep 3, 1981—Robinson; *Post*—Jun 13, 1983—Kessler. See also *Post*—Aug 5, 1981—Lewis and Sherwood; *Post*—May 22, 1981—Piantadosi.

63. DC narcotics detective William Larman quoted in *Post*—May 22, 1981—Piantadosi.

64. *Post*—May 22, 1981—Piantadosi; *Post*—Aug 5, 1981—Lewis and Sherwood; *Post*—Jun 13, 1983—Kessler.

65. *Post*— Sep 27, 1983—Kamen and Lewis; Ruttenber and Luke 1984; *Post*—Sep 28, 1984—Bredemeier.

66. Centers for Disease Control and Prevention 1983.

67. *Post*—March 10, 1985—Milloy and Wheeler; M.J. Alexander et al 2018.

68. *Post*—March 10, 1985—Milloy and Wheeler.

69. *Post*—March 10, 1985—Milloy and Wheeler.

70. Holmberg 1996.

71. P. Rosenberg et al 1992.

72. Bureau of Justice Statistics 1992:28.

73. Friedman et al 1999; Laumann and Youm 1999; Laumann et al 2004; adams et al 2013.

74. Pierce 1999.

75. See also Riley 1997:14 (Table 15) who found that White people in DC were more likely to have a main source for heroin, while Black people had a variety of options.

76. Pierce 1999:2110.

77. J.S. Walker 2018.

78. *Post*—Jun 24, 1979—Tofani.

79. C. Cohen 1999; Friedman et al 1999.

80. US Department of Justice Criminal Division 1991.

81. Empty parentheses were intended for states and the District to fill in as needed; US Department of Justice Criminal Division 1991, Appendix 1, A2.

82. D.C. Law 4-149. Drug Paraphernalia Act of 1982.

83. Strathdee and Vlahov 2001; Hurley et al 1997.

84. Greenberg et al 2009.

85. Ruiz et al 2016.

86. DC HAHSTA 2007:1.

87. Ruiz et al 2016.

88. Ruiz et al 2016.

7. Then Comes Cocaine: Late 1970s–2010s

1. Bowser 1989; Edlin et al 1994; Inciardi 1995.
2. Jonnes 1996; Musto 1999; Inciardi and McElrath 2007; Adler et al 2012.
3. Courtwright 2001; Jonnes 1996; Musto 1999; Inciardi and McElrath 2007.
4. Musto 1999; Jonnes 1996; Reinarman and Levine 1989.
5. Hamid 1992.
6. Hamid 1992; Jonnes 1996; *Post*—June 11, 1980—no author; *Post*—Dec 23, 1984—Mathews (see print newspaper sources at the end of the bibliography).
7. Fishburne et al 1979:33 (Table 6).
8. Voss 1989:38.
9. Bachman et al 1991:373 (Table 2).
10. Bureau of Justice Statistics 1992:28.
11. Kozel et al 1982:266.
12. Colliver and Kopstein 1991:59.
13. Colliver and Kopstein 1991:60 (Table 2).
14. Colliver and Kopstein 1991:62 (Table 4).
15. Pollock et al 1991:2234. (A five-fold increase in National Vital Statistics data.)
16. Miech 2008.
17. Jaffe and Sherwood 2014; *Post*—May 26, 1978—Colen; *Post*—Aug 7, 1984—Engel; Aniline and Ferris 1982.
18. *Post*— Dec 13, 1984—Bruske.
19. *Post*—May 15, 1985—Evans.
20. *Post*—Nov 25, 1986—Walsh; *Post*—Dec 21, 1986—Robinson.
21. *Post*—Sept 15, 1988—Harriston.
22. *Post*—Nov 26, 1989—Buckley.
23. *Post*—Jan 6, 1990—Lewis.
24. Calculated from Colliver and Kopstein 1991:60 (Table 1).
25. Colliver and Kopstein 1991.
26. For NY, https://www.nyc.gov/assets/planning/download/pdf/data-maps/nyc-population/census2010/t_pl_p6_rgn.pdf; For DC, https://planning.dc.gov/sites/default/files/dc/sites/op/publication/attachments/Washington%2520Metropolitan%2520Statistical%2520Area%2520Population%25201900%2520to%25202009.pdf.
27. Colliver and Kopstein 1991:63 (Table 5); Garfield and Drucker 2001:431.
28. Golub and Johnson 1997 (see Exhibit 1 on p. 4 for age-period-cohort analysis; see p. 7 for DC trends); *Post*—May 31, 1993—Gladwell; Dunlap and Johnson 1992; Venkatesh 2000; Bourgois 1995.
29. Reding 2009; Quinones 2015; M.J. Alexander et al 2018.
30. Gorriti 1989.
31. Gorritti 1989; *Post*—May 31, 1980—Krause; *Post*—Nov 8, 1982—Pincus.
32. *Joint Oversight Hearing* 1988:476.

33. Gugliotta and Leen 1989; Agar 2003; Jonnes 1996.

34. *Post*—Mar 30, 1997—Farah and Moore; *Post*—Mar 19, 1986—Thornton; *Post*—May 31, 1993—Robberson; *Post*—Sept 17, 1995—Reding; *Post*—Apr 28, 1996—Moore and Anderson.

35. Gugliotta and Leen 1989; Agar 2003; P. Adler 1985; Drug Enforcement Agency 1994; Jaffe and Sherwood 2014; Reuter and Haaga 1989; *Post*—Mar 26, 1995—McGee.

36. *New York Times*—Oct 1, 1989—Massing; *Post*—June 29, 1988—Churchville; *Post*—Mar 12, 1988—Lait.

37. *Post*—May 21, 1986—Anderson; *Post*—Mar 18, 1987—Lewis; *Post*—Apr 14, 1988—Sanchez; *Post*—Apr 22, 1989—Kurtz.

38. *Post*—Feb 9, 1980—Pichirallo; *Post*—July 11, 1981—Smith; *Post*—May 17, 1989—Thompson.

39. *Post*—Sep 6, 1983—Cody.

40. *Post*—Sep 6, 1983—Cody; *Post*—July 28, 1987—Lewis; Reuter et al 1988.

41. *Post*—May 21, 1981—Knight.

42. *Post*—May 14, 1986—Berg.

43. *Post*—Jun 22, 1986—Melton and Wheeler.

44. *Post*—Sep 10, 1981—Smith and Bohlen.

45. *Post*—Apr 23, 1986—Harris; see also *Post*—May 6, 1987—Hall.

46. *Post*—Sep 2, 1987—Cohn.

47. *Post*—Aug 10, 1987—Evans.

48. *Post*—Aug 10, 1987—Evans; *Post*—July 16, 1986—Arocha; *Post*—Feb 23, 1988—Churchville; Jaffe and Sherwood 2014; Castaneda 2014.

49. T. Williams 1992; Ratner 1993; Riley 1997; Venkatesh 2000; Jacobs 1999; Agar 2003; W. Adler 1995.

50. Anderson 1999; T. Williams 1992. See also Venkatesh 2000; Bourgois 1995; Jacobs 1999 and W. Adler 1995, among many others.

51. Waldorf et al 1991:8.

52. Anderson 1999; Bourgois 1995; W. Adler 1995; Jacobs 1999; Duck 2015; Ralph 2014.

53. Reuter et al 1990:vii. See also Riley 1997. The DC minimum wage was $3.75 in that period (https://fred.stlouisfed.org/series/STTMINWGDC).

54. Levitt and Venkatesh 2000.

55. Reuter et al 1990:ix, 102, 17, 108. See also Kofie 1999.

56. *Post*—Jul 19, 1989—Duke. The article also notes that DC's Edmonds gang took in an estimated $14 million/week, and the IRS estimated DC kingpin Cornell Jones's income at $1 million/week.

57. See also Duck 2015 for Michigan.

58. Rios 2011; Chambliss 1994.

59. Lotke 1998; Chambliss 1994.

60. B. Williams 1988; Kofie 1999; *Post*—Apr 20, 1990—Buckley; Golash-Boza 2023.

61. *Post*—Nov 13, 1988—Milloy.

62. *Post*—Aug 31, 1989—Milloy.

63. *Post*—Dec 22, 1985—Wheeler.

64. *Post*—Dec 22, 1985—Wheeler; *Post*—Dec 4, 1986—Wheeler.

65. *Post*—Sep 19, 1991—Mercer.

66. *Post*—Jul 28, 1987—Lewis; see also *Post*—Aug 2, 1987—Churchville.

67. *Post*—Apr 24, 1988—Horwitz.

68. Kofie 1999; *Post*—Apr 22, 1988—Gaines-Carter and Rupert; *Post*—Apr 23, 1988—Rupert.

69. *Post*—May 8, 1989—Spolar.

70. *Post*—Mar 9, 1987—Editorial.

71. Kofie 1999; see also *Post*—Mar 9, 1987—Editorial.

72. *Post*—Apr 2, 1989—Duke and Price.

73. *Post*—Dec 10, 1987—Duggan; *Post*—Jan 23, 1988—Yorke; *Post*—Feb 10, 1988—Jordan.

74. *Post*—Jul 6, 1988—Meyer; *Post*—Feb 10, 1988—Jordan; *Post*—Feb 28, 1988—Jordan; *Post*—Duke—Feb 26, 1988; *Post*—May 7, 1989—Thomas and Jennings.

75. See Reuter et al 1988 for full report. See *Post*—Feb 26, 1988—Duke for quote.

76. *Post*—Mar 11, 1989—Isikoff.

77. *Post*—Mar 14, 1989—Isikoff and Pianin.

78. *Post*—Aug 17, 1997—Burleigh.

79. *Post*—Nov 26, 1989—Buckley; *Post*—Jan 12, 1996—Smith.

80. See for example Golash-Boza 2023.

81. Brounstein et al 1989. See also *Post*—Aug 31, 1993—Goldstein; Bush and Iannotti 1993.

82. This was an artefact of my sample, as I was conducting snowball sampling. As noted in Chapter 5, this was not a representative sample of trans women in DC.

83. See H. Becker 1953; Friedman et al 1999; Kelly et al 2017.

84. Leshner 1997; Nestler 2005.

85. Dunlap et al 2012; Dash 1996; Pivnick et al 1994.

86. See also Leverentz 2010, 2014.

87. Agrawal and Lynskey 2008; Nestler and Malenka 2004; Nestler 2005.

8. Paying for a Habit: Commercial Sex and Drug Addiction Treatment

1. Reuter et al (1990) estimated that about 30%–40% of crack and powder cocaine dealers retained some drugs for personal use, supporting defendant testing showing that a significant proportion of drug sellers also used.

2. Gugliotta and Leen 1989; W. Adler 1995; P. Adler 1985; Maher and Daly 2017; Maher and Curtis 1992; Maher 2001; Gentry 2008; Sharpe 2005; Elwood et al 1997. Of course men also sell sex (e.g., Aggleton and Parker 2014; T. Logan 2010). But arguably, the gendered economy made women more reliant on commercial sex than men for fast income.

3. Maher and Daly 2017; Maher and Curtis 1992; Maher 2001; Gentry 2008; Sharpe 2005; Elwood et al 1997.

4. Maher and Daly 2017; Maher and Curtis 1992; Maher 2001; Gentry 2008; Sharpe 2005; Elwood et al 1997; Watkins-Hayes 2019.

5. Garnett et al 1996; Astemborski et al 1994; Bowser 1989; Nemoto et al 2004; Elifson et al 1993; Boles and Elifson 1994.

6. Nunley 2021.

7. Nunley 2021:140–141.

8. Nunley 2021:136.

9. Nunley 2021:136.

10. Nunley 2021:136.

11. Nunley 2021:136.

12. Nunley 2021:144.

13. *Post*—Jul 10, 2007—Murray; *Post*—Apr 28, 2007—Kessler; *Post*—Nov 11, 2023—Rosenzweig-Ziff and Salcedo (see print newspaper sources at the end of the bibliography).

14. Vanwesenbeek 2001; Weitzer 2009; Weitzer 2010; Bass 2015; E. Bernstein 2007; Gentry 2008. See M. Scott 2002 for estimate.

15. Weitzer 2009.

16. Quimby and Payne-Jackson 2007:114.

17. Vanwesenbeek 2001; Weitzer 2009, 2010; Bass 2015; M. Scott 2002; E. Bernstein 2007.

18. *Post*—Oct 7, 1980—Stevens.

19. *Post*—Feb 14, 1981—Pichirallo.

20. *Post*—Feb 14, 1981—Pichirallo.

21. *Post*—Mar 4, 1987—Okie and Wheeler; *Post*—Mar 21, 1988—Sanchez.

22. Hail-Jares et al 2017:58–59.

23. *Post*—Mar 21, 1988—Sanchez.

24. *Post*—Jun 17, 1991—Mooar.

25. *Post*—June 17, 1991—Mooar.

26. Hail-Jares et al 2017:62–66. See E. Bernstein 2007 for San Francisco.

27. Dank et al 2014.

28. Dank et al 2014.

29. Quimby and Payne-Jackson 2007:113.

30. He was a long-term nonprogressor (see Part 2).

31. *Post*—Sept 5, 1995—Bowles; Deering et al 2014.

32. Kaye 2020; Whetstone and Gowan. 2017; McKim 2017.

33. Mojtabai et al 2020.

34. For Carter, see Murphy 1994; for Reagan, G. H. W. Bush, and Clinton, see https://trac.syr.edu/tracdea/findings/national/drugbudp.html. I calculated averages for the respective presidencies; the estimate for the Clinton years is until 1998; for G. W. Bush, see https://oig.justice.gov/reports/plus/a0312/intro.htm; for Obama, see https://obamawhitehouse.archives.gov/sites/default/files/ondcp/policy-and-research/fy2017_budget_summary-final.pdf (p. 21, Table 1); for Trump, see https://bipartisanpolicy.org/download/?file=/wp-content/uploads/2019/03/Tracking-Federal-Funding-to-Combat-the-Opioid-Crisis.pdf (p. 15, Figure 3).

35. *Post*—Oct 17, 1984—Greene.

36. *Post*—Oct 17, 1984—Greene.

37. *Post*—January 19, 1986—Feinberg.

38. *Post*—O'Toole—June 15, 1982. See for example Gorman et al 2001.

39. LaVeist and Wallace 2000; Mackenzie 2013; J. P. Lee et al 2020; J. Scott et al 2020.

40. *Post*—Oct 17, 1984—Greene.

41. *Post*—Apr 19, 1989—Abramowitz and LaFraniere.

42. *Post*—June 30, 1986—LaFraniere and Evans; *Post*—Apr 19, 1989—Abramowitz and LaFraniere; *Post*—June 15, 1989—Abramowitz; *Post*—May 10, 1990—Walsh.

43. *Post*—Feb 21, 1988—Abramowitz.

44. *Post*—Dec 27, 1988—Colburn.

45. *Post*—May 16, 1989—Abramowitz.

46. *Post*—Oct 14, 1991—Greene.

47. *Post*—Oct 14, 1991—Greene.

48. *Post*—Dec 27, 1988—Colburn.

49. *Post*—Sep 23, 1996—Goldstein; *Post*—Sep 25, 1997—Harris.

50. *Post*—Aug 25, 1998—Slevin.

51. *Post*—Apr 17, 1999—Horwitz.

9. Homicide Redux and Life in a Syndemic Zone

1. *Post*—Jun 30, 1988—Sklansky and Sanchez; *Post*—Nov 24, 1990—Escobar (see print newspaper sources at the end of the bibliography).

2. *Post*—Nov 25, 1985— Wheeler; *Post*—Nov 27, 1985—Feinberg; Jaffe and Sherwood 2014.

3. *Post*—Nov 25, 1985—Wheeler; *Post*—July 28, 1987—Lewis; *Post*—Nov 8, 1987—Wheeler; *Post*—Nov 19, 1987—Wheeler and Harriston; *Post*—Jan 30, 1988—Horwitz. See also Castenada 2014.

4. Golash-Boza 2023; see also *Post*—Mar 19, 1992—York; *Post*—July 30, 1992—York; *Post*—Jan 7, 1993—York.

5. I first encountered Brad Wye's map in Golash-Boza 2023.

6. *Post*—Oct 28, 1988—Lewis and Horwitz; *Post*—Nov 20, 1988—Horwitz and Lewis (for quote).

7. *Post*—Feb 19, 1988—Churchville; *Post*—Dec 11, 1988—Lewis; *Post*—Aug 18, 1991—Thomas.

8. *Post*—Oct 26, 1988—Horwitz and Lewis; *Post*—Nov 20, 1988—Horwitz and Lewis; *Post*—Nov 24, 1990—Escobar.

9. Papachristos 2009; Papachristos et al 2015.

10. Ralph 2014:121.

11. See Office of Criminal Justice Plans and Analysis 1992:25 (hereafter Homicide Report) for case-closure rates between 1986–1991 which declined from 80% in

1986 to 54% in 1991); *Post*—Oct 24, 1993—Knight; *Post*—Dec 3, 2000—Thompson, Chinoy, and Vobejda.

12. *Post*—Dec 3, 2000—Thompson, Chinoy, and Vobejda.

13. *Post*—Apr 24, 1989—Abramowitz.

14. *Post*—Sep 29, 1996—Harris.

15. *Post*—Mar 9 1989—Horwitz; *Post*—Mar 19, 1989—Isikoff; see Part 5 for budget crisis.

16. *Post*—Dec 5, 2000—Vobejda and Chinoy (for quote); *Post*—Dec 6, 2000—Vobejda and Chinoy.

17. *Post*—Mar 19, 1990—Price.

18. *Post*—Mar 12, 1989—Boodman and Hortwitz.

19. *Post*—Nov 20, 1994—Milloy. See also Forman 2017.

20. Homicide Report, 1992; Lattimore et al 1997:14–16.

21. *Post*—Dec 31, 1992—Harriston and Duggan; *Post*—Dec 31, 1994—Castaneda.

22. *Post*—Mar 14, 1989—Isikoff and Pianin.

23. *Post*—Mar 17, 1989—Lewis.

24. *Post*—Dec 18, 1990—Colburn.

25. Estimates derived from the Homicide Report 1992:8 (Table 2), which reports that in 1990, 82% and 11% of homicides were among Black men and women respectively, while 3% and less than 1% were among White men and women respectively.

26. Homicide Report 1992:18 (Table 10).

27. See Peterson and Krivo 2010 and Braga et al 2010 on the racialized and spatial nature of violent crime nationally.

28. *Post*—Aug 31, 1989—Milloy.

29. Homicide Report 1992:8 (Table 2 and Figure 1). I take the average of 1986–1991 for percent Black. See pp. 9–10 for assailant statistics.

30. Sharkey 2010; Sharkey et al 2012.

31. Ralph 2014.

32. Leibbrand et al 2020; Smith 2015.

33. Goin et al 2019; Koppensteiner and Manacorda 2016; McCormick 1985.

34. G. Miller and Blackwell 2006; Bruce et al 2015; Lloyd et al 2005.

35. *Post*—June 26, 1988—Morin and Allen.

36. Musto 1999; See also *Post*—October 19, 1986—Musto.

37. Forman 2017.

38. Umberson 2017; Umberson et al 2017.

PART 4

Overview

1. President Richard Nixon speech, June 17, 1971, https://www.youtube.com /watch?v=y8TGLLQlD9M.

2. Garland 2001.

3. Schwartz and Nurge 2004:135.

4. Glaze 2010:2 (Table 1).

5. Gramlich 2021.

6. McLaughlin et al 2016. This estimate includes not just justice system costs but also costs to individuals, families and communities.

7. Buehler 2021.

8. Ghandnoosh et al 2023.

9. *Post*—Sep 24, 1987—Wheeler.

10. Lezin 1996.

11. Lotke 1998; see also Chambliss 1994.

12. M. Alexander 2010; Davis 2017; Rehavi and Starr 2014.

13. Ghandnoosh et al 2023.

14. Shannon et al 2017; see also Roehrkasse and Wildeman 2022 who estimated that at its height, Black men's lifetime risk of imprisonment rose as high as 49.6% in 2004. Notably, Hispanic men were also disproportionately impacted by mass incarceration (Roehrkasse and Wildeman 2022); see also https://www.sentencingproject.org/fact-sheet/latinx-disparities-in-youth-incarceration/; for data limitations, see https://www.vera.org/news/we-need-more-data-to-understand-the-impact-of-mass-incarceration-on-latinx-communities; https://apps.urban.org/features/latino-criminal-justice-data/.

15. Wacquant 2000; M. Alexander 2010.

16. American Civil Liberties Union and University of Chicago Law School Global Human Rights Clinic 2022:6.

17. Shannon et al 2017.

18. M. Alexander 2010:2.

19. Pager 2003. See also Pager et al 2009.

20. Asch and Musgrove 2017:404.

21. Schnittker et al 2011.

22. Estelle v. Gamble, 429 U.S. 97 (1976), https://www.loc.gov/item/usrep429097/.

10. Creating Mass Black Incarceration in DC

1. *Post*—Sep 24, 1987—Wheeler (see print newspaper sources at the end of the bibliography).

2. *Post*—Jan 19, 1990—Melton and Abramowitz; *Post*—Feb 16, 1990—York and Walsh.

3. *Post*—Sep 24, 1987—Wheeler.

4. Chambliss 1994:180.

5. Chambliss 1994:183; see also A. Goffman 2009.

6. Forman 2017.

7. Weitzer et al 2008:413.

8. Weitzer 1999:843.

9. *Post*—Aug 28, 1994—Harriston and Flaherty; *Post*—Aug 30, 1994—Harriston and Flaherty; *Post*—Aug 31, 1994—Harriston and Flaherty.

10. *Post*—Jun 14, 1989—Pianin; *Post*—Sep 13, 1989—Abramowitz; *Post*—Aug 28, 1994—Harriston and Flaherty; *Post*—Aug 30, 1994—Harriston and Flaherty; *Post*—Aug 31, 1994—Harriston and Flaherty.

11. *Post*—Dec 16, 1993—Flaherty and Harriston.

12. *Post*—Dec 16, 1993—Flaherty and Harriston.

13. *Post*—Mar 15, 1992—Wilson.

14. *Post*—Aug 28, 1994—Harriston and Flaherty; *Post*—Aug 30, 1994—Harriston and Flaherty; *Post*—Aug 31, 1994—Harriston and Flaherty.

15. *Post*—Nov 15, 1998—Leen, Craven, Jackson, and Horwitz.

16. *Post*—Nov 15, 1998—Leen, Craven, Jackson, and Horwitz.

17. *Post*—Nov 15, 1998—Leen, Craven, Jackson, and Horwitz.

18. *Post*—Nov 15, 1998—Leen, Craven, Jackson, and Horwitz.

19. *Post*—Jun 30, 1991—Horwitz.

20. Hinton 2017.

21. Stevenson 2017; Forman 2017.

22. Forman 2017:155.

23. Staples 2007:647.

24. Wacquant 2000:378.

25. Wacquant 2000:377.

26. *Post*—Milloy and Coleman—Feb 13, 1983.

27. E. Goffman 1958; Clemmer 1960; Irwin and Cressey 1962; Skyes 1958.

28. Comfort 2019; Braman 2004.

29. Weitzer et al 2008; Forman 2017.

30. Forman 2017:11–12.

31. Reuter et al 1990.

32. Western 2006:27 (Figure 1.4). See also Pettit and Western 2004.

33. W. Wilson 1978, 1987; Dawson 1995.

34. Pattillo 1999; Kofie 1999.

35. See for example Anderson 1999; Venkatesh 2000; Braman 2004; Ralph 2014.

36. Forman 2017.

37. Shein 1993; M. Alexander 2010.

38. Shein 1993.

39. *Post*—Feb 20, 1994—Leiby.

40. *Post*—Oct 9, 1996—Flaherty and Casey.

41. Lotke 1998.

42. Braman 2004:3.

43. *Post*—Dec 8, 1988—Lewis and Churchville.

44. *Post*—Dec 8, 1988—Lewis and Churchville.

45. *Post*—Dec 8, 1988—Lewis and Churchville.

46. *Post*—Dec 21 1986—Robinson.

47. *Post*—Jan 26, 1988—Wheeler and Horwitz.

48. Wald and Losen 2003; Hirschfield 2008; Mallett 2016; Rios 2011; Ferguson 2000.

49. Passow 1967:242.

50. Passow 1967:242.

51. Passow 1967:256.

52. Passow 1967:251.

53. Passow 1967:251.

54. Passow 1967:244.

55. See https://dcpsbudget.com/budget-process-timeline-2/; see also pp. 38–172 of the DC Council Code https://code.dccouncil.gov/us/dc/council/code/titles/38/chapters/1A; National Academies of Science 2011.

56. Coleman 1966.

57. Berner 1993:10.

58. Berner 1993:10.

59. Berner 1993.

60. Washington Lawyers' Committee for Civil Rights and Urban Affairs 2010:28. See also Ladner 1997:67 (Figure 8).

61. Washington Lawyers' Committee for Civil Rights and Urban Affairs 2010:2.

62. The racial composition of DC students was obtained from the Office of Data Management in DCs Office of the Superintendent of Education. See also Orfield 1983; Orfield and Ee 2017. Information on DC population sizes by race is in Figure 10.

63. Squires et al 2002; Barrow 2002; Sharkey 2013.

64. Washington Lawyers' Committee for Civil Rights and Urban Affairs 2010:4.

65. Washington Lawyers' Committee for Civil Rights and Urban Affairs 2010:3–4; see also Marvel 2012; National Academies of Science 2011.

66. Ladner 1997.

67. *Post*—July 4 1985—Sargent; *Post*—July 19, 1986—Sargent.

68. *Post*—July 27, 1988—Sanchez.

69. *Post*—July 11, 1990—Sanchez.

70. Education Watch 2002–2003:2.

71. Education Watch 2002–2003:2.

72. Education Watch 2009:4.

73. *Post*—Sept 17, 1992—Horwitz and Jordan.

74. *Post*—Sept 23, 1999—Strauss.

75. Stillwell 2010:7 (Table 2).

76. Pettit and Western 2004.

77. Orfield and Ee 2017:12.

78. Galster and Mikelsons 1995:98.

79. Galster and Mikelsons 1995:101; see also Massey and Denton 1993.

80. B. Jacob 2007; Wilder 2014.

81. E. Goffman 1958.

82. Brounstein et al 1989; *Post*—Jul 28, 1989—Sanchez.

83. During interviews, my respondents and I referred to jails and prisons interchangeably; prison overcrowding meant that sometimes prisoners meant for jail

went to prison or vice versa; however, they and I distinguish between the two where relevant for the story or outcomes discussed.

84. *Post*—Aug 13, 1987—Churchville.

85. *Post*—Jul 22, 1988—Wheeler.

86. *Washington City Paper*—Jul 17, 1998—Park.

87. *Post*—May 5, 1997—Brown.

88. *Post*—May 5, 1997—Brown.

89. *Post*—Sep 3, 1998—Mathews.

90. *Post*—May 7, 1986—Lewis.

91. *Post*—May 7, 1986—Lewis.

92. *Post*—May 7, 1986—Lewis.

93. Hirschfield 2008; Mallett 2016; Rios 2011; Ferguson 2000.

94. Mallett 2016.

95. Hirschfield 2008:83.

96. Hirschfieid 2008; Wald and Losen 2003.

97. Hinton 2017; Hirschfield 2008:92.

98. Wald and Losen 2003:13.

99. Mallett 2016:18.

100. Wald and Losen 2003:10. (There were 48.1 million school-age [6–17 years] kids in 1974 and 49.7 million in 2003. So this was not accounted for by population increase. https://www.childstats.gov/americaschildren/tables /pop1.asp.)

101. Mallett 2016:20.

102. Mallett 2016:20.

103. *Post*—Sep 5, 1986—Wheeler.

104. *Post*—Dec, 1 1986—Fisher.

105. Education Watch: District of Columbia 2002–2003, 2006. See also Marinelli 2022.

106. 2012–2013 DC Equity Report cited in Office of the State Superintendent of Education 2014:15.

107. 2012–2013 DC Equity Report cited in Office of the State Superintendent of Education 2014:15.

108. 2012–2013 DC Equity Report cited in Office of the State Superintendent of Education 2014:7.

109. Office of the State Superintendent of Education 2014:12, 14.

110. *Post*—Sep 11, 1985—Evans.

111. Wald and Losen 2003:10.

112. Wald and Losen 2003:11.

113. Mallett 2016:19.

114. *Post*—Jun 17, 1990—Knight.

115. Sampson and Laub 1995. See also Knight 2024.

116. M. Alexander 2010:95 (quote); see also Western 2018; Harding et al 2019; Wacquant 2000, 2001.

117. *Post*—Apr 9 1989—Webb.

118. *Post*—Aug 13, 1987—Churchville.

119. *Post*—Sep 11, 1998—Slevin.

120. *Washington City Paper*—Jul 17, 1998—Park; *Post*—Sep 11, 1998—Slevin.

121. *Washington City Paper*—Jul 17, 1998—Park.

122. *Post*—Jun 8, 1997—Frankel.

123. Buehler 2021.

124. Wagner and Rabuy 2017.

125. *Magnolia Tribune*—Dec 26, 2022—Summerhays; Harris-Calvin et al 2022.

126. *Post*—Sept 7, 1997—Simon and Burns.

127. See Schwartz and Nurge 2004:133–34.

128. Garland 2001.

129. Schwartz and Nurge 2004:133.

130. Schwartz and Nurge 2004:145.

131. *Post*—May 2, 1986—Lewis.

132. *Post*—May 2, 1986—Lewis.

133. *Post*—Jan 26, 1988—Wheeler and Horwitz.

134. *Post*—Sep 23, 1989—Torry and Horwitz.

135. *Post*—Apr 11, 1989—Horwitz and Spolar.

136. *Post*—Aug 6, 1988—Hockstader and Lewis.

137. *Post*—Dec 8, 1988—Lewis and Churchville.

138. Lezin 1996:170.

139. *Post*—Slevin—May 24, 1998.

140. Hirschfield 2008.

141. Eason 2017.

142. Hirschfield 2008.

143. *Post*—Feb 4, 1997—Miller and Flaherty; *Washington City Paper*—Aug 20, 1999—Ripley.

144. *Post*—Feb 4, 1997—Miller and Flaherty.

145. *Post*—Feb 11, 2001—Lotke.

146. *Post*—Mar 21, 2002—Santana.

147. *Post*—Mar 21, 2002—Santana; Braman 2004; Wildeman 2009.

148. *Post*—Dec 18, 1988—Hockstader.

149. *Post*—Dec 18, 1988—Hockstader.

150. Schwartz and Nurge 2004.

151. Washington Lawyers' Committee for Civil Rights and Urban Affairs 2015:43–44.

152. Washington Lawyers' Committee for Civil Rights and Urban Affairs 2015:44.

153. Schwartz and Nurge 2004:142–43.

154. Schwartz and Nurge 2004:142–43.

155. *Post*—Mar 21, 2002—Santana.

156. Schwartz and Nurge 2004:143.

1. Proportions of prisoners incarcerated for drug use in federal and state prisons were 7.5% (1980s), 24.1% (1990s), 24.2% (2000s). Calculated from https://wayback .archive-it.org/org-652/20231025102502/https://www.albany.edu/sourcebook /tost_6.html#6_b; Snell 1995:11–12 (Tables 1.9–1.10); Harrison and Beck 2002:13–14 (Tables 17, 20).

2. Freudenberg 2001:217.

3. Nunn et al 2009.

4. Merrall et al 2010.

5. National Commission on Acquired Immune Deficiency Syndrome 1991:15.

6. Maruschak 1996–97.

7. Spaulding et al 2002:306.

8. Kunzel 2008.

9. Maruschak 1999:4.

10. Maruschak 1999:6.

11. Maruschak 2001.

12. Maruschak 2009.

13. *Post*—Jan 31, 1993—Mencimer; *Post*—Feb 4, 1991—McCall (see print newspaper sources at the end of the bibliography).

14. *Post*—May 18, 1992—Goldstein; see also *Washington Informer*—May 1, 1996—Peabody; Lezin 1996.

15. Maruschak 2004:2 (Table 1). As noted in Chapter 10, from the late '80s to 2001, DC prisoners were absorbed into the federal prison system due to overcrowding and then due to Lorton prison closing. The federal statistics for DC thus stop after 2000.

16. May and Williams 2002; Buhl 2015.

17. *Post*—Feb 4, 1991—McCall 1991.

18. *Post*—Jan 31, 1993—Mencimer.

19. *Post*—Jan 31, 1993—Mencimer.

20. May and Williams 2002; Bick 2007; Hammett et al 1999.

21. Kunzel 2008.

22. Brien and Harlow 1995:5 (Table 4).

23. Lezin 1995–96:188.

24. Hammett et al 1995:51.

25. Hammett et al 1995:51.

26. American Civil Liberties Union 2013.

27. National Commission on Acquired Immune Deficiency Syndrome 1991; Kunzel 2008; American Civil Liberties Union 2013; Fleury-Steiner 2008.

28. Fleury-Steiner 2008:118.

29. Fleury-Steiner 2008:27.

30. *Post*—May 10, 1988—Colburn.

31. *Post*—May 9, 1986—Engel.

32. *Post*—Jul 12, 1995—Locy.

33. *Post*—Jul 12, 1995—Locy.

34. *Post*—Jul 12, 1995—Locy.

35. *Post*—Jul 12, 1995—Locy.

36. Lezin 1996:194.

37. J. A. Meyer et al 2010.

38. Maruschak 2004:6 (Table 6).

39. Adimora et al 2006; Aral et al 2008; Blankenship et al 2005; R. C. Johnson and Raphael 2009; Friedman et al 1999.

40. *Post*—Jul 4, 1987—Horwitz.

41. *Post*—Apr 26, 1984—Teeley.

42. *Post*—Jul 12, 1997—Thompson.

43. *Post*—Jul 15, 1997—Editorial.

44. Leverentz 2010.

45. *Post*—Jul 3, 1989—Walsh.

46. *Post*—Nov 16, 1993—Miller.

47. *Post*—Jul 3, 1989—Walsh.

48. *Post*—June 10, 1990a—Dash; *Post*—June 10, 1990b—Dash; *Post*—June 11, 1990a—Dash; *Post*—June 11, 1990b—Dash; *Post*—June 12, 1990—Dash; *Post*—June 13, 1990—Dash.

49. Blecker 1990:1208.

50. Blecker 1990:1217.

51. *Post*—Oct 23, 1989—Anderson and Van Atta.

52. *Post*—Oct 22, 1992—Howe; *Post*—June 11, 1990a—Dash.

53. *Post*—Oct 22, 1992—Howe.

54. *Post*—Nov 17, 1993—Miller and Sanchez.

55. *Post*—Nov 17, 1993—Miller and Sanchez; *Post*—June 23, 1990—Howe; *Post*—Mar 18, 1992—Harriston.

56. *Post*—Mar 18, 1992—Harriston.

57. *Post*—Feb 10, 1995—Miller.

58. *Post*—Feb 10, 1995—Miller.

59. *Post*—Sept 28, 1995—Hall; *Post*—Jan 25, 1996—Hall.

60. *Post*—Jan 25, 1996—Hall; *Washington City Paper*—Sept 26, 1997—Peterson.

61. *Post*—Sept 28, 1995—Hall.

62. M. Cohen et al 2011.

63. Mojola et al 2021.

64. Kunzel 2008.

65. See also Jenness and Fenstermaker 2014; J. Greene 2023.

66. See also Kunzel 2008.

67. Kunzel 2008:237.

68. Kunzel 2008:102.

69. Kunzel 2008:237; see also Ward 2015; T. Silva 2017.

70. Mittleman 2023:1272, 1278, 1266 (Table 1).

71. Rupp et al 2014.

72. Pettit and Western 2004; Knight 2024.

73. Mishel et al 2020.

74. Donaldson 2001; Kunzel 2008; Trammell 2011.

75. Hildebrand and Najdowski 2014.

76. Staples 2007; R. C. Johnson and Raphael 2009; Ojikutu et al 2018.

77. R. C. Johnson and Raphael 2009; Ojikutu et al 2018.

78. Ojikutu et al 2018.

79. R. C. Johnson and Raphael 2009:286.

80. *Post*—May 18, 1992—Goldstein.

81. Maruschak 2004:2 (Table 1).

82. Patel et al 2014.

83. See for example Mojola 2011.

84. Thomas and Torrone 2006.

85. Dauria et al 2015; Adimora et al 2006

86. Braman 2004.

87. Wildeman 2009; Wakefield and Wilderman 2013; Turney 2017.

PART 5

Overview

1. Magnus et al 2009.

12. Intersectional Politics and the AIDS Epidemic

1. See for example Shilts 2007; for DC, hear Jim Graham oral history interviews—Rainbow History Project, https://rainbowhistory.org/.

2. Deeks et al 2013:1525.

3. See also https://www.hiv.gov/hiv-basics/overview/history/hiv-and-aids-timeline#year-1998; *Post*—July 23, 2012—Sun (see print newspaper sources at the end of the bibliography).

4. Biehl 2007.

5. Manglos and Trinitapoli 2011.

6. See Koenig et al 2001 and Cotton et al 2006 for reviews of literature on religion and coping with illness, and HIV/AIDS in particular.

7. *Post*—Sep 22, 1983—Engel.

8. https://www.whitman-walker.org/our-history/; *Post*—Aug 8 1988—Boodman; Jim Graham interviews—Rainbow History Project.

9. *Washington City Paper*—Aug 16, 1996—Cloud. See also Jim Graham interviews—Rainbow History Project; https://www.whitman-walker.org/our-history/.

10. https://www.whitman-walker.org/our-history/.

11. https://www.whitman-walker.org/our-history/.

12. *Post*—Jan 25, 1986—Engel.

13. *Post*—April 21, 1987—Barker; *Washington Informer*—Feb 12, 1986—Jackson.

14. *Post*—April 21, 1987—Barker; *Post*—Mar 5, 1987—Sherwood.

15. *Post*—Aug 8, 1988—Boodman.

16. See Watkins-Hayes 2019.

17. DC Law 6-132; *Washington Informer*—May 14, 1986—no author; *Washington Informer*—May 21, 1986–Crawford; *Washington Informer*—Jun 4, 1986—Crawford.

18. *Post*—Oct 5, 1988—Boodman and Pianin.

19. *Post*—Aug 4, 1987—Boodman.

20. *Post*—Sep 6, 1988—Hines and Randal.

21. *Washington Informer*—Sep 16, 1992—no author.

22. See also Dievler and Pappas 1999.

23. Gottlieb et al 1981; Mildvan et al 1982.

24. Mildvan et al 1982.

25. See for example Shilts 2007; Epstein 1996; Andriote 1999; Jim Graham interviews—Rainbow History project (https://rainbowhistory.org/); https://www.whitman-walker.org/our-history). See also PBS—The Age of AIDS, Frontline documentary (https://www.pbs.org/wgbh/frontline/documentary/aids/).

26. Shilts 2007; Epstein 1996; Andriote 1999; Watkins-Hayes 2019; Padamsee 2020.

27. Shilts 2007; Epstein 1996; Andriote 1999; Watkins-Hayes 2019; Padamsee 2020.

28. Shilts 2007; Epstein 1996; Andriote 1999; Watkins-Hayes 2019; Padamsee 2020.

29. Dolinsky 2010, 2013. See also Bost 2015; Andriote 1999.

30. Bost 2015. See also C. Cohen 1999; Hawkeswood 1993, 1996.

31. *Post*—Mar 5, 1987—Sherwood.

32. See also Wright 1993.

33. See also Bost 2015.

34. Dolinsky 2010, 2013; Bost 2015.

35. https://dcblackpride.org/about-us/; Bost 2015.

36. Bost 2015; my key informant interviews.

37. Gates 2022; Levin 1984; Smith et al 2005; Quinn et al 2016; Brewer and Williams 2019.

38. *Post*—Jan 12, 1987—Boodman; *Post*—Aug 4, 1987—Boodman; *Washington Informer*—Mar 30, 1994—no author; *Washington Informer*—Apr 3, 1997—Olds.

39. See also Bost 2015; https://dchistory.org/the-clubhouse/; https://www.ushelpingus.org/history.

40. https://www.nstreetvillage.org/about/.

41. See also C. Cohen 1999; Harris 2010.

42. Fullilove and Fullilove 1999; E. G. Ward 2005; Miller 2007.

43. Greenberg et al 2009.

44. See Watkins-Hayes 2019; https://www.womenscollective.org/our-work/.

45. My analysis of DC Health Department's HIV Surveillance Unit data.

46. *Post*—Jul 11, 1993—Goldstein. Minority groups were defined as non-White groups.

47. *Post*—Aug 8, 1988—Boodman.

48. *Post*—Aug 8, 1988—Boodman.

49. Jim Graham interviews—Rainbow History project, https://rainbowhistory .org/.

50. Jim Graham interviews—Rainbow History project, https://rainbowhistory .org/.

51. *Post*—Aug 8, 1988—Boodman; Andriote 1999.

52. Dievler and Pappas 1999.

53. *Post*—Jul 11, 1993—Goldstein.

54. *Post*—Aug 8, 1988—Boodman.

55. *Washington Informer*—Sep 1, 1993—no author.

56. *Washington Informer*—Sep 1, 1993—no author.

57. *Washington Informer*—June 29, 1994—Peabody.

58. *Washington Informer*—June 29, 1994—Peabody.

59. See also Dievler and Pappas 1999.

60. *Post*—Sep 22, 1983—Engel.

61. Bost 2015:4.

62. Bost 2015:3.

63. Dolinsky 2010; Bost 2015.

64. Dolinsky 2013:1675; Dievler and Pappas 1999.

65. *Post*—Aug 8, 1988—Boodman.

66. C. Cohen 1999.

67. *Post*—Jan 4, 2007—Blanks.

68. *Post*—Dec 13, 2009—Cenziper.

69. *Post*—Dec 13, 2009—Cenziper.

70. *Post*—Dec 13, 2009—Cenziper.

71. *Post*—Dec 13, 2009—Cenziper.

72. See also Dievler and Pappas 1999.

13. Controlling an Epidemic: The Successes and Limits of Technocratic Expertise

1. See Freudenberg et al 2006 and Colgrove 2011 for the New York case.

2. Gillette 1995; Asch and Musgrove 2017; Bouker 2016.

3. *Post*—Jan 13, 1995—Lewis; *Post*—Dec 15, 1989—Twomey (see print newspaper sources at the end of the bibliography).

4. *Post*—Dec 15, 1989—Twomey.

5. *Post*—Mar 25, 1989—Pianin; Lezin 1996.

6. Calculated from *Post*—Nov 4, 1990—Isikoff and Thompson.

7. Lezin 1996.

8. *Post*—Jun 9, 1988—Hockstader.

9. *Post*—Aug 13, 1995—Moore; *Post*—Jun 9, 1988—Hockstader.

10. *Post*—Aug 13, 1995—Moore (Moore was the director of the DC Department of Corrections); *Post*—Dec 6, 1995—Locy.

11. *Post*—Jan 31, 1993—Mencimer.

12. *Post*—May 18, 1992—Goldstein.

13. For 1979, see *Post*—Aug 9, 1988—Hockstader. For 1989, see District of Columbia, Metropolitan Police Department 1989:24. For 1990 and 1995, see Lindgren 1992:9 and Gifford 1999:8 (Bureau of Justice Statistics Bulletins).

14. *Post*—Aug 9, 1988—Hockstader.

15. *Post*—Sep 5, 1990—Abramowitz.

16. *Post*—Feb 2, 1995—Schneider and Vise.

17. Asch and Musgrove 2017; Cook 1997; Bouker 2016.

18. *Post*—Jun 15, 1989—Abramowitz.

19. *Post*—Feb 25, 1989—Abramowitz.

20. *Post*—Feb 25, 1989—Abramowitz.

21. *Post*—Feb 21, 1991—Torry; *Post*—Jun 4, 1991—Henderson.

22. *Post*—May 26, 1998—Goldstein.

23. *Post*—June 4, 1991—Henderson.

24. *Post*—Feb 21, 1991—Torry.

25. *Post*—May 26, 1998—Goldstein.

26. *Post*—Nov 29, 1993—Weinraub.

27. *Post*—Jun 23, 1994—Goldstein.

28. *Washington City Paper*—Aug 16, 1996—Cloud.

29. *Washington City Paper*—Aug 16, 1996—Cloud.

30. *Washington City Paper*—Aug 16, 1996—Cloud.

31. *Washington Informer*—May 8, 1996—Peabody.

32. *Washington City Paper*—Aug 16, 1996—Cloud; *Washington Informer*—Sep 4, 1996—Peabody.

33. *Washington City Paper*—Aug 16, 1996—Cloud.

34. *Washington City Paper*—Aug 16, 1996—Cloud; *Post*—Oct 28, 1997—Goldstein.

35. *Washington Informer*—May 8, 1996—Peabody; *Washington City Paper*—Aug 16, 1996—Cloud.

36. *Washington City Paper*—Aug 16, 1996—Cloud.

37. *Washington City Paper*—Aug 16, 1996—Cloud.

38. *Washington Informer*—May 17, 1995—no author; *Post*—May 12, 1995—Goldstein; *Post*—Jun 18, 1995—Goldstein; DC Appleseed Center 2005.

39. Galvin and Cohen 2004.

40. *Washington City Paper*—Aug 16, 1996—Cloud.

41. https://ryanwhite.hrsa.gov/about/parts-and-initiatives/part-b-adap.

42. *Washington Informer*—Sep 4, 1996—Peabody.

43. Kassaye et al 2016; Gibson et al 2019.

44. Kassaye et al 2016, quote on p. 842. See also Gibson et al 2019. Kassaye et al also found that only "11.4% of the sample had non-B HIV-1 subtypes," underscoring the

likely homegrown nature of the city's epidemic. (A popular thesis I encountered during fieldwork was that the city's epidemic was driven by immigration).

45. Kassaye et al 2016:840–841.

46. Kassaye et al 2016:842.

47. Kassaye et al 2016:842.

48. Lazere and Nickelson 2004.

49. The HIV/AIDS administration grew to incorporate hepatitis, other STIs, and TB, thus becoming HAHSTA. (Surveillance Reports began using HAHSTA in 2009). Here I focus on the HIV/AIDS unit in particular.

50. *GLAA*—Nov 2, 2001—Summersgill; *GLAA*—Mar 6, 2002—Summersgill; *KNH Morning Briefing*—Jan 27, 2003—no author; *GLAA*—July 7, 2004—no author (www.glaa.org).

51. *Post*—Cenziper—Oct 18, 2009. See also *GLAA*—Nov 2, 2001—Summersgill; *GLAA*—Mar 6, 2002—Summersgill; *KNH Morning Briefing*—Jan 27, 2003—no author; *GLAA*—July 7, 2004—no author (www.glaa.org).

52. *Post*—Oct 18, 2009—Cenziper.

53. *Post*—Nov 12, 2009—Cenziper.

54. For interview, see *Post*—Sep 1, 1987—no author. For raising alarm, see *Post*—Mar 5, 1987—Sherwood. For HIV prevention efforts, see for example *Post*—Jul 5, 1988—Boodman; *Post*—Feb 22, 1989—Boodman.

55. Information for individual commissioners and HAHSTA chiefs as listed:

Commissioners

Bennett: *Post*—Jun 8, 2023—Portnot

Lewis: *Washington Informer*—July 27, 2022—WI Web Staff

Nesbitt: *Post*—Dec 30, 2014—DeBonis

Garcia: *Washington Blade*—Jul 24, 2013—Chibbaro Jr.

Levin: *Washington Blade*—May 21, 2013—Chibbaro Jr.

Akhter: *Post*—Jan 8, 2011—Stewart; *Washington Times*—Jun 29, 2012—Howell Jr.

Vigilance: *Post*—Mar 1, 2008—Nakamura

Cano: *Post*—Oct 20, 2007—Nakamura and Woodlee

Pane: *Post*—Aug 5, 2004—Wilgoren

Buford: *Post*—Mar 14, 2002—Goldstein

Walks: *Post*—Aug 20, 1999—Horwitz

Kelly: *Post*—Sep 27, 1998—Vise

Noonan: *Post*—Jul 16, 1997—Goldstein; *Post*—Sep 27, 1998—Vise

Kelly: *Post*—Jul 16, 1997—Goldstein

Sloane: *Post*—Oct 19, 1997—Barry

Akhter: *Post*—Sep 20, 1991—Goldstein

Benjamin: *Post*—Jan 10, 1990—Duke

Tuckson: *Post*—Aug 5, 1986—Engel; *Post*—Sep 1, 1987—no author; *Post*—Jan 10, 1990—Duke

McBride: *Post*—Feb 7, 1986—Engel; *Post*—Aug 5, 1986—Engel

HAHSTA chiefs

Barnes: https://dchealth.dc.gov/page/hivaids-hepatitis-std-and-tb-administration-hahsta

Talwalker: *Washington Blade*—May 5, 2021—Chibbaro Jr.

Kharfen: *Washington Blade*—Jul 31, 2013—Chibbaro Jr.; *Washington Blade*—May 5, 2021—Chibbaro Jr.

Pappas: *Post*—Feb 5, 2011—Stewart; *Washington Blade*—Jul 31, 2013—Chibbaro Jr.

Elias: *Washington Blade*—Jun 9, 2010—Chibbaro Jr.

Hader: *Post*—Aug 9, 2007—Holley; *Washington Blade*—Jun 9, 2010—Chibbaro Jr.

Pane: *Post*—Aug, 9 2007—Holley

Martin: *Post*—Aug 25, 2005—Montgomery; *Post*—Jan 4, 2007—Levine

Watts: *Post*—Aug 5, 2004—Wilgoren; *Post*—Aug 17, 2005—Labbe

Lewis: *Post*—Apr 11, 1998—Horwitz; *Post*—May 16, 2003—Goldstein

Saunders: *Post*—Oct 28, 1997—Goldstein

Wilson: *Post*—Jun 18, 1995—Goldstein

Oldham Jr.: *Post*—Nov 30, 1993—Goldstein; *Post*—Jun 23, 1994

Ryan: *Post*—Jun 4, 1991—Henderson; *Post*—Nov 29, 1993—Weinraub

Lee: *Post*—Feb 18, 1990—Duke

Silver: *Post*—Apr 21, 1987—Barker

Tapscott: *Post*—Mar 25, 2006—Vargas

DeLeon: *Post*—Jan 29, 1986—Engel

56. I drew on information from multiple publicly available sources to construct the table. As such, there may be gaps in the list.

57. See Note 55 references for details.

58. DC Appleseed Center 2005:2.

59. DC Appleseed Center 2005:6.

60. DC Appleseed Center 2005:2.

61. DC Appleseed Center 2005:39.

62. DC Appleseed Center 2005:41 and my interviews.

63. *Post*—Dec 30, 2006—Vargas.

64. *Post*—Dec 30, 2006—Vargas.

65. *Post*—Jun 14, 2008—Stein.

66. Morgan et al 2002.

67. Greenberg et al 2009.

68. For "Know your epidemic," see D. Wilson and Halperin 2008; for testing campaign, see Castel et al 2012b; *Post*—Jan 4, 2007—Levine.

69. Castel et al 2012b; Greenberg et al 2009.

70. DC HAHSTA Report 2007:vii.

71. DC HAHSTA Report 2007, 2008.

72. DC HAHSTA Report 2008:53.

73. DC HAHSTA Report 2008:14.

74. DC HAHSTA Report 2007:2.

75. Octane Public Relations and Advertising 2014.

76. Greenberg et al 2009; Octane Public Relations and Advertising 2014.

77. *Post*—Jul 5, 1988—Boodman; *Post*—Feb 22, 1989—Boodman.

78. The FDA approved PrEP (pre-exposure prophylaxis) in 2012, and the CDC provided guidelines in 2014. (https://www.niaid.nih.gov/diseases-conditions/pre-exposure-prophylaxis-prep#:~:text=The%20Food%20and%20Drug%20Administration,at%20substantial%20risk%20for%20HIV). A city study found that in 2014, there was high PrEP awareness (over 70%) but low use (7.7%) among MSM (Patrick et al 2017). A HAHSTA presentation of the 2017–19 DC Behavioral Surveillance study reported that 94% of MSM were aware of PrEP and 38% reported use. The same study found that in 2019, among high risk heterosexuals, only 49% knew about PrEP and only 0.8% reported use.

79. DC HAHSTA 2017:34 (Table 10).

80. DC HAHSTA 2023:61 (Appendix, Table B8).

81. Castel et al 2012a.

82. DC HAHSTA 2023: Appendix (p. 45, Table A3, living cases), (p. 57, Table B5, newly diagnosed cases), (p. 66, Table B13, AIDS Deaths).

83. DC HAHSTA Report 2023:10.

CONCLUSION

1. See for example Edin et al 2023; Case and Deaton 2020; Metzl 2019.

2. Case and Deaton 2020; Quinones 2015; Macy 2018; Metzl 2019; Devi 2011; Dwyer-Lindgren et al 2022; Goldman and Andrasfay 2022.

3. House 2015.

4. Ryan 1971:25.

5. See for example A. Morris 1999; McCammon et al 2001; Epstein 1996; Ghaziani et al 2016.

6. Edin et al 2023.

7. Department of Housing and Urban Development 1972; Hetzel and Pinsky 1969; Frieden and Kaplan 1987; L. D. Brown 1998; Weber and Wallace 2012; Urban Omnibus 2016; M. Turner 2017; Popkin et al 2009; Gallagher et al 2024; Gelfond and Looney 2018; Eldar and Garber 2022.

8. Hetzel and Pinsky 1969; Frieden and Kaplan 1987; L. D. Brown 1998; Weber and Wallace 2012; Urban Omnibus 2016; M. Turner 2017; Popkin et al 2009; Gallagher et al 2024; Gelfond and Looney 2018; Eldar and Garber 2022.

9. Gillette 1995; Asch and Musgrove 2017.

10. Plummer 1985:218.

APPENDIX: METHODOLOGICAL NOTE

1. See also Anderson 2022.

2. Information to aid accessing the underlying quantitative data for the figures in this book are below:

Figures 1–5 use estimates from the National Vital Statistics Reports, which use data from the National Vital Statistics System.

Figure 1: Arias et al 2024, https://www.cdc.gov/nchs/data/nvsr/nvsr73/nvsr73-07.pdf.

Figures 2–5: 1880: Ruggles 1994:142 (Table 3);
1900–2017: https://www.cdc.gov/nchs/data-visualization/mortality-trends/index.htm;
2018: https://stacks.cdc.gov/view/cdc/97643;
2019: https://www.cdc.gov/nchs/data/nvsr/nvsr70/nvsr70-19.pdf;
2020: https://www.cdc.gov/nchs/data/nvsr/nvsr71/nvsr71-01.pdf;
2021: https://www.cdc.gov/nchs/data/nvsr/nvsr72/nvsr72-12.pdf;
2022: https://www.cdc.gov/nchs/data/nvsr/nvsr74/nvsr74-02.pdf.

Figures 7, 10, 24–28: US Census and American Community Survey data: https://usa.ipums.org/usa/index.shtml; Steven Ruggles, Sarah Flood, Matthew Sobek, Daniel Backman, Grace Cooper, Julia A. Rivera Drew, Stephanie Richards, Renae Rodgers, Jonathan Schroeder, and Kari C. W. Williams, IPUMS USA: Version 16.0 [dataset], Minneapolis, MN: IPUMS, 2025. https://doi.org/10.18128/D010.V16.0

Figure 11: 1880 US Census geocoded data: see Logan et al 2011. Data can be accessed at https://s4.ad.brown.edu/Projects/UTP/index.htm.

Figures 13, 18, 20, 21: US Census Bureau, IPUMS National Historical GIS: https://www.nhgis.org/.

Figure 22: Washington DC and its suburbs: Global Health Data Exchange: https://ghdx.healthdata.org/.

Figures 23, 42: HAHSTA annual reports 2016–2023; DC HIV/AIDS Surveillance data accessed by permission of DC HAHSTA chief and chief epidemiologist.

Figure 29: Data used to construct the MMPI came from IPUMS (US Census Bureau 1950–2000), American Community Survey 5-year data (2010–2020), and the Bureau of Justice Statistics.

Figures 32, 33, 37: Homicide data: Disaster Center: https://www.disastercenter.com/crime/dccrime.htm; DC HIV/AIDS Surveillance data accessed by permission of DC HAHSTA chief and chief epidemiologist. I also relied on the annual HIV/AIDS surveillance reports, which can be accessed at https://dchealth.dc.gov/node/1346196.

3. Mills 1959:3.
4. Elder 1994:10.
5. Reskin 2012.
6. Krieger 1994.
7. Wendland 2022.

BIBLIOGRAPHY

Sources from print newspapers appear in a dedicated section at the end of the bibliography, where they are grouped by publication and arranged by date.

Abraham, Laurie Kaye. 1993. *Mama Might Be Better Off Dead: The Failure of Health Care in Urban America.* University of Chicago Press.

Acciai, Francesco, Aggie J. Noah, and Glenn Firebaugh. 2015. Pinpointing the Sources of the Asian Mortality Advantage in the USA. *Journal of Epidemiology and Community Health* 69(10): 1006–1011.

Acker, Joan. 1990. Hierarchies, Jobs, Bodies: A Theory of Gendered Organizations. *Gender & Society* 4(2): 139–158.

adams, jimi, James Moody, and Martina Morris. 2013. Sex, Drugs, and Race: How Behaviors Differentially Contribute to the Sexually Transmitted Infection Risk Network Structure. *American Journal of Public Health* 103(2): 322–329.

Adimora, Adaora A., and Judith D. Auerbach. 2010. Structural Interventions for HIV Prevention in the United States. *Journal of Acquired Immune Deficiency Syndromes* 55(2): S132–135.

Adimora, Adaora A., Victor J. Schoenbach, Dana M. Bonas, Francis E. A. Martinson, Kathryn H. Donaldson, and Tonya R. Stancil. 2002. Concurrent Sexual Partnerships among Women in the United States. *Epidemiology* 13(3): 320–327.

Adimora, Adaora A., Victor Schoenbach and Irene A. Doherty. 2006. HIV and African Americans in the Southern United States: Sexual Networks and Social Context. *Sexually Transmitted Diseases* 33(7): S39-S45.

Adimora, Adaora A., Victor J. Schoenbach, and Irene A. Doherty. 2007. Concurrent Sexual Partnerships among Men in the United States. *American Journal of Public Health* 97(12): 2230–2237.

Adkins, Judith. 2016. "These People Are Frightened to Death": Congressional Investigations and the Lavender Scare. *Prologue Magazine* 48(2). https://www.archives.gov/publications/prologue/2016/summer/lavender.html.

Adler, Patricia A. 1985. *Wheeling and Dealing: An Ethnography of an Upper-Level Drug Dealing and Smuggling Community.* Columbia University Press.

Adler, Patricia A., Peter Adler, and Patrick K. O'Brien, eds. 2012. *Drugs and the American Dream: An Anthology*. John Wiley & Sons.

Adler, William M. 1995. *Land of Opportunity: One Family's Quest for the American Dream in the Age of Crack*. University of Michigan Press.

Agar, Michael. 2003. The Story of Crack: Towards a Theory of Illicit Drug Trends. *Addiction Research & Theory* 11(1): 3–29.

Aggleton, Peter, and Richard Parker, eds. 2014. *Men Who Sell Sex: Global Perspectives*. Routledge.

Agrawal, Arpana, and Michael T. Lynskey. 2008. Are There Genetic Influences on Addiction: Evidence from Family, Adoption and Twin Studies. *Addiction* 103(7): 1069–1081.

Ahmed, Feroz, Olive Shisana, and Frough Saadatmand. 1991. Leading Causes of Infant Deaths in the District of Columbia. *Journal of the National Medical Association* 83(8): 665–673.

Alba, Richard. 2009. *Blurring the Color Line: The New Chance for a More Integrated America*. Harvard University Press.

Alexander, Michelle. 2010. *The New Jim Crow: Mass Incarceration in the Age of Colorblindness*. New Press.

Alexander, Monica J., Mathew V. Kiang, and Magali Barbieri. 2018. Trends in Black and White Opioid Mortality in the United States, 1979–2015. *Epidemiology* 29(5): 707–715.

Amaro, Hortensia. 1995. Love, Sex, and Power: Considering Women's Realities in HIV Prevention. *American Psychologist* 50(6): 437–447.

Amato, Paul R., and Brett Beattie. 2011. Does the Unemployment Rate Affect the Divorce Rate? An Analysis of State Data 1960–2005. *Social Science Research* 40(3): 705–715.

American Civil Liberties Union. 2013. South Carolina Becomes Final State to End Segregation of Prisoners with HIV. July 10. https://www.aclu.org/press-releases/south-carolina-becomes-final-state-end-segregation-prisoners-hiv.

American Civil Liberties Union and University of Chicago Law School Global Human Rights Clinic. 2022. *Captive Labor: Exploitation of Incarcerated Workers*. https://www.aclu.org/publications/captive-labor-exploitation-incarcerated-workers.

Ammon, Francesca Russello. 2009. Commemoration amid Criticism: The Mixed Legacy of Urban Renewal in Southwest Washington, DC. *Journal of Planning History* 8(3): 175–220.

Anderson, Elijah. 1999. *Code of the Street: Decency, Violence, and the Moral Life of the Inner City*. WW Norton & Company.

Anderson, Elijah. 2022. *Black in White Space: The Enduring Impact of Color in Everyday Life*. University of Chicago Press.

Andrasfay, Theresa, and Noreen Goldman. 2021. Reductions in 2020 US Life Expectancy due to COVID-19 and the Disproportionate Impact on the Black and Latino Populations. *Proceedings of the National Academy of Sciences* 118(5): e2014746118.

Andriote, John-Manuel. 1999. *Victory Deferred: How AIDS Changed Gay Life in America.* University of Chicago Press.

Aniline, Orm, and Ferris N. Pitts. 1982. Phencyclidine (PCP): A Review and Perspectives. *CRC Critical Reviews in Toxicology* 10(2): 145–177.

Aral, Sevgi O., Adaora A. Adimora, and Kevin A. Fenton. 2008. Understanding and Responding to Disparities in HIV and other Sexually Transmitted Infections in African Americans. *The Lancet* 372(9635): 337–340.

Arias, Elizabeth, Jiaquan Xu, Betzaida Tejada-Vera and Brigham Bastian. 2024. U.S. State Life Tables, 2021. 73(7): 1–18. August 21, 2024. *National Vital Statistics Reports.* National Center for Health Statistics.

Asch, Chris Myers, and George Derek Musgrove. 2017. *Chocolate City: A History of Race and Democracy in the Nation's Capital.* University of North Carolina Press.

Ashforth, Adam. 1999. Weighing Manhood in Soweto. *Codesria Bulletin* 3(4): 51–58.

Astemborski, Jacquie, David Vlahov, Dora Warren, Liza Solomon, and Kenrad E. Nelson. 1994. The Trading of Sex for Drugs or Money and HIV Seropositivity among Female Intravenous Drug Users. *American Journal of Public Health* 84(3): 382–387.

Auerbach, Judith D. 2019. Getting to Zero Begins with Getting to Ten. *Journal of Acquired Immune Deficiency Syndromes* 82(2): S99-S103.

Auerbach, Judith D., Justin O. Parkhurst, and Carlos F. Cáceres. 2011. Addressing Social Drivers of HIV/AIDS for the Long-Term Response: Conceptual and Methodological Considerations. *Global Public Health* 6(Suppl 3): S293-S309.

Aultman, B. 2014. Cisgender. *Transgender Studies Quarterly* 1(1–2): 61–62.

Bachman, Jerald G., John M. Wallace Jr., Patrick M. O'Malley, Lloyd D. Johnston, Candace L. Kurth, and Harold W. Neighbors. 1991. Racial/Ethnic Differences in Smoking, Drinking, and Illicit Drug Use among American High School Seniors, 1976–89. *American Journal of Public Health* 81(3): 372–377.

Badgett, M. V. Lee, Soon Kyu Choi, and Bianca D. M. Wilson. 2019. *LGBT Poverty in the United States: A Study of Differences between Sexual Orientation and Gender Identity Groups.* The Williams Institute, UCLA School of Law.

Baker, Robert B., Harriet A. Washington, Ololade Olakanmi, Todd L. Savitt, Elizabeth A. Jacobs, Eddie Hoover, and Matthew K. Wynia. 2008. African American Physicians and Organized Medicine, 1846–1968: Origins of a Racial Divide. *JAMA* 300(3): 306–313.

Bailey, Zinzi D., Nancy Krieger, Madina Agénor, Jasmine Graves, Natalia Linos, and Mary T. Bassett. 2017. Structural Racism and Health Inequities in the USA: Evidence and Interventions. *The Lancet* 389(10077): 1453–1463.

Barker, David J. 1990. The Fetal and Infant Origins of Adult Disease. *British Medical Journal* 301(6761): 1111.

Barlas, Stephen. 2017. US and States Ramp Up Response to Opioid Crisis: Regulatory, Legislative, and Legal Tools Brought to Bear. *Pharmacy and Therapeutics* 42(9): 569–571, 592.

Barnes, William R. 1980. A Battle for Washington: Ideology, Racism, and Self-Interest in the Controversy over Public Housing, 1943–1946. *Records of the Columbia Historical Society* 50(1980): 452–483.

Barrow, Lisa. 2002. School Choice through Relocation: Evidence from the Washington D.C. Area. *Journal of Public Economics* 86(2): 155–189.

Bass, Alison. 2015. *Getting Screwed: Sex Workers and the Law.* University Press of New England.

Bauermeister, José A. 2008. Latino Gay Men's Drug Functionality. *Journal of Ethnicity in Substance Abuse* 7(1): 41–65.

Bearman, Peter S., James Moody, and Katherine Stovel. 2004. Chains of Affection: The Structure of Adolescent Romantic and Sexual Networks. *American Journal of Sociology* 110(1): 44–91.

Becasen, Jeffrey S., Christa L. Denard, Mary M. Mullins, Darrel H. Higa, and Theresa Ann Sipe. 2019. Estimating the Prevalence of HIV and Sexual Behaviors among the US Transgender Population: A Systematic Review and Meta-Analysis, 2006–2017. *American Journal of Public Health* 109(1): e1–e8.

Becker, Howard S. 1953. Becoming a Marihuana User. *American Journal of Sociology* 59(3): 235–242.

Becker, Jill B., Michele L. McClellan, and Beth Glover Reed. 2017. Sex Differences, Gender and Addiction. *Journal of Neuroscience Research* 95(1–2): 136–147.

Beemyn, Genny. 2014. *A Queer Capital: A History of Gay Life in Washington DC.* Routledge.

Beer, Linda, Christine L. Mattson, Heather Bradley, and Jacek Skarbinski. 2016. Understanding Cross-Sectional Racial, Ethnic, and Gender Disparities in Antiretroviral Use and Viral Suppression among HIV Patients in the United States. *Medicine* 95(13): 1–9.

Benjamin Ruha. 2019. *Race After Technology: Abolitionist Tools for the New Jim Code.* John Wiley & Sons.

Berkman, Lisa F., and Ichiro Kawachi, eds. 2000. *Social Epidemiology.* Oxford University Press.

Berner, Maureen M. 1993. Building Conditions, Parental Involvement, and Student Achievement in the District of Columbia Public School System. *Urban Education* 28(1): 6–29.

Bernstein, Elizabeth. 2007. *Temporarily Yours: Intimacy, Authenticity, and the Commerce of Sex.* University of Chicago Press.

Bernstein, Jared, Elizabeth McNichol, and Karen Lyons. 2006. *Pulling Apart: A State-by-State Analysis of Income Trends.* Center on Budget and Policy Priorities.

Bérubé, Allan. 1990. *Coming Out Under Fire: The History of Gay Men and Women in World War II.* Free Press.

Bethencourt, Francisco. 2014. *Racisms: From the Crusades to the Twentieth Century.* Princeton University Press.

Bick, Joseph A. 2007. Infection Control in Jails and Prisons. *Clinical Infectious Diseases* 45(8): 1047–1055.

Biehl, João. 2007. *Will to Live: AIDS Therapies and the Politics of Survival.* Princeton University Press.

Biles, Roger. 1992. Black Mayors: A Historical Assessment. *The Journal of Negro History* 77(3): 109–125.

Bingham, Trista A., Nina T. Harawa, Denise F. Johnson, Gina M. Secura, Duncan A. Mackellar, and Linda A. Valleroy. 2003. The Effect of Partner Characteristics on HIV Infection among African American Men Who Have Sex with Men in the Young Men's Survey, Los Angeles, 1999–2000. *AIDS Education and Prevention* 15(Supp A): 39–52.

Bird, Chloe E., and Patricia P. Rieker. 1999. Gender Matters: An Integrated Model for Understanding Men's and Women's Health. *Social Science & Medicine* 48(6): 745–755.

Bischoff, Kendra, and Sean F. Reardon. 2014. Residential Segregation by Income, 1970–2009. In John R. Logan, ed., *Diversity and Disparities: America Enters a New Century,* pp. 208–234. Russell Sage.

Blackhawk, Ned. 2023. *The Rediscovery of America: Native Peoples and the Unmaking of US History.* Yale University Press.

Blackwell, Debra L., and Daniel T. Lichter. 2004. Homogamy among Dating, Cohabiting, and Married Couples. *The Sociological Quarterly* 45(4): 719–737.

Blankenship, Kim M., Amy B. Smoyer, Sarah J. Bray, and Kristin Mattocks. 2005. Black-White Disparities in HIV/AIDS: The Role of Drug Policy and the Corrections System. *Journal of Health Care for the Poor and Underserved* 16(4 Suppl B): 140–146.

Blecker, Robert. 1990. Haven or Hell? Inside Lorton Central Prison: Experiences of Punishment Justified. *Stanford Law Review* 42(5): 1149–1249.

Board of Health.
    1872   *Annual Report of the Commissioners of the District of Columbia.*
    1875   *Annual Report of the Commissioners of the District of Columbia.*
    1876   *Annual Report of the Commissioners of the District of Columbia.*
    1877   *Annual Report of the Commissioners of the District of Columbia.*
    1890   *Annual Report of the Commissioners of the District of Columbia.*
    1900   *Annual Report of the Commissioners of the District of Columbia.*
    1910   *Annual Report of the Commissioners of the District of Columbia.*
    1920   *Annual Report of the Commissioners of the District of Columbia.*
    1930   *Annual Report of the Commissioners of the District of Columbia.*
    1940   *Annual Report of the Commissioners of the District of Columbia.*
    1950   *Annual Report of the Commissioners of the District of Columbia.*
    1960   *Annual Report of the Commissioners of the District of Columbia.*

Boardman, Jason D., Brian Karl Finch, Christopher G. Ellison, David R. Williams, and James S. Jackson. 2001. Neighborhood Disadvantage, Stress, and Drug Use among Adults. *Journal of Health and Social Behavior* 42(2): 151–165.

Boardman, Jason D., Jarron M. Saint Onge, Richard G. Rogers, and Justin T. Denney. 2005. Race Differentials in Obesity: The Impact of Place. *Journal of Health and Social Behavior* 46(3): 229–243.

Bockting, Walter, B. E. Robinson, and B. R. Simon Rosser. 1998. Transgender HIV Prevention: A Qualitative Needs Assessment. *AIDS Care* 10(4): 505–525.

Boles, Jacqueline, and Kirk W. Elifson. 1994. The Social Organization of Transvestite Prostitution and AIDS. *Social Science & Medicine* 39(1): 85–93.

Bonilla-Silva, Eduardo. 1997. Rethinking Racism: Toward a Structural Interpretation. *American Sociological Review* 62(3): 465–480.

Bonilla-Silva, Eduardo. 2004. From Bi-Racial to Tri-Racial: Towards a New System of Racial Stratification in the USA. *Ethnic and Racial Studies* 27(6): 931–950.

Bonilla-Silva, Eduardo. 2006. *Racism without Racists: Color-Blind Racism and the Persistence of Racial Inequality in the United States.* Rowman & Littlefield Publishers.

Bonilla-Silva, Eduardo. 2021. What Makes Systemic Racism Systemic? *Sociological Inquiry* 91(3): 513–533.

Bontempi, Jean M. Breny, Eugenia Eng, and Sandra Crouse Quinn. 2008. Our Men Are Grinding Out: A Qualitative Examination of Sex Ratio Imbalances, Relationship Power, and Low-Income African American Women's Health. *Women & Health* 48(1): 63–81.

Borchert, James. 1971/1972. The Rise and Fall of Washington's Inhabited Alleys: 1852–1972. *Records of the Columbia Historical Society, Washington, D.C.* 71/72: 267–288.

Borchert, James. 1973/1974. Alley Life in Washington: An Analysis of 600 Photographs. *Records of the Columbia Historical Society, Washington, D.C.* 49: 244–259.

Borchert, James. 1980. *Alley Life in Washington: Family, Community, Religion, and Folklife in the City, 1850–1970.* University of Illinois Press.

Bost, Darius. 2015. At the Club: Locating Early Black Gay AIDS Activism in Washington, DC. *Occasion* 8: 1–9.

Bouker, Jon. 2016. *The DC Revitalization Act: History, Provisions, and Promises.* Brookings Institution.

Bourgois, Phillipe. 1995. *In Search of Respect.* Cambridge University Press.

Boutyline, Andrei, and Laura K. Soter. 2021. Cultural Schemas: What They Are, How to Find Them, and What to Do Once You've Caught One. *American Sociological Review* 86(4): 728–758.

Bowleg, Lisa. 2004. Love, Sex, and Masculinity in Sociocultural Context: HIV Concerns and Condom Use among African American Men in Heterosexual Relationships. *Men and Masculinities* 7(2): 166–186.

Bowleg, Lisa, Kenya J. Lucas, and Jeanne M. Tschann. 2004. "The Ball Was Always in His Court": An Exploratory Analysis of Relationship Scripts, Sexual Scripts, and Condom Use among African American Women. *Psychology of Women Quarterly* 28: 70–82.

Bowleg, Lisa, Michelle Teti, Jenné S. Massie, Aditi Patel, David J. Malebranche, and Jeanne M. Tschann. 2011. "What Does It Take to Be a Man? What Is a Real Man?": Ideologies of Masculinity and HIV Sexual Risk among Black Heterosexual Men. *Culture, Health & Sexuality* 13(5): 545–559.

Bowser, Benjamin P. 1989. Crack and AIDS: An Ethnographic Impression. *Journal of the National Medical Association* 81(5): 538–540.

Bowser, Benjamin P., Ernest Quimby, and Merrill Singer, eds. 2007. *When Communities Assess their AIDS Epidemics. Results of Rapid Assessment of HIV/AIDS in Eleven US Cities.* Lexington Books.

Boykin, Keith. 1996. *One More River to Cross: Black and Gay in America.* Anchor Books.

Brabner-Smith, John W. 1936. The Government's Housing Program to Date. *American Bar Association Journal* 22(9): 631–637.

Brabner-Smith, John W. 1937. The Wagner Act: A Definite Housing Program. *American Bar Association Journal* 23: 681–682.

Braga, Anthony A., Andrew V. Papachristos, and David M. Hureau. 2010. The Concentration and Stability of Gun Violence at Micro Places in Boston, 1980–2008. *Journal of Quantitative Criminology* 26: 33–53.

Braman, Donald. 2004. *Doing Time on the Outside: Incarceration and Family Life in Urban America.* University of Michigan Press.

Braveman, Paula A., Catherine Cubbin, Susan Egerter, David R. Williams, and Elsie Pamuk. 2010. Socioeconomic Disparities in Health in the United States: What the Patterns Tell Us. *American Journal of Public Health* 100(S1): S186-S196.

Brekhus, Wayne. 2003. *Peacocks, Chameleons, Centaurs: Gay Suburbia and the Grammar of Social Identity.* University of Chicago Press.

Brewer, LaPrincess C., and David R. Williams. 2019. We've Come This Far by Faith: The Role of The Black Church in Public Health. *American Journal of Public Health* 109(3): 385–386.

Brien, Peter M., and Caroline Wolf Harlow. 1995. *HIV in Prisons and Jails, 1993.* Bureau of Justice Statistics Bulletin, NCJ 152765. US Department of Justice.

Brounstein, Paul J., Harry P. Hatry, David M. Altschuler and Louis H. Blair. 1989. *Patterns of Substance Use and Delinquency among Inner City Adolescents.* The Urban Institute. Prepared for the U.S. Department of Justice.

Brown, Lawrence D. 1998. Urban Health Policy. *Journal of Urban Health: Bulletin of the New York Academy of Medicine* 75(2): 273–280.

Brown, Letitia Woods. 1972. *Free Negroes in the District of Columbia, 1790–1846.* Oxford University Press.

Brown, Tyson H., and Patricia Homan. 2024. Structural Racism and Health Stratification: Connecting Theory to Measurement. *Journal of Health and Social Behavior* 65(1): 141–160.

Bruce, Marino A., Derek M. Griffith, and Roland J. Thorpe Jr. 2015. Stress and the Kidney. *Advances in Chronic Kidney Disease* 22(1): 46–53.

Buehler, Emily D. 2021. *Justice Expenditures and Employment in the United States, 2017.* Bureau of Justice Statistics Bulletin, NCJ 256093. US Department of Justice.

Buhl, Larry. 2015. Condoms and Corrections. *America's AIDS Magazine.*

Bullard, Robert D. 1990. *Dumping in Dixie: Race, Class, and Environmental Quality.* Westview Press.

Bullard, Robert D., Paul Mohai, Robin Saha, and Beverly Wright. 2008. Toxic Wastes and Race at Twenty: Why Race Still Matters After All of These Years. *Environmental Law* 38: 371–411.

Bureau of Justice Statistics. 1992. *Drugs, Crime and the Criminal Justice System.* NCJ 133652. US Department of Justice.

Bush, Patricia J., and Ronald J. Iannotti. 1993. Alcohol, Cigarette, and Marijuana Use among Fourth-Grade Urban Schoolchildren in 1988/89 and 1990/91. *American Journal of Public Health* 83(1): 111–114.

Byrand, Karl John. 1999. *Changing Race, Changing Place: Racial, Occupational, and Residential Patterns in Shaw, Washington, DC, 1880–1920.* Doctoral Dissertation. Geography. University of Maryland, College Park.

Candipan, Jennifer, Nolan Edward Phillips, Robert J. Sampson, and Mario Small. 2021. From Residence to Movement: The Nature of Racial Segregation in Everyday Urban Mobility. *Urban Studies* 58(15): 3095–3117.

Carey, Michael P., Theresa E. Senn, Derek X. Seward, and Peter A. Vanable. 2010. Urban African-American Men Speak Out on Sexual Partner Concurrency: Findings from a Qualitative Study. *AIDS and Behavior* 14(1): 38–47.

Case, Anne, and Angus Deaton. 2015. Rising Morbidity and Mortality in Midlife among White Non-Hispanic Americans in the 21st Century. *Proceedings of the National Academy of Sciences* 112(49): 15078–15083.

Case, Anne, and Angus Deaton. 2020. *Deaths of Despair and the Future of Capitalism.* Princeton University Press.

Case, Anne, and Christina Paxson. 2005. Sex Differences in Morbidity and Mortality. *Demography* 42(2): 189–214.

Castaneda, Ruben. 2014. *S Street Rising: Crack, Murder, and Redemption in DC.* Bloomsbury Publishing.

Castel, Amanda D., Montina Befus, Sarah Willis, Angelique Griffin, Tiffany West, Shannon Hader, and Alan E. Greenberg. 2012a. Use of the Community Viral Load as a Population-Based Biomarker of HIV Burden. *AIDS* 26(3): 345–353.

Castel, Amanda D., Manya Magnus, James Peterson, Karishma Anand, Charles Wu, Marsha Martin, Marie Sansone, Nestor Rocha, Titilola Jolaosho, Tiffany West, Shannon Hader, and Alan E. Greenberg. 2012b. Implementing a Novel Citywide Rapid HIV Testing Campaign in Washington, DC: Findings and Lessons Learned. *Public Health Reports* 127(4): 422–431.

Centers for Disease Control and Prevention. 2024a. *HIV Surveillance Report: Supplemental Report. Estimated HIV Incidence and Prevalence in the United States, 2018–2022.*

Centers for Disease Control and Prevention. 2024b. *HIV Surveillance Report: Diagnoses, Deaths, and Prevalence of HIV in the United States and 6 territories and Freely Associated States, 2022.*

Centers for Disease Control and Prevention. 1983. Heroin-Related Deaths—District of Columbia, 1980–1982. *Morbidity and Mortality Weekly Report* 32(25): 321–324.

Chambliss, William J. 1994. Policing the Ghetto Underclass: The Policing of Law and Law Enforcement. *Social Problems* 41(2): 177–194.

Chan, Shirley K., Lupita R. Thornton, Karen J. Chronister, Jeffrey Meyer, Marcia Wolverton, Cynthia K. Johnson, Raouf R. Arafat, Patricia M. Joyce, William M. Switzer, Walid Heneine, Anupama Shankar, Timothy Granade, Michele S. Owen, Patrick Sprinkle, and Vickie Sullivan. 2014. Likely Female-to-Female Sexual Transmission of HIV—Texas, 2012. *Morbidity and Mortality Weekly Report* 63(10): 209–212.

Chauncey, George. 1994. *Gay New York: Gender, Urban Culture, and the Making of the Gay Male World. 1890–1940.* Hachette UK.

Chesson, Harrell W., Ian H. Spicknall, Adrienna Bingham, Marc Brisson, Samuel T. Eppink, Paul G. Farnham, Kristen M. Kreisel, Sagar Kumar, Jean-François Laprise, Thomas A. Peterman, Henry Roberts, and Thomas L. Gift. 2021. The Estimated Direct Lifetime Medical Costs of Sexually Transmitted Infections Acquired in the United States in 2018. *Sexually Transmitted Diseases* 48(4): 215–221.

Chetty, Raj, Michael Stepner, Sarah Abraham, Shelby Lin, Benjamin Scuderi, Nicholas Turner, Augustin Bergeron, and David Cutler. 2016. The Association Between Income and Life Expectancy in the United States, 2001–2014. *JAMA* 315(16): 1750–1766.

Choi, Kyung-Hee, Joseph A. Catania, and M. Margaret Dolcini. 1994. Extramarital Sex and HIV Risk Behavior among US Adults: Results from the National AIDS Behavioral Survey. *American Journal of Public Health* 84(12): 2003–2007.

Chowkwanyun, Merlin. 2011. The Strange Disappearance of History from Racial Health Disparities Research. *Du Bois Review: Social Science Research on Race* 8(1): 253–270.

Chu, Susan Y., Lisa Conti, Barbara A. Schable, and Theresa Diaz. 1994. Female-to-Female Sexual Contact and HIV transmission. *JAMA* 272(6): 433.

Ciccarone, Daniel, and Philippe Bourgois. 2003. Explaining the Geographical Variation of HIV among Injection Drug Users in the United States. *Substance Use & Misuse* 38(14): 2049–2063.

Clark, Kenneth B. 1965. *Dark Ghetto: Dilemmas of Social Power.* Harper TorchBooks.

Clark, Shelley. 2004. Early Marriage and HIV Risks in Sub-Saharan Africa. *Studies in Family Planning* 35(3): 149–160.

Clark-Lewis, Elizabeth. 1994. *Living In, Living Out: African American Domestics in Washington, D.C., 1910–1940.* Smithsonian Institution Press.

Clements-Nolle, Kristen, Rani Marx, Robert Guzman, and Mitchell Katz. 2001. HIV Prevalence, Risk Behaviors, Health Care Use, and Mental Health Status of Transgender Persons: Implications for Public Health Intervention. *American Journal of Public Health* 91(6): 915–921.

Clemmer, Donald. 1960. *The Prison Community.* Holt, Rinehart and Winston.

Cohen, Cathy. J. 1999. *The Boundaries of Blackness: AIDS and the Breakdown of Black Politics.* University of Chicago Press.

Cohen, Dov, and Richard E. Nisbett. 1994. Self-Protection and the Culture of Honor: Explaining Southern Violence. *Personality and Social Psychology Bulletin* 20(5): 551–567.

Cohen, Myron S., Ying Q. Chen, Marybeth McCauley, Theresa Gamble, Mina C. Hosseinipour, Nagalingeswaran Kumarasamy, James G. Hakim, Johnstone Kumwenda, Beatriz Grinsztejn, Jose H. S. Pilotto, Sheela V. Godbole, Sanjay Mehendale, Suwat Chariyalertsak, Breno R. Santos, Kenneth H. Mayer, Irving F. Hoffman, Susan H. Eshleman, Estelle Piwowar-Manning, Lei Wang, Joseph Makhema, Lisa A. Mills, Guy de Bruyn, Ian Sanne, Joseph Eron, Joel Gallant, Diane Havlir, Susan Swindells, Heather Ribaudo, Vanessa Elharrar, David Burns, Taha E. Taha, Karin Nielsen-Saines, David Celentano, Max Essex, and Thomas R. Fleming. 2011. Prevention of HIV-1 infection with Early Antiretroviral Therapy. *The New England Journal of Medicine* 365(6): 493–505.

Cohen, Philip N., and Joanna R. Pepin. 2018. Unequal Marriage Markets: Sex Ratios and First Marriage among Black and White Women. *Socius* 4: 1–10.

Cohn, D'Vera. 2010. *Race and the Census: The "Negro" Controversy.* Pew Research Center. January 21.

Coleman, James S. 1966. *Equality of Educational Opportunity Study.* Inter-University Consortium for Political and Social Research.

Colgrove, James. 2011. *Epidemic City: The Politics of Public Health in New York.* Russell Sage Foundation.

Collins, James W., Jr., Shou-Yien Wu, and Richard J. David. 2002. Differing Intergenerational Birth Weights among the Descendants of US-Born and Foreign-Born Whites and African Americans in Illinois. *American Journal of Epidemiology* 155(3): 210–216.

Collins, Patricia Hill. 1990. *Black Feminist Thought: Knowledge, Consciousness, and the Politics of Empowerment.* Routledge.

Collins, Patricia Hill. 2004. *Black Sexual Politics: African Americans, Gender, and the New Racism.* Routledge.

Colliver, James D. and Andrea N. Kopstein. 1991. Trends in Cocaine Abuse Reflected in Emergency Room Episodes Reported to DAWN. *Public Health Reports* 106(1): 59–68.

Comfort, Megan. 2019. *Doing Time Together: Love and Family in the Shadow of the Prison.* University of Chicago Press.

Commission for Racial Justice. 1987. *Toxic Wastes and Race in the United States. A National Report on the Racial and Socio-Economic Characteristics of Communities with Hazardous Waste Sites.* United Church of Christ.

Connell, R. W. 2005. The Social Organization of Masculinity. In *Masculinities,* pp. 67–86. University of California Press.

Connell, Raewyn. 2012. Gender, Health and Theory: Conceptualizing the Issue in Local and World Perspective. *Social Science & Medicine* 74(11): 1675–1683.

Cook, Stephen R. 1997. Tough Love in the District: Management Reform under the District of Columbia Financial Responsibility and Management Assistance Act. *The American University Law Review* 47: 993–1028.

Copen, Casey E. 2017. Condom Use During Sexual Intercourse Among Women and Men Aged 15–44 in the United States: 2011–2015 National Survey of Family Growth. *National Health Statistics Reports* 105 (August 10): 1–17.

Cotton, Sian, Christina M. Puchalski, Susan N. Sherman, Joseph M. Mrus, Amy H. Peterman, Judith Feinberg, Kenneth I. Pargament, Amy C. Justice, Anthony C. Leonard, and Joel Tsevat. 2006. Spirituality and Religion in Patients with HIV/AIDS. *Journal of General Internal Medicine* 21(S5): S5-S13.

Courtenay, Will H. 2000. Constructions of Masculinity and Their Influence on Men's Well-Being: A Theory of Gender and Health. *Social Science & Medicine* 50(10): 1385–1401.

Courtwright, David T. 2001 (1982). *Dark Paradise: A History of Opiate Addiction in America*. Harvard University Press.

Craig, Richard B. 1978. La Campaña Permanente: Mexico's Antidrug Campaign. *Journal of Interamerican Studies and World Affairs* 20(2): 107–131.

Crenshaw, Kimberle. 1991. Mapping the Margins: Intersectionality, Identity Politics, and Violence Against Women of Color. *Stanford Law Review* 43(6): 1241–1299.

Crowder, Kyle, and Liam Downey. 2010. Inter-Neighborhood Migration, Race, and Environmental Hazards: Modeling Microlevel Processes of Environmental Inequality. *American Journal of Sociology* 115(4): 1110–1149.

Crum, Rosa M., Marsha Lillie-Blanton, and James C. Anthony. 1996. Neighborhood Environment and Opportunity to Use Cocaine and Other Drugs in Late Childhood and Early Adolescence. *Drug and Alcohol Dependence* 43(3): 155–161.

Cunningham, Lynn E. 1999. Washington, DC's Successful Public Housing Receivership. *Journal of Affordable Housing & Community Development Law* 9(1): 74–91.

Curington, Celeste Vaughan, Jennifer Hickes Lundquist, and Ken-Hou Lin. 2021. *The Dating Divide: Race and Desire in the Era of Online Romance*. University of California Press.

Curran, Laura, and Laura S. Abrams. 2000. Making Men into Dads: Fatherhood, the State, and Welfare Reform. *Gender & Society* 14(5): 662–678.

Currie, Janet, Joshua Graff Zivin, Jamie Mullins, and Matthew Neidell. 2014. What Do We Know about Short- and Long-Term Effects of Early-Life Exposure to Pollution? *Annual Review of Resource Economics.* 6(1): 217–247.

Dank, Meredith, Bilal Khan, P. Mitchell Downey, Cybele Kotonias, Deborah Mayer, Colleen Owens, Laura Pacifici, and Lilly Yu. 2014. *Estimating the Size and Structure of the Underground Commercial Sex Economy in Eight Major US Cities*. Urban Institute.

Daly, Martin, and Margo Wilson. 1988. *Homicide*. De Gruyter.

Dash, Leon. 1996. *Rosa Lee: A Generational Tale of Poverty and Survival in Urban America*. Basic Books.

Dauria, Emily F., Lisa Oakley, Kimberly Jacob Arriola, Kirk Elifson, Gina Wingood, and Hannah L. F. Cooper. 2015. Collateral Consequences: Implications of Male Incarceration Rates, Imbalanced Sex Ratios and Partner Availability for Heterosexual Black Women. *Culture, Health & Sexuality* 17(10): 1190–1206.

Davis, Angela J., ed. 2017. *Policing the Black Man.* Pantheon Books.

Dawson, Michael C. 1995. *Behind the Mule: Race and Class in African-American Politics.* Princeton University Press.

DC Appleseed Center. 2005. *HIV/AIDS in the Nation's Capital: Improving the District of Columbia's Response to a Public Health Crisis.* DC Appleseed Center and Hogan & Hartson, LLP.

DC Fiscal Policy Institute. 2011. *New Census Data Show that One in Five DC Residents Lived in Poverty in 2010.* September 22, 2011.

DC Law 4–149. Drug Paraphernalia Act of 1982.

DC Policy Center. 2021. *DC Racial Equity Profile for Economic Outcomes.* Council Office of Racial Equity.

De Boo, Hendrina A., and Jane E. Harding. 2006. The Developmental Origins of Adult Disease (Barker) Hypothesis. *Australian and New Zealand Journal of Obstetrics and Gynaecology* 46(1): 4–14.

Deeks, Steven G., Sharon R. Lewin, and Diane V. Havlir. 2013. The End of AIDS: HIV Infection as a Chronic Disease. *The Lancet* 382(9903): 1525–1533.

Deering, Kathleen N., Avni Amin, Jean Shoveller, Ariel Nesbitt, Claudia Garcia-Moreno, Putu Duff, Elena Argento, and Kate Shannon. 2014. A Systematic Review of the Correlates of Violence Against Sex Workers. *American Journal of Public Health* 104(5): e42-e54.

De Graffenried, Mary Clare. 1896. Typical Alley Houses in Washington, November 14, 1896. *The Woman's Anthropological Society Bulletin* 7: 5–15.

D'Emilio, John. 1998. *The Making of a Homosexual Minority in the United States, 1940–1970.* University of Chicago Press.

Denizet-Lewis, Benoit. 2003. Double Lives on the Down Low. *New York Times Magazine* 3: 28–33.

Department of Housing and Urban Development. 1972. *The Model Cities Program: A Comparative Analysis of Participating Cities Process, Product, Performance and Prediction.* Office of Community Development Evaluation Division.

Department of Justice. 2003. *Audit Report: Department of Justice Drug Demand Reduction Activities.* Office of the Inspector General. https://oig.justice.gov/reports/plus/a0312/final.pdf.

Des Jarlais, Don C., Samuel R. Friedman, David M. Novick, Jo L. Sotheran, Pauline Thomas, Stanley R. Yancovitz, Donna Mildvan, John Weber, Mary Jeanne Kreek, Robert Maslansky, Sarah Bartelme, Thomas Spira, and Michael Marmor. 1989. HIV-1 Infection among Intravenous Drug Users in Manhattan, New York City, from 1977 through 1987. *JAMA* 261(7): 1008–1012.

Desmond, Matthew. 2016. *Evicted: Poverty and Profit in the American City.* Crown.

Desmond, Matthew. 2023. *Poverty, by America.* Crown.

Devi, Sharmila. 2011. Native American Health Left Out in the Cold. *The Lancet* 377(9776): 1481–1482.

Dievler, Anne, and Gregory Pappas. 1999. Implications of Social Class and Race for Urban Public Health Policy Making: A Case Study of HIV/AIDS and TB Policy in Washington D.C. *Social Science and Medicine* 48: 1095–1102.

Diez Roux, Ana V., and Christina Mair. 2010. Neighborhoods and Health. *Annals of the New York Academy of Sciences* 1186(1): 125–145.

DiMaggio, Paul. 1997. Culture as Cognition. *Annual Review of Sociology* 23: 263–287.

District of Columbia Department of Health. 2014. *District Of Columbia Community Health Needs Assessment,* Volume 1.

District of Columbia Department of Health. 2019. *Health Equity Summary Report: District of Columbia 2018.*

District of Columbia HIV/AIDS, Hepatitis, STD, and TB Administration (HAHSTA). Department of Health, Government of the District of Columbia.

    2007 *Annual Epidemiology and Surveillance Report.*
    2008 *Annual Epidemiology and Surveillance Report.*
    2009 *Annual Epidemiology and Surveillance Report.*
    2010 *Annual Epidemiology and Surveillance Report.*
    2011 *Annual Epidemiology and Surveillance Report.*
    2012 *Annual Epidemiology and Surveillance Report.*
    2013 *Annual Epidemiology and Surveillance Report.*
    2014 *Annual Epidemiology and Surveillance Report.*
    2015 *Annual Epidemiology and Surveillance Report.*
    2016 *Annual Epidemiology and Surveillance Report.*
    2017 *Annual Epidemiology and Surveillance Report.*
    2018 *Annual Epidemiology and Surveillance Report.*
    2019 *Annual Epidemiology and Surveillance Report.*
    2020 *Annual Epidemiology and Surveillance Report.*
    2021 *Annual Epidemiology and Surveillance Report.*
    2022 *Annual Epidemiology and Surveillance Report.*
    2023 *Annual Epidemiology and Surveillance Report.*

District of Columbia Department of Human Services. Government of the District of Columbia.

    1974 *Vital Statistics Summary.*
    1980 *Vital Statistics Summary.*
    1985 *Vital Statistics Summary.*

District of Columbia, Metropolitan Police Department. 1989. *Annual Report.*

Dole, Vincent P., and Marie Nyswander. 1965. A Medical Treatment for Diacetylmorphine (Heroin) Addiction: A Clinical Trial with Methadone Hydrochloride. *JAMA* 193(8): 646–650.

Dole, Vincent P., and Marie E. Nyswander. 1976. Methadone Maintenance Treatment: A Ten-Year Perspective. *JAMA* 235(19): 2117–2119.

Dolinsky, Rebecca C. 2010. *Lesbian And Gay DC: Identity, Emotion, And Experience in Washington, DC's Social and Activist Communities (1961–1986).* Doctoral Dissertation. Sociology. University of California, Santa Cruz.

Dolinsky, Rebecca C. 2013. Emotional Memories Stemming From a Crisis: A Snapshot of AIDS Activism in Washington, DC (1981–1986). *Journal of Homosexuality,* 60(12): 1666–1694.

Donaldson Stephen. 2001. A Million Jockers, Punks, and Queens. In Don Sabo, Terry A. Kupers, and Willie London, *Prison Masculinities*, pp. 118–126. Temple University Press.

Dovel, Kathryn, Sara Yeatman, Susan Watkins, and Michelle Poulin. 2015. Men's Heightened Risk of AIDS-Related Death: The Legacy of Gendered HIV Testing and Treatment Strategies. *AIDS* 29(10): 1123–1125.

Dow, Dawn Marie. 2019. *Mothering While Black: Boundaries and Burdens of Middle-Class Parenthood.* University of California Press.

Downs, Jim. 2012. *Sick from Freedom: African-American Illness and Suffering During the Civil War and Reconstruction.* Oxford University Press.

Drake, St. Clair, and Horace R. Cayton. 1945. *Black Metropolis: A Study of Negro Life in a Northern City.* University of Chicago Press.

Drug Enforcement Agency. 1994. *The Cali Cartel: The New Kings of Cocaine; Drug Intelligence Report.* US Department of Justice, Drug Enforcement Agency.

Du Bois, William Edward Burghardt. 1899. *The Philadelphia Negro: A Social Study.* Published for the University.

Du Bois, William Edward Burghardt. 1904. *The Souls of Black Folk: Essays and Sketches.* Fourth Edition. A. C. McClurg & Co.

Du Bois, William Edward Burghardt. 1935 *Black Reconstruction: An Essay Toward a History of the Part Which Black Folk Played in the Attempt to Reconstruct Democracy in America, 1860–1880.* Russell and Russell.

Duck, Waverly. 2015. *No Way Out: Precarious Living in the Shadow of Poverty and Drug Dealing.* University of Chicago Press.

Dula, Annette. 1994. African American Suspicion of the Healthcare System Is Justified: What Do We Do About It? *Cambridge Quarterly of Healthcare Ethics* 3(3): 347–357.

Duneier, Mitchell. 2016. *Ghetto: The Invention of a Place, the History of an Idea.* Farrar, Strauss and Giroux.

Dunlap, Eloise, Andrew Golub, and Bruce D. Johnson. 2012. The Severely Distressed African American Family in the Crack Era: Empowerment Is Not Enough. In Adler et al 2012, pp. 102–111.

Dunlap, Eloise, and Bruce D. Johnson. 1992. The Setting for the Crack Era: Macro Forces, Micro Consequences (1960–1992). *Journal of Psychoactive Drugs* 24(4): 307–321.

DuPont, Robert L. 1971. Profile of a Heroin-Addiction Epidemic. *The New England Journal of Medicine,* 285(6), 320–324.

DuPont, Robert L., and Mark H. Greene. 1973. The Dynamics of a Heroin Addiction Epidemic: Heroin Abuse has Declined in Washington, DC. *Science* 181(4101): 716–722.

Dworkin, Shari L. 2005. Who Is Epidemiologically Fathomable in the HIV/AIDS Epidemic? Gender, Sexuality, and Intersectionality in Public Health. *Culture, Health & Sexuality* 7(6): 615–623.

Dworkin, Shari L. 2015. *Men at Risk: Masculinity, Heterosexuality and HIV Prevention.* New York University Press.

Dwyer-Lindgren, Laura, Parkes Kendrick, Yekaterina O. Kelly, Dillon O. Sylte, Chris Schmidt, Brigette F. Blacker, Farah Daoud, Amal A. Abdi, Mathew Baumann, Farah Mouhanna, Ethan Kahn, Simon I. Hay, George A. Mensah, Anna M. Nápoles, Eliseo J. Pérez-Stable, Meredith Shiels, Neal Freedman, Elizabeth Arias, Stephanie A. George, David M. Murray, John W. R. Phillips, Michael L. Spittel, Christopher J. L. Murray, and Ali H. Mokdad. 2022. Life Expectancy by County, Race, and Ethnicity in the USA, 2000–19: A Systematic Analysis of Health Disparities. *The Lancet* 400(10345): 25–38.

Eason, John M. 2017. *Big House on the Prairie: Rise of the Rural Ghetto and Prison Proliferation.* University of Chicago Press.

Edin, Kathryn, and Maria Kefalas. 2011. *Promises I Can Keep: Why Poor Women Put Motherhood Before Marriage.* University of California Press.

Edin, Kathryn, and Timothy J. Nelson. 2013. *Doing the Best I Can: Fatherhood in the Inner City.* University of California Press.

Edin, Kathryn, H. Luke Shaefer, and Timothy J. Nelson. 2023. *The Injustice of Place: Uncovering the Legacy of Poverty in America.* Harper Collins.

Edlin, Brian R., Kathleen L. Irwin, Sairus Faruque, Clyde B. McCoy, Carl Word, Yolanda Serrano, James A. Inciardi, Benjamin P. Bowser, Robert F. Schilling, and Scott D. Holmberg. 1994. Intersecting Epidemics: Crack Cocaine Use and HIV Infection among Inner-City Young Adults. *New England Journal of Medicine* 331(21): 1422–1427.

Education Watch: District of Columbia. The Education Trust, Inc.

2002–2003   *Key Education Facts and Figures.*

2006   *Key Education Facts and Figures.*

2009   *State Report. District of Columbia.*

Edwards, Marc, Simoni Triantafyllidou, and Dana Best. 2009. Elevated Blood Lead in Young Children Due to Lead-Contaminated Drinking Water: Washington, DC, 2001–2004. *Environmental Science & Technology* 43(5): 1618–1623.

Egan, James E., Victoria Frye, Steven P. Kurtz, Carl Latkin, Minxing Chen, Karin Tobin, Cui Yang, and Beryl A. Koblin. 2011. Migration, Neighborhoods, and Networks: Approaches to Understanding How Urban Environmental Conditions Affect Syndemic Adverse Health Outcomes among Gay, Bisexual and Other Men Who Have Sex with Men. *AIDS and Behavior* 15(1): 35–50.

Elbers, Benjamin. 2021. Trends in US Residential Racial Segregation, 1990 to 2020. *Socius* 7.

Eldar, Ofer, and Chelsea Garber. 2022. Opportunity Zones: A Program in Search of a Purpose. *Boston University Law Review* 102: 1397–1440.

Elder, Glen H., Jr. 1994. Time, Human Agency, and Social Change: Perspectives on the Life Course. *Social Psychology Quarterly* 57(1): 4–15.

Elifson, Kirk W., Jacqueline Boles, Ellen Posey, Mike Sweat, William Darrow, and William Elsea. 1993. Male Transvestite Prostitutes and HIV Risk. *American Journal of Public Health* 83(2): 260–262.

Ellingson, Stephen, and Kirby Schroeder. 2004. Race and the Construction of Same-Sex Sex Markets in Four Chicago Neighborhoods. In Laumann et al 2004, pp. 93–123.

Elo, Irma T., Hiram Beltrán-Sánchez, and James Macinko. 2014a. The Contribution of Health Care and Other Interventions to Black–White Disparities in Life Expectancy, 1980–2007. *Population Research and Policy Review* 33: 97–126.

Elo, Irma T., Zoua Vang, and Jennifer F. Culhane. 2014b. Variation in Birth Outcomes by Mother's Country of Birth among Non-Hispanic Black Women in the United States. *Maternal and Child Health Journal* 18: 2371–2381.

Elwood, W. N., M. L. Williams, D. C. Bell, and A. J. Richard. 1997. Powerlessness and HIV Prevention among People who Trade Sex for Drugs ('strawberries'). *AIDS Care* 9(3): 273–284.

Engels, Friedrich, and Clemens Palme Dutt. 1872. *The Housing Question.* Foreign Languages Press.

England, Paula, Andrew Levine, and Emma Mishel. 2020. Progress toward Gender Equality in the United States has Slowed or Stalled. *Proceedings of the National Academy of Sciences* 117(13): 6990–6997.

Epstein, Steven. 1996. *Impure Science: AIDS, Activism, and the Politics of Knowledge.* University of California Press.

Everett, Bethany G., Aubrey Limburg, Patricia Homan, and Morgan M. Philbin. 2022. Structural Heteropatriarchy and Birth Outcomes in the United States. *Demography* 59(1): 89–110.

Faber, Jacob W. 2020. We Built This: Consequences of New Deal Era Intervention in America's Racial Geography. *American Sociological Review* 85(5): 739–775.

Feagin, Joe. 2013. *Systemic Racism: A Theory of Oppression.* Routledge.

Feagin, Joe, and Zinobia Bennefield. 2014. Systemic Racism and US Health Care. *Social Science & Medicine* 103: 7–14.

Feldman, Justin M., and Mary T. Bassett. 2021. Variation in COVID-19 Mortality in the US by Race and Ethnicity and Educational Attainment. *JAMA Network Open* 4(11): e2135967.

Ferguson, Ann Arnett. 2000. *Bad Boys: Public Schools in the Making of Black Masculinity.* University of Michigan Press.

Fernández-Kelly, Patricia. 2015. *The Hero's Fight: African Americans in West Baltimore and the Shadow of the State.* Princeton University Press.

Fielding-Miller, Rebecca K., Maria E. Sundaram, and Kimberly Brouwer. 2020. Social Determinants of COVID-19 Mortality at the County Level. *PloS One* 15(10): e0240151.

Fiscella, Kevin, Peter Franks, Marthe R. Gold, and Carolyn M. Clancy. 2000. Inequality in Quality: Addressing Socioeconomic, Racial, and Ethnic Disparities in Health Care. *JAMA* 283(19): 2579–2584.

Fishburne, Patricia M., Herbert I. Abelson, and Ira Cisin. 1979. *National Survey on Drug Abuse—Main Findings: 1979.* NCJ 72696. Office of Justice Programs.

Fishman, Samuel H., Robert A. Hummer, Gracia Sierra, Taylor Hargrove, Daniel A. Powers, and Richard G. Rogers. 2021. Race/Ethnicity, Maternal Educational

Attainment, and Infant Mortality in the United States. *Biodemography and Social Biology* 66(1): 1–26.

Fitzpatrick, Kevin M., and Mark LaGory. 2003. "Placing" Health in an Urban Sociology: Cities as Mosaics of Risk and Protection. *City & Community* 2(1)2: 33–46.

Fletcher, Kenneth, R. 2008. A Brief History of Pierre L'Enfant and Washington, D.C. How One Frenchman's Vision Became Our Capital City. *Smithsonian Magazine*. April 30.

Fleury-Steiner, Benjamin. 2008. *Dying Inside: The HIV/AIDS Ward at Limestone Prison*. University of Michigan Press.

Flores, Andrew R., Jody L. Herman, Gary J. Gates and Taylor N. T. Brown. 2016a. *How Many Adults Identify as Transgender in the United States*. The Williams Institute, UCLA School of Law.

Flores, Andrew R., Taylor N. T. Brown, and Jody L. Herman. 2016b. *Race and Ethnicity of Adults Who Identify as Transgender in the United States*. The Williams Institute, UCLA School of Law.

Ford, Chandra L., Kathryn D. Whetten, Susan A. Hall, Jay S. Kaufman, and Angela D. Thrasher. 2007. Black Sexuality, Social Construction, and Research Targeting 'The Down Low' ('The DL'). *Annals of Epidemiology* 17(3): 209–216.

Forman, James, Jr. 2017. *Locking Up Our Own: Crime and Punishment in Black America*. Farrar, Straus and Giroux.

Friedland, Roger, and Robert R. Alford. 1991. Bringing Society Back In: Symbols, Practices and Institutional Contradictions. In Walter W. Powell and Paul J. DiMaggio, eds., *The New Institutionalism of Organizational Analysis*, pp. 232–263. University of Chicago Press.

Friedman, Samuel R., Hannah L. F. Cooper, and Andrew H. Osborne. 2009. Structural and Social Contexts of HIV Risk among African Americans. *American Journal of Public Health* 99(6): 1002–1008.

Friedman, Samuel R., Richard Curtis, Alan Neaigus, Benny Jose, and Don C. Des Jarlais. 1999. *Social Networks, Drug Injectors' Lives and HIV/AIDS*. Kluwer Academic Publishers.

Friedman, Joseph R., and Helena Hansen. 2022. Evaluation of Increases in Drug Overdose Mortality Rates in the US by Race and Ethnicity Before and During the COVID-19 Pandemic. *JAMA Psychiatry* 79(4): 379–381.

Freudenberg, Nicholas. 2001. Jails, Prisons, and the Health of Urban Populations: A Review of the Impact of the Correctional System on Community Health. *Journal of Urban Health* 78(2): 214–235.

Freudenberg, Nicholas, Marianne Fahs, Sandro Galea, and Andrew Greenberg. 2006. The Impact of New York City's 1975 Fiscal Crisis on the Tuberculosis, HIV, and Homicide Syndemic. *American Journal of Public Health* 96(3): 424–434.

Frieden, Bernard J., and Marshall Kaplan. 1987. Model Cities and Project Renewal: Adjusting the Strategy to the 1980s. *Policy Studies Journal.* 16(2): 377–383.

Friesema, H. Paul. 1969. Black Control of Central Cities: The Hollow Prize. *American Institute of Planners Journal* 35(2): 75–79.

Fry, Richard, and Kim Parker. 2021. *Rising Share of US Adults Are Living without a Spouse or Partner.* Pew Research Center.

Fuchs, Victor. R. 2016. Black Gains in Life Expectancy. *JAMA* 316: 1869–1870.

Fullilove, Mindy Thompson. 2004. *Root Shock: How Tearing Up City Neighborhoods Hurts America, and What We Can Do about It.* Ballantine Books.

Fullilove, Mindy Thompson, and Robert E. Fullilove III. 1999. Stigma as an Obstacle to AIDS Action: The Case of The African American Community. *American Behavioral Scientist* 42(7): 1117–1129.

Fullilove, Mindy Thompson, Robert E. Fullilove III, Katherine Haynes, and Shirley Gross. 1990. Black Women and AIDS Prevention: A View towards Understanding the Gender Rules. *Journal of Sex Research* 27(1): 47–64.

Galvin, Shannon R., and Myron S. Cohen. 2004. The Role of Sexually Transmitted Diseases in HIV Transmission. *Nature Reviews Microbiology* 2(1): 33–42.

Gallagher, Megan, Lori Nathanson, Peter Tatian, and Jarle Crocker. 2024. *Making the Case for Promise Neighborhoods.* Urban Institute.

Galster, George C., and Maris Mikelsons. 1995. The Geography of Metropolitan Opportunity: A Case Study of Neighborhood Conditions Confronting Youth in Washington, DC. *Housing Policy Debate* 6(1): 73–102.

Garber, Eric. 1989. A Spectacle in Color: The Lesbian and Gay Subculture of Jazz Age Harlem. In Martin Duberman, Martha Vicinus, and George Chauncey Jr., *Hidden from History: Reclaiming the Gay and Lesbian Past*, pp. 318–331. Penguin Random House.

Garfield, Jamie, and Ernest Drucker. 2001. Fatal Overdose Trends in Major US Cities: 1990–1997. *Addiction Research & Theory* 9(5): 425–436.

Garland, David. 2001. *The Culture of Control: Crime and the Social Order in Contemporary Society.* Oxford University Press.

Gardner Edward M., Margaret P. McLees, John F. Steiner, Carlos Del Rio, and William J. Burman. 2011. The Spectrum of Engagement in HIV Care and Its Relevance to Test-and-Treat Strategies for Prevention of HIV Infection. *Clinical Infectious Diseases* 52(6): 793–800.

Garnett, Geoffrey P., James P. Hughes, Roy M. Anderson, Bradley P. Stoner, Sevgi O. Aral, William L. Whittington, H. Hunter Handsfield, and King K. Holmes. 1996. Sexual Mixing Patterns of Patients Attending Sexually Transmitted Diseases Clinics. *Sexually Transmitted Diseases* 23(3): 248–257.

Gates, Henry Louis, Jr. 2022. *The Black Church: This Is Our Story, This Is Our Song.* Penguin.

Gatewood, Willard B., Jr. 1988. Aristocrats of Color: South and North—The Black Elite, 1880–1920. *The Journal of Southern History* 54(1): 3–20.

Gatewood, Willard B., Jr. 1990. *Aristocrats of Color: The Black Elite 1880–1920.* Indiana University Press.

Gelfond, Hilary, and Adam Looney. 2018. *Learning from Opportunity Zones: How to Improve Place-Based Policies.* Brookings Institution.

Gentry, Quinn M. 2008. *Black Women's Risk for HIV: Rough Living.* Routledge.

Georgetown University. 2016. *The Health of the African American Community in the District of Columbia: Disparities and Recommendations.* Prepared for the DC Commission on African American Affairs.

Geronimus, Arline T. 1992. The Weathering Hypothesis and the Health of African-American Women and Infants: Evidence and Speculations. *Ethnicity & Disease* 2(3): 207–221.

Ghandnoosh, Nazgol, Celeste Barry, and Luke Trinka. 2023. *One in Five: Racial Disparity in Imprisonment; Causes and Remedies.* The Sentencing Project.

Ghaziani, Amin. 2014. *There Goes The Gayborhood?* Princeton University Press.

Ghaziani, Amin, Verta Taylor, and Amy Stone. 2016. Cycles of Sameness and Difference in LGBT Social Movements. *Annual Review of Sociology* 42(1): 165–183.

Gibson, Keylie M., Margaret C. Steiner, Seble Kassaye, Frank Maldarelli, Zehava Grossman, Marcos Pérez-Losada, and Keith A. Crandall. 2019. A 28-year History of HIV-1 Drug Resistance and Transmission in Washington, DC. *Frontiers in Microbiology* 10: 369.

Gieryn, Thomas F. 2000. A Space for Place in Sociology. *Annual Review of Sociology* 26(1): 463–496.

Gifford, Lea A. 1999. *Justice Expenditure and Employment in the United States, 1995.* Bureau of Justice Statistics Bulletin, NCJ 178235. US Department of Justice.

Gilbert, Ben W. 1968. *Ten Blocks from the White House: Anatomy of the Washington Riots of 1968.* FA Praeger.

Gillette, Howard, Jr. 1985. A National Workshop for Urban Policy: The Metropolitanization of Washington, 1946–1968. *The Public Historian* 7(1): 7–27.

Gillette, Howard, Jr. 1995. *Between Justice and Beauty: Race, Planning, and the Failure of Urban Policy in Washington, D.C.* Johns Hopkins University Press.

Glaze, Lauren E. 2010. *Correctional Populations in the United States, 2009.* Bureau of Justice Statistics Bulletin, NCJ 236319. US Department of Justice.

Goffman, Alice. 2009. On the Run: Wanted Men in a Philadelphia Ghetto. *American Sociological Review* 74(3): 339–357.

Goffman, Erving. 1958. Characteristics of Total Institutions. In *Symposium on Preventive and Social Psychiatry,* pp. 43–84. US Government Printing Office.

Goin, Dana E., Anu Manchikanti Gomez, Kriszta Farkas, Scott Zimmerman, Ellicott C. Matthay, and Jennifer Ahern. 2019. Exposure to Community Homicide During Pregnancy and Adverse Birth Outcomes: A Within-Community Matched Design. *Epidemiology* 30(5): 713–722.

Golash-Boza, Tanya Maria. 2023. *Before Gentrification: The Creation of DC's Racial Wealth Gap.* University of California Press.

Goldfield, David R. 1980. Private Neighborhood Redevelopment and Displacement: The Case of Washington D.C. *Urban Affairs Quarterly.* 15(4): 453–468.

Goldman, Noreen, and Theresa Andrasfay. 2022. Life Expectancy Loss among Native Americans During the COVID-19 Pandemic. *Demographic Research* 47: 233–246.

Golub, Andrew Lang, and Bruce D. Johnson. 1997. *Crack's Decline: Some Surprises Across US Cities.* US Department of Justice, Office of Justice Programs, National Institute of Justice.

Goosby, Bridget J., Jacob E. Cheadle, and Colter Mitchell. 2018. Stress-Related Biosocial Mechanisms of Discrimination and African American Health Inequities. *Annual Review of Sociology* 44: 319–40.

Gorman, Dennis M., Paul W. Speer, Paul J. Gruenewald, and Erich W. Labouvie. 2001. Spatial Dynamics of Alcohol Availability, Neighborhood Structure and Violent Crime. *Journal of Studies on Alcohol* 62(5): 628–636.

Gorriti, Gustavo A. 1989. How to Fight the Drug War. *The Atlantic Monthly* 263: 70–76.

Gottlieb, Michael S., Robert Schroff, Howard M. Schanker, Joel D. Weisman, Peng Thim Fan, Robert A. Wolf, and Andrew Saxon. 1981. Pneumocystis Carinii Pneumonia and Mucosal Candidiasis in Previously Healthy Homosexual Men: Evidence of a New Acquired Cellular Immunodeficiency. *The New England Journal of Medicine* 305(24): 1425–1431.

Gramlich, John. 2021. *America's Incarceration Rate Falls to Lowest Level Since 1995.* Pew Research Center.

Green, Adam Isaiah. 2007. On the Horns of a Dilemma: Institutional Dimensions of the Sexual Career in a Sample of Middle-Class, Urban, Black, Gay Men. *Journal of Black Studies* 37(5): 753–774.

Green, Adam Isaiah. 2008. The Social Organization of Desire: The Sexual Fields Approach. *Sociological Theory* 26(1): 25–50.

Green, Constance McLaughlin. 1962. *Washington: A History of the Capital, 1800–1950.* Princeton University Press.

Green, Constance McLaughlin, 1967. *The Secret City: A History of Race Relations in the Nation's Capital.* Princeton University Press.

Greenberg, Alan E., Shannon L. Hader, Henry Masur, A. Toni Young, Jennifer Skillicorn, and Carl W. Dieffenbach. 2009. Fighting HIV/AIDS in Washington, DC. *Health Affairs* 28(6): 1677–1687.

Greene, Joss. 2023. Gender Bound: Making, Managing, and Navigating Prison Gender Boundaries, 1941–2018. *American Journal of Sociology* 128(4): 993–1030.

Greene, Mark H. 1974. An Epidemiologic Assessment of Heroin Use. *American Journal of Public Health* 64(12 Suppl): 1–10.

Grigoryeva, Angelina, and Martin Ruef. 2015. The Historical Demography of Racial Segregation. *American Sociological Review* 80(4): 814–842.

Groves, Paul A. 1973. The Development of a Black Residential Community in Southwest Washington: 1860–1897. *Records of the Columbia Historical Society, Washington, DC* 49: 260–275.

Groves, Paul A. 1974. The "Hidden" Population: Washington Alley Dwellers in the Late Nineteenth Century. *The Professional Geographer.* 26(3): 270–276.

Groves, Paul A., and Edward K. Muller. 1975. The Evolution of Black Residential Areas in Late Nineteenth-Century Cities. *Journal of Historical Geography* 1(2): 169–191.

Gugliotta, Guy, and Jeff Leen. 1989. *Kings of Cocaine: Inside the Medellín Cartel; An Astonishing True Story of Murder, Money and International Corruption.* Simon and Schuster.

Gutin, Iliya, and Robert A. Hummer. 2021. Social Inequality and the Future of US Life Expectancy. *Annual Review of Sociology* 47: 501–20.

Guttmacher Institute. 2019. *Unintended Pregnancy in the United States.*

Hail-Jares, Katie, Corey S. Shdaimah, and Chrysanthi S. Leon. 2017. *Challenging Perspectives on Street-Based Sex Work.* Temple University Press.

Hall, Matthew, John Iceland, and Youngmin Yi. 2019. Racial Separation at Home and Work: Segregation in Residential and Workplace Settings. *Population Research and Policy Review* 38: 671–694.

Hallfors, Denise Dion, Bonita J. Iritani, William C. Miller, and Daniel J. Bauer. 2007. Sexual and Drug Behavior Patterns and HIV and STD Racial Disparities: The Need for New Directions. *American Journal of Public Health* 97(1): 125–132.

Hamid, Ansley. 1992. The Developmental Cycle of a Drug Epidemic: The Cocaine Smoking Epidemic of 1981–1991. *Journal of Psychoactive Drugs* 24(4): 337–348.

Hamilton, Tod G. 2019. *Immigration and the Remaking of Black America.* Russell Sage Foundation.

Hamilton, Tod G., and Tiffany L. Green. 2018. From the West Indies to Africa: A Universal Generational Decline in Health among Blacks in the United States. *Social Science Research* 73: 163–174.

Hamilton, Tod G., and Robert A. Hummer. 2011. Immigration and the Health of US Black Adults: Does Country of Origin Matter? *Social Science & Medicine* 73(10): 1551–1560.

Hammett, Theodore. M., Patricia Harmon, and Laura M. Maruschak. 1999. *1996–1997 Update: HIV/AIDS, STDs, and TB in Correctional Facilities.* National Institute of Justice.

Hammett, Theodore M., Rebecca Widom, Joel Epstein, Michael Gross, Santiago Sifre, and Tammy Enos. 1995. *1994 Update: HIV/AIDS and STDs in Correctional Facilities.* US Department of Justice.

Hammonds, Evelynn M., and Susan M. Reverby. 2019. Toward a Historically Informed Analysis of Racial Health Disparities Since 1619. *American Journal of Public Health* 109(10): 1348–1349.

Hanna-Attisha, Mona, Jenny LaChance, Richard Casey Sadler, and Allison Champney Schnepp. 2016. Elevated Blood Lead Levels in Children Associated with the Flint Drinking Water Crisis: A Spatial Analysis of Risk and Public Health Response. *American Journal of Public Health* 106(2): 283–290.

Hannerz, Ulf. 1969. *Soulside: Inquiries into Ghetto Culture and Community.* Columbia University Press.

Harawa, Nina T., Sander Greenland, Trista A. Bingham, Denise F. Johnson, Susan D. Cochran, William E. Cunningham, David D. Celentano, Beryl A. Koblin, Marlene LaLota, Duncan A. MacKellar, William McFarland, Douglas Shehan, Sue Stoyanoff, Hanne Thiede, Lucia Torian, and Lucia A. Valleroy. 2004. Associations of Race/Ethnicity with HIV Prevalence and HIV-Related Behaviors among Young Men Who Have Sex with Men in 7 Urban Centers in the United States. *JAIDS Journal of Acquired Immune Deficiency Syndromes* 35(5): 526–536.

Harding, David J., Jeffrey D. Morenoff, and Jessica J. B. Wyse. 2019. *On the Outside: Prisoner Reentry and Reintegration.* University of Chicago Press.

Harris, Angelique C. 2010. Sex, Stigma, and The Holy Ghost: The Black Church and The Construction of AIDS in New York City. *Journal of African American Studies* 14: 21–43.

Harris-Calvin, Jullian, Sebastian Solomon, Benjamin Heller, and Brian King. 2022. *The Cost of Incarceration in New York State.* Vera Institute.

Harrison, Paige M. and Allen J. Beck. 2002. *Prisoners in 2001.* Bureau of Justice Statistics Bulletin, NCJ 195189. US Department of Justice.

Harper, Sam, John Lynch, Scott Burris, George Davey Smith. 2007. Trends in the Black-White Life Expectancy Gap in the United States, 1983–2003. *JAMA* 297(11): 1224–1232.

Harper, Sam, Richard F. MacLehose, and Jay S. Kaufman. 2014. Trends in the Black-White Life Expectancy Gap among US States, 1990–2009. *Health Affairs* 33(8): 1375–1382.

Harper, Sam, Dinela Rushani, Jay. S. Kaufman. 2012. Trends in the Black-White Life Expectancy Gap, 2003–2008. *JAMA* 307(21): 2257–2259.

Havlir, Diane, and Chris Beyrer. 2012. The Beginning of the End of AIDS? *The New England Journal of Medicine* 367(8): 685–687.

Hawkeswood, William G. 1993. AIDS Ain't a Gay Thing: The Impact of AIDS on Gay Black Men. *Transforming Anthropology* 4(1–2): 27–38.

Hawkeswood, William G. 1996. *One of the Children: Gay Black Men in Harlem.* University of California Press.

Hendi, Arun S. 2024. Where Does the Black–White Life Expectancy Gap Come From? The Deadly Consequences of Residential Segregation. *Population and Development Review* 50(2): 403–436.

Herbst, Jeffrey H., Elizabeth D. Jacobs, Teresa J. Finlayson, Vel S. McKleroy, Mary Spink Neumann, and Nicole Crepaz. 2008. Estimating HIV Prevalence and Risk Behaviors of Transgender Persons in the United States: A Systematic Review. *AIDS and Behavior* 12(1): 1–17.

Herman, Jody L., Andrew R. Flores, and Kathryn K. O'Neill. 2022. *How Many Adults and Youth Identify as Transgender in the United States?* The Williams Institute, UCLA School of Law.

Hersker, Alan L., II, 2002, *The Landscape From Within: Citizenship, Locale and The Construction of Place in Dupont Circle.* Doctoral Dissertation. Anthropology. American University.

Hess, Kristen L., Xiaohong Hu, Amy Lansky, Jonathan Mermin, and Hildegard Irene Hall. 2017. Lifetime Risk of a Diagnosis of HIV Infection in the United States. *Annals of Epidemiology* 27(4): 238–243.

Hetzel, Otto J., and David E. Pinsky. 1969. The Model Cities Program. *Vanderbilt Law Review.* 22(4): 727–756.

Higginbotham, Evelyn Brooks. 1994. *Righteous Discontent: The Women's Movement in the Black Baptist Church, 1880–1920.* Harvard University Press.

Higgins, Jenny A., Susie Hoffman, and Shari L. Dworkin. 2010. Rethinking Gender, Heterosexual Men, and Women's Vulnerability to HIV/AIDS. *American Journal of Public Health* 100(3): 435–445.

Hildebrand, Meagen M., and Cynthia J. Najdowski. 2014. The Potential Impact of Rape Culture on Juror Decision Making: Implications for Wrongful Acquittals in Sexual Assault Trials. *Albany Law Review* 78(3): 1059–1086.

Hinton, Elizabeth. 2017. *From the War on Poverty to the War on Crime.* Harvard University Press.

Hirsch, Arnold R. 1998 (1983). *Making the Second Ghetto: Race and Housing in Chicago, 1940–1960.* University of Chicago Press.

Hirsch, Jennifer S., and Shamus Khan. 2020. *Sexual Citizens: A Landmark Study of Sex, Power, and Assault on Campus.* WW Norton & Company.

Hirsch, Jennifer S., Holly Wardlow, Daniel Jordan Smith, Harriet M. Phinney, Shanti Parikh, and Constance A. Nathanson. 2009. *The Secret: Love, Marriage, and HIV.* Vanderbilt University Press.

Hirschfield, Paul J. 2008. Preparing for Prison? The Criminalization of School Discipline in the USA. *Theoretical Criminology* 12(1): 79–101.

Hochschild, Arlie, with Anne Machung. 1989. *The Second Shift.* Viking Press.

Hodder, Frank Heywood. 1936. The Authorship of the Compromise of 1850. *The Mississippi Valley Historical Review* 22(4): 525–536.

Holland, Kristin M., Christopher Jones, Alana M. Vivolo-Kantor, Nimi Idaikkadar, Marissa Zwald, Brooke Hoots, Ellen Yard, Ashley D'Inverno, Elizabeth Swedo, May S. Chen, Emiko Petrosky, Amy Board, Pedro Martinez, Deborah M. Stone, Royal Law, Michael A. Coletta, Jennifer Adjemian, Craig Thomas, Richard W. Puddy, Georgina Peacock, Nicole F. Dowling, and Debra Houry. 2021. Trends in US Emergency Department Visits for Mental Health, Overdose, and Violence Outcomes Before and During the COVID-19 Pandemic. *JAMA Psychiatry* 78(4): 372–379.

Hollingsworth, T. Déirdre, Roy M. Anderson, and Christophe Fraser. 2008. HIV-1 Transmission, by Stage of Infection. *The Journal of Infectious Diseases* 198(5): 687–693.

Holmberg, Scott D. 1996. The Estimated Prevalence and Incidence of HIV in 96 Large US Metropolitan Areas. *American Journal of Public Health* 86(5): 642–654.

Holmes, Kwame A. 2011. *Chocolate to Rainbow City: The Dialectics of Black and Gay Community Formation in Postwar Washington, D.C., 1946–1978.* Doctoral Dissertation. History. University of Illinois at Urbana-Champaign.

Holmes, Kwame. 2016. Beyond the Flames: Queering the History of the 1968 DC Riot. In E. Patrick Johnson, ed., *No Tea, No Shade: New Writings in Black Queer Studies,* pp. 304–320. Duke University Press.

Homan, Patricia. 2019. Structural Sexism and Health in the United States: A New Perspective on Health Inequality and the Gender System. *American Sociological Review* 84(3): 486–516.

Hopkins, Daniel J., and Katherine T. McCabe. 2012. After It's Too Late: Estimating the Policy Impacts of Black Mayoralties in US Cities. *American Politics Research* 40(4): 665–700.

House, James S. 2015. *Beyond Obamacare: Life, Death, and Social Policy*. Russell Sage Foundation.

Hser, Yih-Ing, Valerie Hoffman, Christine E. Grella, and M. Douglas Anglin. 2001. A 33-year Follow-up of Narcotics Addicts. *Archives of General Psychiatry* 58(5): 503–508.

Hurley, Susan F., Damien J. Jolley, and John M. Kaldor. 1997. Effectiveness of Needle-Exchange Programmes for Prevention of HIV Infection. *The Lancet* 349(9068): 1797–1800.

Hyra, Derek S. 2017. *Race, Class, and Politics in the Cappuccino City*. University of Chicago Press.

Hyra, Derek, and Sabiyha Prince, eds. 2016. *Capital Dilemma: Growth and Inequality in Washington, DC*. Routledge.

Ifatunji, Mosi Adesina, Yanica Faustin, Wendy Lee, and Deshira Wallace. 2022. Black Nativity and Health Disparities: A Research Paradigm for Understanding the Social Determinants of Health. *International Journal of Environmental Research and Public Health* 19(15): 9166.

Inciardi, James A. 1995. Crack, Crack House Sex, and HIV Risk. *Archives of Sexual Behavior* 24(3): 249–269.

Inciardi, James A., and Karen McElrath. 2007. *American Drug Scene*. Roxbury.

Irwin, John, and Donald R. Cressey. 1962. Thieves, Convicts and the Inmate Culture. *Social Problems* 10(2): 142–155.

Islam, Nazrul, Ben Lacey, Sharmin Shabnam, A. Mesut Erzurumluoglu, Hajira Dambha-Miller, Gerardo Chowell, Ichiro Kawachi, and Michael Marmot. 2021. Social Inequality and the Syndemic of Chronic Disease and COVID-19: County-level Analysis in the USA. *Journal of Epidemiology and Community Health* 75(6): 496–500.

Jackson, Kenneth T. 1987. *Crabgrass Frontier: The Suburbanization of the United States*. Oxford University Press.

Jacob, Brian A. 2007. The Challenges of Staffing Urban Schools with Effective Teachers. *The Future of Children* 17(1): 129–153.

Jacobs, Bruce A. 1999. *Dealing Crack: The Social World of Street Selling*. Northeastern Press.

Jaffe, Harry S., and Tom Sherwood. 2014. *Dream City: Race, Power, and the Decline Revival? of Washington, D.C.*, 20th Anniversary Edition. Simon & Schuster.

Jenness, Valerie, and Sarah Fenstermaker. 2014. Agnes Goes to Prison: Gender Authenticity, Transgender Inmates in Prisons for Men, and Pursuit of "the Real Deal." *Gender & Society* 28(1): 5–31.

Jensen, Eric, Nicholas Jones, Kimberly Orozco, Lauren Medina, Marc Perry, Ben Bolender, and Karen Battle. 2021. *Measuring Racial and Ethnic Diversity for the 2020 Census*. August 4, 2021.

Johnson, Catherine O., Alexandra S. Boon-Dooley, Nicole K. DeCleene, Kiana F. Henny, Brigette F. Blacker, Jason A. Anderson, Ashkan Afshin, Aleksandr Aravkin, Matthew W. Cunningham, Joseph L. Dieleman, Rachel G. Feldman, Emmanuela Gakidou, Ali H. Mokdad, Mohsen Naghavi, Cory N. Spencer, Joanna L. Whisnant, Hunter Wade York, Rahul R. Zende, Peng Zheng, Christopher J. L. Murray, and Gregory A. Roth. 2022. Life Expectancy for White, Black, and Hispanic Race/Ethnicity in US States: Trends and Disparities, 1990 to 2019. *Annals of Internal Medicine* 175(8): 1057–1064.

Johnson, Kecia R., and Karyn Loscocco. 2015. Black Marriage Through the Prism of Gender, Race, and Class. *Journal of Black Studies* 46(2): 142–171.

Johnson, E. Patrick. 2011. *Sweet Tea: Black Gay Men of the South.* University of North Carolina Press.

Johnson, Ronald M. 1984. From Romantic Suburb to Racial Enclave: LeDroit Park, Washington, DC, 1880–1920. *Phylon* 45(4): 264–270.

Johnson, Rucker C., and Steven Raphael. 2009. The Effects of Male Incarceration Dynamics on Acquired Immune Deficiency Syndrome Infection Rates among African American Women and Men. *Journal of Law and Economics* 52(2): 251–293.

Joint Oversight Hearing Before the Subcommittee on Fiscal Affairs and Health of the Committee on the District of Columbia and the Select Committee on Narcotics Abuse and Control, House of Representatives, One Hundredth Congress, Second Session on Interstate Drug Trafficking in the Washington Metropolitan Area. 1988. US Government Printing Office, Serial No. 100–12. April 20, 1988.

Jones, Mark R., Matthew B. Novitch, Syena Sarrafpour, Ken P. Ehrhardt, Benjamin B. Scott, Vwaire Orhurhu, Omar Viswanath, Alan D. Kaye, Jatinder Gill, and Thomas T. Simopoulos. 2019. Government Legislation in Response to the Opioid Epidemic. *Current Pain and Headache Reports* 23: 1–7.

Jonnes, Jill. 1996. *Hep-Cats, Narcs, and Pipe Dreams: A History of America's Romance with Illegal Drugs.* Johns Hopkins University Press.

Kanazawa, Satoshi, and Mary C. Still. 2000. Why Men Commit Crimes (and Why They Desist). *Sociological Theory* 18(3): 434–447.

Kanny, Dafna, William L. Jeffries IV, Johanna Chapin-Bardales, Paul Denning, Susan Cha, Teresa Finlayson, Cyprian Wejnert (National HIV Behavioral Surveillance Study Group). 2019. Racial/Ethnic Disparities in HIV Preexposure Prophylaxis among Men Who Have Sex with Men—23 Urban Areas. *Morbidity and Mortality Weekly Report* 68(37): 801–806.

Karmakar, Monita, Paula M. Lantz, and Renuka Tipirneni. 2021. Association of Social and Demographic Factors with COVID-19 Incidence and Death Rates in the US. *JAMA Network Open* 4(1).

Kassaye, Seble G., Zehava Grossman, Maya Balamane, Betsy Johnston-White, Chenglong Liu, Princy Kumar, Mary Young, Michael C. Sneller, Irini Sereti, Robin Dewar, Catherine Rehm, William Meyer, III, Robert Shafer, David Katzenstein, and Frank Maldarelli. 2016. Transmitted HIV Drug Resistance Is High and Longstanding in Metropolitan Washington, DC. *Clinical Infectious Diseases* 63(6): 836–843.

Kawachi, Ichiro, and Lisa F. Berkman, eds. 2003. *Neighborhoods and Health.* Oxford University Press.

Kaye, Kerwin. 2020. *Enforcing Freedom: Drug Courts, Therapeutic Communities, and the Intimacies of the State.* Columbia University Press.

Keller, Edmond J. 1978. The Impact of Black Mayors on Urban Policy. *Annals of the American Academy of Political and Social Science* 439: 40–52.

Kelly, Brian C., Mike Vuolo, and Alexandra C. Marin. 2017. Multiple Dimensions of Peer Effects and Deviance: The Case of Prescription Drug Misuse among Young Adults. *Socius* 3: 2378023117706819.

Kerrigan, Deanna, Katherine Andrinopoulous, Shang-en Chung, Barbara Glass, and Jonathan Ellen. 2008 Gender Ideologies, Socio-Economic Opportunities, and HIV/STI Related Vulnerability among Female African-American Adolescents. *Journal of Urban Health* 85(5): 717–726.

Kiang, Mathew V., Alexander C. Tsai, Monica J. Alexander, David H. Rehkopf, and Sanjay Basu. 2021. Racial/Ethnic Disparities in Opioid-Related Mortality in the USA, 1999–2019: The Extreme Case of Washington, DC. *Journal of Urban Health* 98: 589–595.

Killewald, Alexandra, Fabian T. Pfeffer, and Jared N. Schachner. 2017. Wealth Inequality and Accumulation. *Annual Review of Sociology* 43(1): 379–404.

King, Christopher J., Bryan O. Buckley, Riya Maheshwari, and Derek M. Griffith. 2022. Race, Place, and Structural Racism: A Review of Health and History in Washington, DC. *Health Affairs* 41(2): 273–280.

King, J. L., with Karen Hunter. 2004. *On the Down Low: A Journey into the Lives of 'Straight' Black Men Who Sleep with Men.* Harlem Moon, Broadways Books.

Kirby, James B., Gregg Taliaferro, and Samuel H. Zuvekas. 2006. Explaining Racial and Ethnic Disparities in Health Care. *Medical Care* 44(5): 164–172.

Knight, David Jonathan. 2024. Carceral Passages: Coming of Age in Prison America. *American Journal of Sociology* 129(5): 1359–1408.

Kochanek, Kenneth D., Jeffrey D. Maurer, Harry M. Rosenberg. 1994. Why Did Black Life Expectancy Decline from 1984 through 1989 in the United States? *American Journal of Public Health* 84: 938–944.

Kofie, Nelson F. 1999. *Race, Class, and The Struggle for Neighborhood in Washington, DC.* Taylor & Francis.

Koenig, Harold G., David B. Larson, and Susan S. Larson. 2001. Religion and Coping with Serious Medical Illness. *Annals of Pharmacotherapy* 35(3): 352–359.

Koppensteiner, Martin Foureaux, and Marco Manacorda. 2016. Violence and Birth Outcomes: Evidence from Homicides in Brazil. *Journal of Development Economics* 119: 16–33.

Kosten, Thomas R., and Tony P. George. 2002. The Neurobiology of Opioid Dependence: Implications for Treatment. *Science & Practice Perspectives* 1(1): 13–20.

Kosten, Thomas R., and David A. Gorelick. 2002. The Lexington Narcotic Farm. *American Journal of Psychiatry* 159(1): 22.

Kozel, N. J., R. A. Crider, and E. H. Adams. 1982. National Surveillance of Cocaine Use and Related Health Consequences. *Morbidity and Mortality Weekly Report* 31(20): 265–273.

Kposowa, Augustine J. 2013. Marital Status and HIV/AIDS Mortality: Evidence from the US National Longitudinal Mortality Study. *International Journal of Infectious Diseases* 17(10): e868-e874.

Kraus, Neil, and Todd Swanstrom. 2001. Minority Mayors and the Hollow-Prize Problem. *PS: Political Science & Politics* 34(1): 99–105.

Kreisel, Kristen M., Ian H. Spicknall, Julia W. Gargano, Felicia M. T. Lewis, Rayleen M. Lewis, Lauri E. Markowitz, Henry Roberts, Anna Satcher Johnson, Ruiguang Song, Sancta B. St. Cyr, Emily J. Weston, Elizabeth A. Torrone, and Hillard S. Weinstock. 2021. Sexually Transmitted Infections among US Women and Men: Prevalence and Incidence Estimates, 2018. *Sexually Transmitted Diseases* 48(4): 208–214.

Krieger, Nancy. 1994. Epidemiology and the Web of Causation: Has Anyone Seen the Spider? *Social Science & Medicine* 39(7): 887–903.

Krieger, Nancy. 2000. Discrimination and Health. In Berkman and Kawachi 2000, pp. 36–75.

Krieger, Nancy. 2021. *Ecosocial Theory, Embodied Truths, and the People's Health.* Oxford University Press.

Kunzel, Regina. 2008. *Criminal Intimacy: Prison and the Uneven History of Modern American Sexuality.* University of Chicago Press.

Kuo, Irene, Alan E. Greenberg, Manya Magnus, Gregory Phillips II, Anthony Rawls, James Peterson, Flora Hamilton, Tiffany West-Ojo, and Shannon Hader. 2011. High Prevalence of Substance Use among Heterosexuals Living in Communities with High Rates of AIDS and Poverty in Washington, DC. *Drug and Alcohol Dependence* 117(2–3): 139–144.

Kuzawa, Christopher W., and Elizabeth Sweet. 2009. Epigenetics and the Embodiment of Race: Developmental Origins of US Racial Disparities in Cardiovascular Health. *American Journal of Human Biology* 21(1): 2–15.

Kwan, Candice K., and Joel D. Ernst. 2011. HIV and Tuberculosis: A Deadly Human Syndemic. *Clinical Microbiology Reviews* 24(2): 351–376.

Lacy, Karyn. 2007. *Blue-Chip Black: Race, Class, and Status in the New Black Middle Class.* University of California Press.

Ladner, Joyce A. 1986. Black Women Face The 21st Century: Major Issues and Problems. *The Black Scholar* 17(5): 12–19.

Ladner, Joyce A. 1997. Financing Education in the District of Columbia from the Perspective of the Financial Authority. In William J. Fowler, ed., *Developments in School Finance: 1997. Fiscal Proceedings from the Annual State Data Conference (July 1997),* pp. 59–74. National Center for Education Statistics.

Lait, Jack, and Mortimer Lee. 1951. *Washington Confidential.* Crown Publishers.

Landry, Bart. 2002. *Black Working Wives: Pioneers of the American Family Revolution.* University of California Press.

Lattimore, Pamela K., James Trudeau, K. Jack Riley, Jordan Leiter, and Steven Edwards. 1997. *Homicide in Eight US Cities: Trends, Context, and Policy Implications; An Intramural Research Project.* US Department of Justice, Office of Justice Programs, National Institute of Justice.

Laumann, Edward O., Stephen Ellingson, Jenna Mahay, Anthony Paik, and Yoosik Youm. 2004. *The Sexual Organization of the City.* University of Chicago Press.

Laumann, Edward O., John H. Gagnon, Robert T. Michael, and Stuart Michaels. 1994. *The Social Organization of Sexuality: Sexual Practices in the United States.* University of Chicago Press.

Laumann, Edward O., and Yoosik Youm. 1999. Racial/Ethnic Group Differences in the Prevalence of Sexually Transmitted Diseases in the United States: A Network Explanation. *Sexually Transmitted Diseases* 26(5): 250–261.

LaVeist, Thomas, Keshia Pollack, Roland Thorpe Jr., Ruth Fesahazion, and Darrell Gaskin. 2011. Place, Not Race: Disparities Dissipate in Southwest Baltimore When Blacks and Whites Live Under Similar Conditions. *Health Affairs* 30(10): 1880–1887.

LaVeist, Thomas A., and John M. Wallace Jr. 2000. Health Risk and Inequitable Distribution of Liquor Stores in African American Neighborhoods. *Social Science & Medicine* 51(4): 613–617.

Lavine, Amy. 2010. Urban Renewal and the Story of Berman v Parker. *The Urban Lawyer* 42(2): 423–475.

Lazere, Ed, and Idara Nickelson. 2004. *The Untold Story of the DC Budget: Overall Spending Has Grown Only Modestly Since 1990 but Support for Services to Low-Income Residents Has Fallen Sharply.* DC Fiscal Policy Institute. March 16, 2004.

Leap, William L. 2009. Professional Baseball, Urban Restructuring, and (Changing) Gay Geographies in Washington, DC. In Ellen Lewin and William L. Leap, eds., *Out in Public: Reinventing Lesbian/Gay Anthropology in a Globalizing World*, pp. 202–222. Wiley-Blackwell.

Lee, Jennifer, and Frank D. Bean. 2004. America's Changing Color Lines: Immigration, Race/Ethnicity and Multiracial Identification. *Annual Review of Sociology* 30: 221–242.

Lee, Juliet P., William Ponicki, Christina Mair, Paul Gruenewald, and Lina Ghanem. 2020. What Explains the Concentration of Off-Premise Alcohol Outlets in Black Neighborhoods? *SSM-Population Health* 12: 100669.

Lee, Sharon M. 1993. Racial Classifications in the US Census: 1890–1990, *Ethnic and Racial Studies,* 16(1): 75–94.

Leibbrand, Christine, Heather Hill, Ali Rowhani-Rahbar, and Frederick Rivara. 2020. Invisible Wounds: Community Exposure to Gun Homicides and Adolescents' Mental Health and Behavioral Outcomes. *SSM-Population Health* 12: 100689.

Lerner, Steve. 2010. *Sacrifice Zones: The Front Lines of Toxic Chemical Exposure in the United States.* MIT Press.

Leshner, Alan I. 1997. Addiction Is a Brain Disease, and It Matters. *Science* 278(5335) 45–47.

Leung-Gagné, Josh, and Sean F. Reardon. 2023. It Is Surprisingly Difficult to Measure Income Segregation. *Demography* 60(5): 1387–1413.

Leverentz, Andrea. 2010. People, Places, and Things: How Female Ex-Prisoners Negotiate Their Neighborhood Context. *Journal of Contemporary Ethnography* 39(6): 646–681.

Leverentz, Andrea M. 2014. *The Ex-Prisoner's Dilemma: How Women Negotiate Competing Narratives of Reentry and Desistance.* Rutgers University Press.

Levin, Jeffrey S. 1984. The Role of the Black Church in Community Medicine. *Journal of the National Medical Association* 76(5): 477–483.

Levine, Martin P. 1979. Gay Ghetto. *Journal of Homosexuality* 4(4): 363–377.

Levitt, Steven D., and Sudhir Alladi Venkatesh. 2000. An Economic Analysis of a Drug-Selling Gang's Finances. *The Quarterly Journal of Economics* 115(3): 755–789.

Lewis, Nathaniel M. 2010 Grappling with Governance: The Emergence of Business Improvement Districts in a National Capital. *Urban Affairs Review* 46(2): 180–217.

Lezin, Katya. 1996. Life At Lorton: An Examination of Prisoners Rights at the District of Columbia Correctional Facilities. *Public Interest Law Journal* 5(2): 165–211.

Liebow, Elliot. 1967. *Tally's Corner: A Study of Negro Streetcorner Men.* Rowman & Littlefield.

Limerick, Patricia Nelson. 1987. *Legacy of Conquest: The Unbroken Past of the American West.* WW Norton & Company.

Linas, Benjamin P., Alexandra Savinkina, Carolina Barbosa, Peter P. Mueller, Magdalena Cerdá, Katherine Keyes, and Jagpreet Chhatwal. 2021. A Clash of Epidemics: Impact of the COVID-19 Pandemic Response on Opioid Overdose. *Journal of Substance Abuse Treatment* 120: 108158.

Lindgren, Sue A. 1992. *Justice Expenditure and Employment in the United States, 1990.* Bureau of Justice Statistics Bulletin, NCJ 135777. US Department of Justice.

Link, Bruce G., and Jo Phelan. 1995. Social Conditions as Fundamental Causes of Disease. *Journal of Health and Social Behavior* (1995): 80–94.

Lipka, Michael. 2014. *Many U.S. Congregations Are Still Racially Segregated, but Things Are Changing.* Pew Research Center.

Lloyd, Cathy, Julie Smith, and Katie Weinger. 2005. Stress and Diabetes: A Review of the Links. *Diabetes Spectrum* 18(2): 121–127.

Lo, Celia C., Ratonia C. Runnels, and Tyrone C. Cheng. 2018. Racial/Ethnic Differences in HIV Testing: An Application of the Health Services Utilization Model. *SAGE Open Medicine* 6.

Logan, John R., Jason Jindrich, Hyoungjin Shin, and Weiwei Zhang. 2011. Mapping America in 1880: The Urban Transition Historical GIS Project. *Historical Methods* 44(1): 49–60.

Logan, John R., and Harvey Molotch. 1987. *Urban Fortunes: The Political Economy of Place.* University of California Press.

Logan, Trevon D. 2010. Personal Characteristics, Sexual Behaviors, and Male Sex Work: A Quantitative Approach. *American Sociological Review* 75(5): 679–704.

Lotke, Eric. 1998. Hobbling a Generation: Young African American Men in Washington, DC's Criminal Justice System—Five Years Later. *Crime & Delinquency* 44(3): 355–366.

Mackenzie, Sonja. 2013. *Structural Intimacies: Sexual Stories in the Black AIDS Epidemic*. Rutgers University Press.

Macy, Beth. 2018. *Dopesick: Dealers, Doctors, and the Drug Company that Addicted America*. Little, Brown and Company.

Madfis, Eric. 2014. Triple Entitlement and Homicidal Anger: An Exploration of the Intersectional Identities of American Mass Murderers. *Men and Masculinities* 17(1): 67–86.

Magnus, Manya, Irene Kuo, Katharine Shelley, Anthony Rawls, James Peterson, Luz Montanez, Tiffany West-Ojo, Shannon Hader, Flora Hamilton, and Alan E. Greenberg. 2009. Risk Factors Driving the Emergence of a Generalized Heterosexual HIV Epidemic in Washington, District of Columbia Networks at Risk. *AIDS* 23(10): 1277–1284.

Maher Lisa. 2001, *Sexed Work: Gender, Race and Resistance in a Brooklyn Drug Market*. Oxford University Press.

Maher, Lisa, and Richard Curtis. 1992. Women on the Edge of Crime: Crack Cocaine and the Changing Contexts of Street-Level Sex Work in New York City. *Crime, Law and Social Change* 18(3): 221–258.

Maher, Lisa, and Kathleen Daly. 2017. Women in the Street-Level Drug Economy: Continuity or Change? In Meda Chesney-Lind and Morash Merry, eds., *Feminist Theories of Crime*, pp. 69–95. Routledge.

Majors, Richard, and Janet Mancini Billson. 1993. *Cool Pose: The Dilemma of Black Manhood in America*. Simon and Schuster.

Malebranche, David J., Kimberly Jacob Arriola, Tyrrell R. Jenkins, Emily Dauria, and Shilpa N. Patel. 2010. Exploring the "Bisexual Bridge": A Qualitative Study of Risk Behavior and Disclosure of Same-Sex Behavior among Black Bisexual Men. *American Journal of Public Health* 100(1): 159–164.

Mallett, Christopher A. 2016. The School-to-Prison Pipeline: A Critical Review of the Punitive Paradigm Shift. *Child and Adolescent Social Work Journal* 33(1): 15–24.

Manglos, Nicolette D., and Jenny Trinitapoli. 2011. The Third Therapeutic System: Faith Healing Strategies in the Context of a Generalized AIDS Epidemic. *Journal of Health and Social Behavior* 52(1): 107–122.

Manning, Robert D. 1998. Multicultural Washington DC: The Changing Social and Economic Landscape of a Post-Industrial Metropolis. *Ethnic and Racial Studies*. 21(2): 328–355.

Marinelli, John. 2022. Education Under Armed Guard: An Analysis of the School-to-Prison Pipeline in Washington, DC. *American Criminal Law Review*. 59: 1697–1727.

Markides, Kyriakos S., and Karl Eschbach. 2005. Aging, Migration, and Mortality: Current Status of Research on the Hispanic Paradox. *The Journals of Gerontology Series B: Psychological Sciences and Social Sciences* 60 (2, Special Issue): S68-S75.

Marsh, Kris. 2023. *The Love Jones Cohort: Single and Living Alone in the Black Middle Class.* Cambridge University Press.

Maruschak, Laura M. Bureau of Justice Statistics Bulletin.

1999 *HIV in Prisons and Jails.*
2001 *HIV in Prisons and Jails.*
2004 *HIV in Prisons and Jails.*
2009 *HIV in Prisons and Jails.*

Maruschak, Laura M. 1996–97. HIV in Prisons and Jails, 1996. In *HIV/AIDS, STDs, and TB in Correctional Facilities, 1996–1997 Update,* pp. 5–19. NCJ 176344. National Institute of Justice.

Marvel, John D. 2012. *Should I Stay or Should I Go? Turnover among Public School Teachers and Principals.* Dissertation. School of Public Affairs. American University.

Massey, Douglas, and Nancy A. Denton. 1993. *American Apartheid: Segregation and the Making of the Underclass.* Harvard University Press.

May, John P., and Earnest L. Williams Jr. 2002. Acceptability of Condom Availability in a US Jail. *AIDS Education and Prevention* 14(5 Suppl): 85–91.

Mbembe, Achille. 2019. *Necropolitics.* Duke University Press.

McBride, David. 1991. *From TB to AIDS: Epidemics among Urban Blacks Since 1900.* State University of New York Press.

McCammon, Holly J., Karen E. Campbell, Ellen M. Granberg, and Christine Mowery. 2001. How Movements Win: Gendered Opportunity Structures and US Women's Suffrage Movements, 1866 to 1919. *American Sociological Review* 66(1): 49–70.

McConnell, Bailey and Yesim Sayin. 2023. D.C.'s Household Growth Is Predominantly Driven by Singles Aged 25 to 34. D.C. Policy Center.

McCormick, Marie C. 1985. The Contribution of Low Birth Weight to Infant Mortality and Childhood Morbidity. *The New England Journal of Medicine* 312(2): 82–90.

McKay, Tara, Nathaniel M. Tran, Harry Barbee, and Judy K. Min. 2023. Association of Affirming Care with Chronic Disease and Preventive Care Outcomes among Lesbian, Gay, Bisexual, Transgender, and Queer Older Adults. *American Journal of Preventive Medicine* 64(3): 305–314.

McKim, Allison. 2017. *Addicted to Rehab: Race, Gender, and Drugs in the Era of Mass Incarceration.* Rutgers University Press.

McLaughlin, Michael, Carrie Pettus-Davis, Derek Brown, Chris Veeh and Tanya Renn. 2016. *The Economic Burden of Incarceration in the United States.* Institute for Justice Research and Development, Florida State University.

Meier, August, and Elliott Rudwick. 1967. The Rise of Segregation in the Federal Bureaucracy, 1900–1930. *Phylon* 28(2): 178–184.

Melendez, Rita M., and Rogério Pinto. 2007. 'It's Really a Hard Life': Love, Gender and HIV Risk among Male-to-Female Transgender Persons. *Culture, Health & Sexuality* 9(3): 233–245.

Merrall, Elizabeth L. C., Azar Kariminia, Ingrid A. Binswanger, Michael S. Hobbs, Michael Farrell, John Marsden, Sharon J. Hutchinson, and Sheila M. Bird. 2010. Meta-Analysis of Drug-Related Deaths Soon After Release from Prison. *Addiction* 105(9): 1545–1554.

Merton, Robert K. 1968. The Matthew Effect in Science: The Reward and Communication Systems of Science Are Considered. *Science* 159(3810): 56–63.

Metzl, Jonathan M. 2019. *Dying of Whiteness: How the Politics of Racial Resentment Is Killing America's Heartland.* Basic Books.

Meyer, Jack A., Randall R. Bovbjerg, Barbara A. Ormond, and Gina M. Lagomarsino. 2010. *Expanding Health Coverage in the District of Columbia: D.C.'s Shift from Providing Services to Subsidizing Individuals and Its Continuing Challenges in Promoting Health, 1999–2009.* Brookings Institution and the Rockefeller Foundation.

Meyer, Jaimie P., Sandra A. Springer, and Frederick L. Altice. 2011. Substance Abuse, Violence, and HIV in Women: A Literature Review of the Syndemic. *Journal of Women's Health* 20(7): 991–1006.

Meyers, Edward M. 1996. *Public Opinion and the Political Future of the Nation's Capital.* Georgetown University Press.

Michney, Todd. M., and LaDale Winling. 2020. New Perspectives on New Deal Housing Policy: Explicating and Mapping HOLC Loans to African Americans. *Journal of Urban History,* 46(1): 150–180.

Miech, Richard. 2008. The Formation of a Socioeconomic Health Disparity: The Case of Cocaine Use During the 1980s and 1990s. *Journal of Health and Social Behavior* 49(3): 352–366.

Mildvan, D., U. Mathur, R. W. Enlow, D. Armstrong, J. Gold, C. Sears, B. Wong, A. Brown, S. Henry, and B. Safai. 1982. Persistent, Generalized Lymphadenopathy among Homosexual Males. *Morbidity and Mortality Weekly Report* 31(19): 249–251.

Miller, Gregory E., and Ekin Blackwell. 2006. Turning Up the Heat: Inflammation as a Mechanism Linking Chronic Stress, Depression, and Heart Disease. *Current Directions in Psychological Science* 15(6): 269–272.

Miller, Lisa R., and Eric Anthony Grollman. 2015. The Social Costs of Gender Nonconformity for Transgender Adults: Implications for Discrimination and Health. *Sociological Forum* 30(3): 809–831.

Miller, Robert L., Jr. 2007. Legacy Denied: African American Gay Men, AIDS, and The Black Church. *Social Work* 52(1): 51–61.

Millett, Gregorio A., Stephen A. Flores, John L. Peterson, and Roger Bakeman. 2007. Explaining Disparities in HIV Infection among Black and White Men Who Have Sex With Men: A Meta-Analysis of HIV Risk Behaviors. *AIDS* 21(15): 2083–2091.

Millett, Gregorio A., Brian Honermann, Austin Jones, Elise Lankiewicz, Jennifer Sherwood, Susan Blumenthal, and Asal Sayas. 2020. White Counties Stand Apart: The Primacy of Residential Segregation in COVID-19 and HIV diagnoses. *AIDS Patient Care and STDs* 34(10): 417–424.

Millett, Gregorio, David Malebranche, Byron Mason, and Pilgrim Spikes. 2005. Focusing "Down Low": Bisexual Black Men, HIV Risk and Heterosexual Transmission. *Journal of the National Medical Association* 97(7 Suppl): 52S–59S.

Mills, C. Wright. 1959. *The Sociological Imagination*. Oxford University Press.

Milstein, Bobby. 2001. *Introduction to the Syndemics Prevention Network*. Centers for Disease Control and Prevention.

Miniño, Arialdi M., Elizabeth Arias, Kenneth D. Kochanek, Sherry L. Murphy, and Betty L. Smith. 2002. Deaths: Final Data for 2000. *National Vital Statistics Reports*. 50(15).

Mishel, Emma, Paula England, Jessie Ford, and Mónica L. Caudillo. 2020. Cohort Increases in Sex with Same-Sex Partners: Do Trends Vary by Gender, Race, and Class? *Gender & Society* 34(2): 178–209.

Mittleman, Joel. 2023. Sexual Fluidity: Implications for Population Research. *Demography* 60(4): 1257–1282.

Moen, Phyllis. 2001. The Gendered Life Course. In Robert H. Binstock and Linda K. George, eds., *Handbook of Aging and the Social Sciences,* pp. 179–196. Academic Press.

Mojola, Sanyu A. 2011. Fishing in Dangerous Waters: Ecology, Gender and Economy in HIV Risk. *Social Science & Medicine* 72(2): 149–156.

Mojola, Sanyu A., Nicole Angotti, Enid Schatz, and Brian Houle. 2021. "A Nowadays Disease": HIV/AIDS and Social Change in a Rural South African Community. *American Journal of Sociology* 127(3): 950–1000.

Mojola, Sanyu A., Erin Ice, Enid Schatz, Nicole Angotti, Brian Houle, and F. Xavier Gómez-Olivé. 2022. The Meaning of Health in Rural South Africa: Gender, the Life Course, and the Socio-epidemiological Context. *Population and Development Review* 48(4): 1061–1095.

Mojtabai, Ramin, Christine Mauro, Melanie M. Wall, Colleen L. Barry, and Mark Olfson. 2020. Private Health Insurance Coverage of Drug Use Disorder Treatment: 2005–2018. *PLos One* 15(10): e0240298.

Monk, Ellis P., Jr. 2021. Colorism and Physical Health: Evidence from a National Survey. *Journal of Health and Social Behavior* 62(1): 37–52.

Montez, Jennifer Karas, Jason Beckfield, Julene Kemp Cooney, Jacob M. Grumbach, Mark D. Hayward, Huseyin Zeyd Koytak, Steven H. Woolf, and Anna Zajacova. 2020. US State Policies, Politics, and Life Expectancy. *The Milbank Quarterly* 98(3): 668–699.

Moore, Jacqueline M., 1999. *Leading the Race: The Transformation of the Black Elite in the Nation's Capital, 1880–1920*. University Press of Virginia.

Morenoff, Jeffrey D. 2003. Neighborhood Mechanisms and the Spatial Dynamics of Birth Weight. *American Journal of Sociology* 108(5): 976–1017.

Morgan, Dilys, Cedric Mahe, Billy Mayanja, J. Martin Okongo, Rosemary Lubega, and James A. G. Whitworth. 2002. HIV-1 Infection in Rural Africa: Is There a Difference in Median Time to AIDS and Survival Compared with That in Industrialized Countries? *AIDS* 16(4): 597–603.

Morris, Aldon D. 1999. A Retrospective on the Civil Rights Movement: Political and Intellectual Landmarks. *Annual Review of Sociology* 25(1): 517–539.

Morris, Aldon. 2015. *The Scholar Denied: W. E. B. Du Bois and the Birth of Modern Sociology.* University of California Press.

Morris, Martina, ed. 2004. *Network Epidemiology: A Handbook for Survey Design and Data Collection.* Oxford University Press.

Morris, Martina, and Mirjam Kretzschmar. 1997. Concurrent Partnerships and The Spread of HIV. *AIDS* 11(5): 641–648.

Morris, Martina, Ann E. Kurth, Deven T. Hamilton, James Moody, and Steve Wakefield. 2009. Concurrent Partnerships and HIV Prevalence Disparities by Race: Linking Science and Public Health Practice. *American Journal of Public Health* 99(6): 1023–1031.

Mumola, Christopher J. 2007. *Medical Causes of Death in State Prisons, 2001–2004.* Bureau of Justice Statistics Bulletin, NCJ 216340. US Department of Justice.

Murphy, Patrick. 1994. *Keeping Score: The Frailties of the Federal Drug Budget.* APRC Issue Paper. RAND Drug Policy Research Center.

Musgrove, George Derek. 2017. Statehood Is Far More Difficult: The Struggle for D.C. Self-Determination, 1980–2017. *Washington History.* 29(2): 3–17.

Musto, David F. 1999 (1973). *The American Disease: Origins of Narcotic Control.* New York: Oxford University Press. Third Edition.

National Academies of Science. 2011. *A Plan for Evaluating the District of Columbia's Public Schools: From Impressions to Evidence.* Committee on the Independent Evaluation of DC Public Schools.

National Advisory Commission On Civil Disorders. 1967. *Kerner Commission Report on the Causes, Events, and Aftermaths of the Civil Disorders of 1967.* NCJ Number 8073.

National Capital Housing Authority. 1944. *Report of the National Capital Housing Authority for the Ten-Year Period 1934–1944.*

National Center for Health Statistics. US Department of Health, Education and Human Welfare.

    1963   *Vital Statistics of the United States. 1960.* Volume II-*Mortality.* Part A.

    1966   *U.S. Decennial Life Tables. State Life Tables: 1959–61.* Volume II, Numbers 27–51.

    1974   *Vital Statistics of the United States. 1970.* Volume II-*Mortality.* Part A.

    1975   *U.S. Decennial Life Tables. State Life Tables: 1969–71.* Volume II, Numbers 1–26.

National Center for Health Statistics. US Department of Health and Human Services.

    1985   *U.S. Decennial Life Tables for 1979–81,* Volume II, *State Life Tables.* Number 9, District of Columbia.

1998   *U.S. Decennial Life Tables for 1989–91*, Volume II, *State Life Tables*. Number 9, District of Columbia.

National Center for Transgender Equality. 2017. *U.S. Transgender Survey 2015: Washington, D.C. Report*.

National Commission on Acquired Immune Deficiency Syndrome. 1991. *HIV Disease in Correctional Facilities*. March 1991.

National Committee on Segregation in the Nation's Capitol. 1948. *Segregation in Washington: A Report*.

Naveed, Minahil. 2017. *Income Inequality in DC Highest in the Country. Dec 12. 2017. The District's Time: Going Beyond the Budget Book*. DC Fiscal Policy Institute.

Nemoto, Tooru, Don Operario, JoAnne Keatley, Lei Han, and Toho Soma. 2004. HIV Risk Behaviors among Male-to-Female Transgender Persons of Color in San Francisco. *American Journal of Public Health* 94(7): 1193–1199.

Nero, Charles I. 2005. Why Are All the Gay Ghettoes White? In E. Patrick Johnson, Mae G. Henderson, Sharon Patricia Holland, and Cathy J. Cohen, eds. *Black Queer Studies: A Critical Anthology*, pp. 228–245. Duke University Press.

Nestler, Eric J. 2005. The Neurobiology of Cocaine Addiction. *Science & Practice Perspectives* 3(1): 4–10.

Nestler, Eric J., and Robert C. Malenka. 2004. The Addicted Brain. *Scientific American* 290(3): 78–85.

Newell, Marie-Louise. 1998. Mechanisms and Timing of Mother-to-Child Transmission of HIV-1. *AIDS* 12(8): 831–837.

Nicolosi, Alfredo, Maria Lea Correa Leite, Massimo Musicco, Claudio Arid, Giovanna Gavazzeni, and Adriano Lazzarin. 1994. The Efficiency of Male-to Female and Female-to-Male Sexual Transmission of the Human Immunodeficiency Virus: A Study of 730 Stable Couples. *Epidemiology* 5(6): 570–575.

Noonan, Douglas S. 2005. Neighbours, Barriers and Urban Environments: Are Things Different on the Other Side of the Tracks? *Urban Studies* 42(10): 1817–1835.

Nunley, Tamika, Y. 2021. *At the Threshold of Liberty: Women, Slavery and Shifting Identities in Washington D.C.* UNC-Chapel Hill Press.

Nunn, Amy, Nickolas Zaller, Samuel Dickman, Catherine Trimbur, Ank Nijhawan, and Josiah D. Rich. 2009. Methadone and Buprenorphine Prescribing and Referral Practices in US Prison Systems: Results from a Nationwide Survey. *Drug and Alcohol Dependence* 105(1–2): 83–88.

Octane Public Relations and Advertising. 2014. *DC Takes On HIV: Public Awareness, Resident Engagement and a Call to Action. A Research Report Prepared for the DC Department of Health; HIV/AIDS, Hepatitis, STD and TB Administration (HAHSTA)*.

Office of Criminal Justice Plans and Analysis. 1992. *Homicide Report*. US Department of Justice, National Institute of Justice. April 1992.

Office of the State Superintendent of Education. 2014. *Reducing Out-of-School Suspensions and Expulsions in District of Columbia Public and Public Charter Schools*.

Ojikutu, Bisola O., Sumeeta Srinivasan, Laura M. Bogart, S. V. Subramanian, and Kenneth H. Mayer. 2018. Mass Incarceration and The Impact of Prison Release on HIV Diagnoses in the US South. *PloS One* 13(6).

Oliver, Melvin, and Thomas Shapiro. 2006 (1995). *Black Wealth/White Wealth: A New Perspective on Racial Inequality*. Routledge.

Omi, Michael, and Howard Winant. 1994. *Racial Formation in the United States*. Routledge.

Operario, Don, Jennifer Burton, Kristen Underhill, and Jae Sevelius. 2008. Men Who Have Sex with Transgender Women: Challenges to Category-based HIV Prevention. *AIDS and Behavior* 12(1): 18–26.

Orfield, Gary. 1983. *Public School Desegregation in the United States, 1968–1980*. Joint Center for Political Studies, Washington D.C.

Orfield, Gary, and Jongyeon Ee. 2017. *Our Segregated Capital: An Increasingly Diverse City with Racially Polarized Schools*. The Civil Rights Project.

Orne, Jason. 2017. *Boystown: Sex and Community in Chicago*. University of Chicago Press.

Osofsky, Gilbert. 1971. *Harlem: The Making of a Ghetto; Negro New York, 1890–1930*. Harper & Row.

Oster, Alexandra M., Joel O. Wertheim, Angela L. Hernandez, M. Cheryl Bañez Ocfemia, Neeraja Saduvala, and H. Irene Hall. 2015. Using Molecular HIV Surveillance Data to Understand Transmission Between Subpopulations in the United States. *Journal of Acquired Immune Deficiency Syndromes* 70(4): 444–451.

Padamsee, Tasleem J. 2020. Fighting an Epidemic in Political Context: Thirty-Five Years of HIV/AIDS Policy Making in the United States. *Social History of Medicine* 33(3): 1001–1028.

Pager, Devah. 2003. The Mark of a Criminal Record. *American Journal of Sociology* 108(5): 937–975.

Pager, Devah, Bruce Western, and Naomi Sugie. 2009. Sequencing Disadvantage: Barriers to Employment Facing Young Black and White Men with Criminal Records. *The Annals of the American Academy of Political and Social Science* 623(1): 195–213.

Papachristos, Andrew V. 2009. Murder by Structure: Dominance Relations and the Social Structure of Gang Homicide. *American Journal of Sociology* 115(1): 74–128.

Papachristos, Andrew V., Christopher Wildeman, and Elizabeth Roberto. 2015. Tragic, but not Random: The Social Contagion of Nonfatal Gunshot Injuries. *Social Science & Medicine* 125: 139–150.

Parker, Kim, Juliana Menasce Horowitz, Rich Morin, and Mark Hugo Lopez. 2015. *Multiracial in America: Proud, Diverse and Growing in Numbers*. Pew Research Center.

Parsons, Jeffrey T., Christian Grov, and Brian C. Kelly. 2009. Club Drug Use and Dependence among Young Adults Recruited through Time-Space Sampling. *Public Health Reports* 124(2): 246–254.

Passow, A. Harry. 1967. *Toward Creating a Model Urban School System: A Study of the Washington D.C. Public Schools.* US Department of Health, Education and Welfare. Office of Education.

Patel, Pragna, Craig B. Borkowf, John T. Brooks, Arielle Lasry, Amy Lansky, and Jonathan Mermin. 2014. Estimating Per-Act HIV Transmission Risk: A Systematic Review. *AIDS* 28(10): 1509–1519.

Patrick, Rudy, David Forrest, Gabriel Cardenas et al. 2017. Awareness, Willingness, and Use of Pre-exposure Prophylaxis among Men Who Have Sex with Men in Washington, DC and Miami-Dade County, FL: National HIV Behavioral Surveillance, 2011 and 2014. *Journal of Acquired Immune Deficiency Syndrome* 75(Suppl 3): 375–82.

Pattillo, Mary. 1999. *Black Picket Fences: Privilege and Peril among the Black Middle Class.* University of Chicago Press.

Pedulla, David S., and Sarah Thébaud. 2015. Can We Finish the Revolution? Gender, Work-Family Ideals, and Institutional Constraint. *American Sociological Review* 80(1): 116–139.

Peralta, Carmen A., Ronit Katz, Ian DeBoer, Joachim Ix, Mark Sarnak, Holly Kramer, David Siscovick, Steven Shea, Moyses Szklo, and Michael Shlipak. 2011. Racial and Ethnic Differences in Kidney Function Decline Among Persons without Chronic Kidney Disease. *Journal of the American Society of Nephrology* 22(7): 1327–1334.

Perry, Andre M., Regina Seo, Anthony Barr, Carl Romer, and Kristen Broady. 2022. *Black-Owned Businesses in U.S. Cities: The Challenges, Solutions, and Opportunities for Prosperity.* Brookings Metro.

Peterson, Ruth D., and Lauren J. Krivo. 2010. *Divergent Social Worlds: Neighborhood Crime and the Racial-Spatial Divide.* Russell Sage Foundation.

Pettit, Becky, and Bruce Western. 2004. Mass Imprisonment and the Life Course: Race and Class Inequality in US Incarceration. *American Sociological Review* 69(2): 151–169.

Phelan, Jo C., and Bruce G. Link. 2015. Is Racism a Fundamental Cause of Inequalities in Health? *Annual Review of Sociology* 41: 311–330.

Philpot, Steven P., Duane Duncan, Jeanne Ellard, Benjamin R. Bavinton, Jeffrey Grierson, and Garrett Prestage. 2018. Negotiating Gay Men's Relationships: How Are Monogamy and Non-Monogamy Experienced and Practised over Time? *Culture, Health & Sexuality* 20(8): 915–928.

Pierce, Todd G. 1999. Gen-X Junkie: Ethnographic Research with Young White Heroin Users in Washington, DC. *Substance Use & Misuse* 34(14): 2095–2114.

Pinderhughes, Elaine B. 2002. African American Marriage in the 20th Century. *Family Process* 41(2): 269–282.

Piquero, Alex R., and John K. Roman. 2024. Firearm Homicide Demographics Before and After the COVID-19 Pandemic. *JAMA Network Open* 7(5) (2024): e2412946-e2412946.

Pivnick, Anitra, Audrey Jacobson, Kathleen Eric, Lynda Doll, and Ernest Drucker. 1994. AIDS, HIV Infection, and Illicit Drug Use within Inner-City Families and Social Networks. *American Journal of Public Health* 84(2): 271–274.

Plummer, Betty L. 1985 *A History of Public Health in Washington D.C. 1800–1890.* Doctoral Dissertation. History. University of Maryland, College Park.

Pollock, Daniel A., Patricia Holmgreen, Kung-Jong Lui, and Marilyn L. Kirk. 1991. Discrepancies in the Reported Frequency of Cocaine-Related Deaths, United States, 1983 through 1988. *JAMA* 266(16): 2233–2237.

Popkin, Susan J., Diane K. Levy, and Larry Buron. 2009. Has HOPE VI Transformed Residents' Lives? New Evidence from the HOPE VI Panel Study. *Housing Studies* 24(4): 477–502.

Post, Wendy S., Karol E. Watson, Spencer Hansen, Aaron R. Folsom, Moyses Szklo, Steven Shea, R. Graham Barr et al. 2022. Racial and Ethnic Differences in All-Cause and Cardiovascular Disease Mortality: The MESA Study. *Circulation* 146(3): 229–239.

Prewitt, Kenneth. 2005. Racial Classification in America: Where Do We Go From Here? *Daedalus* 134(1): 5–17.

Prince, Sabiyha. 2014. *African Americans and Gentrification in Washington, DC: Race, Class and Social Justice in the Nation's Capital.* Ashgate Publishing.

Pritchett, Wendell E. 2005. A National Issue: Segregation in the District of Columbia and the Civil Rights Movement at Mid-Century. *Georgetown Law Journal* 93(4): 1321–1334.

Public Law 89-793, Nov 8, 1966 [H.R.9167]. Narcotic Addict Rehabilitation Act of 1966.

Quimby, Ernest, and Arvilla Payne-Jackson. 2007. AIDS in the Shadow of Power: Washington D.C. In Bowser et al 2007, pp. 103–128.

Quinn, Katherine, Julia Dickson-Gomez, and Jeffrey A. Kelly. 2016. The Role of the Black Church in The Lives of Young Black Men Who Have Sex with Men. *Culture, Health & Sexuality* 18(5): 524–537.

Quinones, Sam. 2015. *Dreamland: The True Tale of America's Opiate Epidemic.* Bloomsbury Publishing USA.

Raley, R. Kelly, Megan M. Sweeney, and Danielle Wondra. 2015. The Growing Racial and Ethnic Divide in US Marriage Patterns. *The Future of Children* 25(2): 89–109.

Ralph, Laurence. 2014. *Renegade Dreams: Living through Injury in Gangland Chicago.* University of Chicago Press.

Ratner, Mitchell S., ed. 1993. *Crack Pipe as Pimp: An Ethnographic Investigation of Sex-for-Crack Exchanges.* Lexington Books.

Ray, Victor. 2019. A Theory of Racialized Organizations. *American Sociological Review* 84(1): 26–53.

Read, Jen'nan Ghazal, and Bridget K. Gorman. 2010. Gender and Health Inequality. *Annual Review of Sociology* 36(1): 371–386.

Reardon, Sean F., Kendra Bischoff, Ann Owens, and Joseph B. Townsend. 2018. Has Income Segregation Really Increased? Bias and Bias Correction in Sample-Based Segregation Estimates. *Demography* 55(6): 2129–2160.

Reding, Nick. 2009. *Methland: The Death and Life of An American Small Town.* Bloomsbury Publishing USA.

Rehavi, M. Marit, and Sonja B. Starr. 2014. Racial Disparity in Federal Criminal Sentences. *Journal of Political Economy* 122(6): 1320–1354.

Reinarman, Craig, and Harry G. Levine. 1989. Crack in Context: Politics and Media in the Making of a Drug Scare. *Contemporary Drug Problems* 16: 535–577.

Reinarman, Craig, and Harry Gene Levine, eds. 1997. *Crack in America: Demon Drugs and Social Justice.* University of California Press.

Reskin, Barbara. 2012. The Race Discrimination System. *Annual Review of Sociology* 38: 17–35.

Reuter, Peter, and John Haaga. 1989. *The Organization of High-Level Drug Markets: An Exploratory Study.* RAND Corporation.

Reuter, Peter, John Haaga, Patrick Murphy, and Amy Praskac. 1988. *Drug Use and Drug Programs in the Washington Metropolitan Area.* RAND Corporation.

Reuter, Peter, Robert MacCoun, and Patrick Murphy. 1990. *Money From Crime: A Study of the Economics of Drug Dealing in Washington D.C.* RAND Corporation.

Rhodes, Tim, Merrill Singer, Philippe Bourgois, Samuel R. Friedman, and Steffanie A. Strathdee. 2005. The Social Structural Production of HIV Risk Among Injecting Drug Users. *Social Science & Medicine* 61(5): 1026–1044.

Ridgeway, Cecilia L., and Shelley J. Correll. 2004. Unpacking the Gender System: A Theoretical Perspective on Gender Beliefs and Social Relations. *Gender & Society* 18(4): 510–531.

Riley, K. Jack. 1997. *Crack, Powder Cocaine, and Heroin: Drug Purchase and Use Patterns in Six U.S. Cities.* NCJ 167265. National Institute of Justice and Office of National Drug Control Policy.

Rios, Victor M. 2011. *Punished: Policing the Lives of Black and Latino Boys.* New York University Press.

Riosmena, Fernando, Rebeca Wong, and Alberto Palloni. 2013. Migration Selection, Protection, and Acculturation in Health: A Binational Perspective on Older Adults. *Demography* 50(3): 1039–1064.

Risman, Barbara J. 2004. Gender as a Social Structure: Theory Wrestling with Activism. *Gender & Society* 18(4): 429–450.

Roberts, Dorothy. 2017. *Killing the Black Body: Race, Reproduction, and the Meaning of Liberty.* 20th anniversary ed. Vintage.

Roberts, Eric T., Samuel R. Friedman, Joanne E. Brady, Enrique R. Pouget, Barbara Tempalski, and Sandro Galea. 2010. Environmental Conditions, Political Economy, and Rates of Injection Drug Use in Large US Metropolitan Areas 1992–2002. *Drug and Alcohol Dependence* 106(2–3): 142–153.

Roberts, Max, Eric N. Reither, and Sojung Lim. 2020. Contributors to the Black-White Life Expectancy Gap in Washington D.C. *Nature Research. Scientific Reports* 10: 13416.

Roberts, Samuel. 2009. *Infectious Fear: Politics, Disease, and the Health Effects of Segregation.* University of North Carolina Press.

Robins, Lee N., Darlene H. Davis, and Donald W. Goodwin. 1974. Drug Use by US Army Enlisted Men in Vietnam: A Follow-Up on their Return Home. *American Journal of Epidemiology* 99(4): 235–249.

Roehrkasse, Alexander F., and Christopher Wildeman. 2022. Lifetime Risk of Imprisonment in the United States Remains High and Starkly Unequal. *Science Advances* 8(48).

Rogers, Richard G. 1992. Living and Dying in the USA: Sociodemographic Determinants of Death Among Blacks and Whites. *Demography* 29(2): 287–303.

Rosenberg, Charles. 1962. *The Cholera Years: The United States in 1832, 1849, and 1866.* University of Chicago Press.

Rosenberg, P. S. and R. J. Biggar. 1993. Portrait of the HIV/AIDS Epidemic in Washington D.C. *JAIDS* 6(6): 747.

Rosenberg, Philip S., Martin E. Levy, John F. Brundage, Lyle R. Petersen, John M. Karon, Thomas R. Fears, Lytt I. Gardner et al. 1992. Population-Based Monitoring of an Urban HIV/AIDS Epidemic: Magnitude and Trends in the District of Columbia. *JAMA* 268(4): 495–503.

Rosenfeld, Michael J. 2007. *The Age of Independence: Interracial Unions, Same-Sex Unions, and the Changing American Family.* Harvard University Press.

Ross, Catherine E., and John Mirowsky. 2001. Neighborhood Disadvantage, Disorder, and Health. *Journal of Health and Social Behavior* 42(3): 258–276.

Rothstein, Richard. 2017. *The Color of Law: A Forgotten History of How Our Government Segregated America.* Liveright Publishing.

Rubin, Gayle. 1993 [1984]. Thinking Sex: Notes for a Radical Theory of the Politics of Sexuality. In H. Abelove, M. Barale, and D. Halperin, eds. *The Lesbian and Gay Studies Reader*, pp. 3–44. Routledge.

Ruble, Blair. 2010. *Washington's U Street: A Biography.* Johns Hopkins University Press.

Ruggles, Steve. 1994. The Origins of African-American Family Structure. *American Sociological Review* 59(1): 136–151.

Ruggles, Steven, Sarah Flood, Matthew Sobek, Daniel Backman, Grace Cooper, Julia A. Rivera Drew, Stephanie Richards, Renae Rodgers, Jonathan Schroeder, and Kari C.W. Williams. IPUMS USA: Version 16.0 [dataset]. Minneapolis, MN: IPUMS, 2025.

Ruiz, Monica S., Allison O'Rourke, and Sean T. Allen. 2016. Impact Evaluation of a Policy Intervention for HIV Prevention in Washington, DC. *AIDS and Behavior* 20(1): 22–28.

Rupp, Leila J., Verta Taylor, Shiri Regev-Messalem, Alison C. K. Fogarty, and Paula England. 2014. Queer Women in the Hookup Scene: Beyond the Closet? *Gender & Society* 28(2): 212–235.

Ruttenber, A. James, and James L. Luke. 1984. Heroin-Related Deaths: New Epidemiologic Insights. *Science* 226(4670): 14–20.

Ryan, William. 1971. *Blaming the Victim.* Vintage Books.

Saleh, Lena Denise, and Don Operario. 2009. Moving Beyond "The Down Low": A Critical Analysis of Terminology Guiding HIV Prevention Efforts for African American Men Who Have Secretive Sex with Men. *Social Science & Medicine* 68(2): 390–395.

Sampson, Robert J. 2012. *Great American City: Chicago and the Enduring Neighborhood Effect.* University of Chicago Press.

Sampson, Robert J., and John H. Laub. 1995. *Crime in the Making: Pathways and Turning Points through Life.* Harvard University Press.

Sampson, Robert J., and William Julius Wilson. 2005. Toward a Theory of Race, Crime, and Urban Inequality. In Shaun L. Gabbidon and Helen Taylor Greene, eds., *Race, Crime, and Justice: A Reader,* pp. 177–190. Routledge.

Saperstein, Aliya, Andrew M. Penner, and Ryan Light. 2013. Racial Formation in Perspective: Connecting Individuals, Institutions, and Power Relations. *Annual Review of Sociology.* 39(1): 359–378.

Sawyer, Noah, and Peter Tatian. 2003. *Segregation Patterns in the District of Columbia: 1980 to 2000.* The Urban Institute.

Schilt, Kristen, and Laurel Westbrook. 2009. Doing Gender, Doing Heteronormativity: "Gender Normals," Transgender People, and the Social Maintenance of Heterosexuality. *Gender & Society* 23(4): 440–464.

Schneider, Eric C. 2008. *Smack: Heroin and the American City.* University of Pennsylvania Press.

Schnittker, Jason, Michael Massoglia, and Christopher Uggen. 2011. Incarceration and the Health of the African American Community. *Du Bois Review* 8(1): 133–141.

Schoendorf, Kenneth C., Carol J. R. Hogue, Joel C. Kleinman, and Diane Rowley. 1992. Mortality among Infants of Black as Compared with White College-Educated Parents. *New England Journal of Medicine* 326(23): 1522–1526.

Schwandt, Hannes, Janet Currie, Marlies Bär, James Banks, Paola Bertoli, Aline Bütikofer, Sarah Cattan et al. 2021. Inequality in Mortality Between Black and White Americans by Age, Place, and Cause and in Comparison to Europe, 1990 to 2018. *Proceedings of the National Academy of Sciences* 118(40).

Schwartz, Martin D., and Dana M. Nurge. 2004. Capitalist Punishment: Ethics and Private Prisons. *Critical Criminology* 12(2): 133–156.

Scott, James C. 1998. *Seeing Like a State: How Certain Schemes to Improve the Human Condition Have Failed.* Yale University Press.

Scott, Jennifer, Denise Danos, Robert Collins, Neal Simonsen, Claudia Leonardi, Richard Scribner, and Denise Herd. 2020. Structural Racism in the Built Environment: Segregation and the Overconcentration of Alcohol Outlets. *Health & Place* 64: 102385.

Scott, Michael S. 2002. *Street Prostitution. Problem-Oriented Guides for Police Series.* No.2. US Department of Justice: Office of Community Oriented Policing Services.

Seidman, Steven, Chet Meeks, and Francie Traschen. 1999. Beyond the Closet? The Changing Social Meaning of Homosexuality in the United States. *Sexualities* 2(1): 9–34.

Service, S. K. and S. M. Blower. 1995. HIV Transmission in Sexual Networks: An Empirical Analysis. *Proceedings: Biological Sciences* 260(1359): 237–244.

Shannon, Sarah K. S., Christopher Uggen, Jason Schnittker, Melissa Thompson, Sara Wakefield, and Michael Massoglia. 2017. The Growth, Scope, and Spatial

Distribution of People with Felony Records in the United States, 1948–2010. *Demography* 54(5): 1795–1818.

Shapiro, Justin. 2020. *Decent, Safe and Sanitary? Public Housing and the Environment of Eastern Washington, D.C. 1940–1965.* Doctoral Dissertation. History. University of Maryland.

Shapiro, Justin. 2024. Infrastructure and Inequality in Washington, DC: Environmental Change and Federal Management of the District's Forgotten River. *Journal of Urban History* (2024): 00961442241286454.

Sharkey, Patrick. 2008. The Intergenerational Transmission of Context. *American Journal of Sociology* 113(4): 931–969.

Sharkey, Patrick. 2010. The Acute Effect of Local Homicides on Children's Cognitive Performance. *Proceedings of the National Academy of Sciences* 107(26): 11733–11738.

Sharkey, Patrick. 2013. *Stuck in Place: Urban Neighborhoods and the End of Progress towards Racial Inequality.* University of Chicago Press.

Sharkey, Patrick, and Michael Friedson. 2019. The Impact of the Homicide Decline on Life Expectancy of African American Males. *Demography* 56: 645–663.

Sharkey, Patrick T., Nicole Tirado-Strayer, Andrew V. Papachristos, and C. Cybele Raver. 2012. The Effect of Local Violence on Children's Attention and Impulse Control. *American Journal of Public Health* 102(12): 2287–2293.

Sharpe, Tanya Telfair. 2005. *Behind the Eight Ball: Sex for Crack Exchange and Poor Black Women.* Haworth.

Shein, Marcia G. 1993. Racial Disparity in Crack Cocaine Sentencing. *Criminal Justice* 8(2): 28–62.

Shilts, Randy. 2007. *And The Band Played On: Politics, People, and the AIDS Epidemic.* St. Martin's Griffin.

Shoenfeld, Sarah. 2019a. The History and Evolution of Anacostia's Barry Farm. DC Policy Center.

Shoenfeld, Sarah. 2019b. Mapping Segregation in D.C. DC Policy Center. April 23, 2019.

Shoenfeld, Sarah Jane, and Mara Cherkasky. 2017. "A Strictly White Residential Section": The Rise and Demise of Racially Restrictive Covenants in Bloomingdale. *Washington History* 29(1): 24–41.

Silva, Abigail, Nazia S. Saiyed, Emma Canty, and Maureen R. Benjamins. 2023. Pre-Pandemic Trends and Black-White Inequities in Life Expectancy Across the 30 Most Populous US Cities: A Population-Based Study. *BMC Public Health* 23(1): 2310.

Silva, Tony. 2017. Bud-Sex: Constructing Normative Masculinity Among Rural Straight Men That Have Sex with Men. *Gender & Society* 31(1): 51–73.

Silva, Tony J. 2019. Straight Identity and Same-Sex Desire: Conservatism, Homophobia, and Straight Culture. *Social Forces* 97(3): 1067–1094.

Singer, Merrill. 1994. AIDS and the Health Crisis of the US Urban Poor: The Perspective of Critical Medical Anthropology. *Social Science & Medicine* 39(7): 931–948.

Singer, Merrill. 2011. Down Cancer Alley: The Lived Experience of Health and Environmental Suffering in Louisiana's Chemical Corridor. *Medical Anthropology Quarterly* 25 (2): 141–163.

Singer, Merrill, and the Hispanic Health Council. 2000. A Dose of Drugs, A Touch of Violence, A Case of AIDS: Conceptualizing the SAVA Syndemic. *Free Inquiry in Creative Sociology* 28(1): 13–24.

Singer, Merill, and Scott Clair. 2003. Syndemics and Public Health: Reconceptualizing Disease in Bio-Social Context. *Medical Anthropology Quarterly* 17(4): 423–441.

Singer, Merrill, Nicola Bulled, Bayla Ostrach, and Emily Mendenhall. 2017. Syndemics and the Biosocial Conception of Health. *The Lancet* 389(10072): 941–950.

Skyes, Gresham. 1958. *The Society of Captives: A Study of a Maximum Security Prison.* Princeton University Press.

Smith, Jocelyn R. 2015. Unequal Burdens of Loss: Examining the Frequency and Timing of Homicide Deaths Experienced by Young Black Men Across the Life Course. *American Journal of Public Health* 105(S3): S483–S490.

Smith, Justin, Emma Simmons, and Kenneth H. Mayer. 2005. HIV/AIDS and the Black Church: What Are the Barriers to Prevention Services? *Journal of the National Medical Association* 97(12): 1682–1685.

Snell, Tracy L. 1995. *Correctional Populations in the United States, 1993.* Bureau of Justice Statistics Bulletin, NCJ 156241. US Department of Justice.

Snorton, C. Riley. 2014. *Nobody Is Supposed to Know: Black Sexuality on the Down Low.* University of Minnesota Press.

Sobo, Elisa J. 1995. *Choosing Unsafe Sex: AIDS Risk Denial among Disadvantaged Women.* University of Pennsylvania Press.

Spain, Daphne. 2014. Gender and Urban Space. *Annual Review of Sociology* 40: 581–598.

Spanakis, Elias K., and Sherita Hill Golden. 2013. Race/Ethnic Difference in Diabetes and Diabetic Complications. *Current Diabetes Reports* 13: 814–823.

Spaulding, Anne, Becky Stephenson, Grace Macalino, William Ruby, Jennifer G. Clarke, and Timothy P. Flanigan. 2002. Human Immunodeficiency Virus in Correctional Facilities: A Review. *Clinical Infectious Diseases* 35(3): 305–312.

Squires, Gregory D., Samantha Friedman, and Catherine E. Saidat. 2002. Experiencing Residential Segregation: A Contemporary Study of Washington, DC. *Urban Affairs Review* 38(2): 155–183.

Stall, Ron, Mark Friedman, and Joseph A. Catania. 2008. Interacting Epidemics and Gay Men's Health: A Theory of Syndemic Production Among Urban Gay Men. In Richard J. Wolitski, Ron Stall, and Ronald O. Valdiserri, eds., *Unequal Opportunity: Health Disparities Affecting Gay and Bisexual Men in the United States*, pp. 251–274. Oxford University Press.

Staples, Brent. 2007. Introduction: Defining Decarceration. *Social Research: An International Quarterly* 74(2): 647–650.

Starr, Paul. 2019. *Entrenchment: Wealth, Power, and the Constitution of Democratic Societies.* Yale University Press.

Stevenson, Bryan. 2017. A Presumption of Guilt: The Legacy of America's History of Racial Injustice. In Davis, ed.

Stillwell, Robert. 2010. *Public School Graduates and Dropouts from the Common Core of Data: School Year 2007–08. First Look*. National Center for Education Statistics, NCES 2010-341. US Department of Education.

Strathdee, Stephanie A., and David Vlahov. 2001. The Effectiveness of Needle Exchange Programs: A Review of the Science and Policy. *AIDScience* 1(16): 1–33.

Sturtevant, Lisa. 2014. The New District of Columbia: What Population Growth and Demographic Change Mean for the City. *Journal of Urban Affairs* 36(2): 276–299.

Sugano, Eiko, Tooru Nemoto, and Don Operario. 2006. The Impact of Exposure to Transphobia on HIV Risk Behavior in a Sample of Transgendered Women of Color in San Francisco. *AIDS and Behavior* 10(2): 217–225.

Swope, Carolyn. 2018. The Problematic Role of Public Health in Washington DC's Urban Renewal. *Public Health Reports*. 133(6): 707–714.

Taylor, Elizabeth Dowling. 2017. *The Original Black Elite: Daniel Murray and the Story of a Forgotten Era*. Harper Collins.

Taylor, Keeanga-Yamahtta. 2019. *Race for Profit: How Banks and the Real Estate Industry Undermined Black Homeownership*. University of North Carolina Press.

Thomas, James C. and Elizabeth Torrone. 2006. Incarceration as Forced Migration: Effects on Selected Community Health Outcomes. *American Journal of Public Health* 96: 1762–1765.

Tilly, Charles. 1998. *Durable Inequality*. University of California Press.

Tilly, Charles. 2000. Relational Studies of Inequality. *Contemporary Sociology* 29(6): 782–785.

Trammell, Rebecca. 2011. Symbolic Violence and Prison Wives: Gender Roles and Protective Pairing in Men's Prisons. *The Prison Journal* 91(3): 305–324.

Treitler, Vilna Bashi. 2013. *The Ethnic Project: Transforming Racial Fiction into Ethnic Factions*. Stanford University Press.

Turner, Margery Austin. 2017. *History of Place-Based Interventions*. US Partnership on Mobility and Poverty. Urban Institute.

Turner, Nick, Kaveh Danesh, and Kelsey Moran. 2020. The Evolution of Infant Mortality Inequality in the United States, 1960–2016. *Science Advances* 6(29): 3–8.

Turney, Kristin. 2017. The Unequal Consequences of Mass Incarceration for Children. *Demography* 54(1): 361–389.

Umberson, Debra. 2017. Black Deaths Matter: Race, Relationship Loss, and Effects on Survivors. *Journal of Health and Social Behavior* 58(4): 405–420.

Umberson, Debra, Julie Skalamera Olson, Robert Crosnoe, Hui Liu, Tetyana Pudrovska, and Rachel Donnelly. 2017. Death of Family Members as an Overlooked Source of Racial Disadvantage in the United States. *Proceedings of the National Academy of Sciences* 114(5): 915–920.

United States Government Accountability Office. 2022. *K–12 Education. Student Population Has Significantly Diversified, But Many Schools Remain Divided Along Racial, Ethnic and Economic Lines.* Report to the Chairman, Committee on Education and Labor, House of Representatives.

Urban Omnibus. 2016. *Making Sense of Model Cities.* Architectural League of New York.

US Department of Health and Human Services. 2024. *Healthy People 2030: Building a Healthier Future for All.*

US Department of Justice Criminal Division. 1991. *Drug Paraphernalia: Federal Prosecution Manual.* National Institute of Justice.

van Eeden-Moorefield, Brad, Kevin Malloy, and Kristen Benson. 2016. Gay Men's (Non) Monogamy Ideals and Lived Experience *Sex Roles* 75(1): 43–55.

Vanwesenbeek, Ine. 2001. Another Decade of Social Scientific Work on Sex Work: A Review of Research 1990–2000. *Annual Review of Sex Research* 12(1): 242–289.

Venkatesh, Sudhir Alladi. 2000. *American Project: The Rise and Fall of a Modern Ghetto.* Harvard University Press.

Verbrugge, Lois M. 1985. Gender and Health: An Update on Hypotheses and Evidence. *Journal of Health and Social Behavior* 26: 156–182.

Verbrugge, Lois M. 1989. The Twain Meet: Empirical Explanations of Sex Differences in Health and Mortality. *Journal of Health and Social Behavior* 30(3): 282–304.

Voss, Harwin L. 1989. Patterns of Drug Use: Data from the 1985 National Household Survey. Drugs in the Workplace: Research and Evaluation Data. *NIDA Research Monograph* 91: 33–46.

Vyas, Darshali A., Leo G. Eisenstein, and David S. Jones. 2020. Hidden in Plain Sight: Reconsidering the Use of Race Correction in Clinical Algorithms. *New England Journal of Medicine* 383(9): 874–882.

Wacquant, Loïc. 2000. 'The New Peculiar Institution': On the Prison as Surrogate Ghetto. *Theoretical Criminology* 4(3): 377–389.

Wacquant, Loïc. 2001. Deadly Symbiosis: When Ghetto and Prison Meet and Mesh. *Punishment and Society* 3(1): 95–134.

Wagner, Peter, and Bernadette Rabuy. 2017. *Following the Money of Mass Incarceration.* Prison Policy Initiative.

Wailoo, Keith. 2001. *Dying in the City of the Blues: Sickle Cell Anemia and the Politics of Race and Health.* University of North Carolina Press.

Waidmann, Timothy, Kristen Brown, Karishma Furtado, and Vincent Pancini. 2025. *State Variation in Black and White Life Expectancy and Evolving Disparities.* Urban Institute.

Waite, Linda J. 1995. Does Marriage Matter?. *Demography* 32(4): 483–507.

Wakefield, Sara, and Christopher Wildeman. 2013. *Children of the Prison Boom: Mass Incarceration and the Future of American Inequality.* Oxford University Press.

Wald, Johanna, and Daniel J. Losen. 2003. Defining and Redirecting a School-to-Prison Pipeline. *New Directions for Youth Development* 2003(99): 9–15.

Waldorf, Dan, Craig Reinarman, and Sheigla Murphy. 1991. *Cocaine Changes: The Experience of Using and Quitting.* Temple University Press.

Walker, J. Samuel. 2018. *Most of 14th Street Is Gone: The Washington, DC Riots of 1968.* Oxford University Press.

Walker, Renee E., Christopher R. Keane, and Jessica G. Burke. 2010. Disparities and Access to Healthy Food in the United States: A Review of Food Deserts Literature. *Health & Place* 16(5): 876–884.

Wallace, Deborah, and Rodrick Wallace. 1998. *A Plague on Your Houses: How New York Was Burned Down and National Public Health Crumbled.* Verso.

Wallace, Rodrick. 1990. Urban Desertification, Public Health and Public Order: 'Planned Shrinkage', Violent Death, Substance Abuse and AIDS in the Bronx. *Social Science & Medicine* 31(7): 801–813.

Ward, Elijah G. 2005. Homophobia, Hypermasculinity and the US Black Church. *Culture, Health & Sexuality* 7(5): 493–504.

Ward, Jane. 2015. *Not Gay: Sex Between Straight White Men.* New York University Press.

Washington, Harriet A. 2006. *Medical Apartheid: The Dark History of Medical Experimentation on Black Americans from Colonial Times to the Present.* Doubleday Books.

Washington Lawyers' Committee for Civil Rights and Urban Affairs. 2010. *The State of the District of Columbia Public Schools 2010: A Five Year Update.*

Washington Lawyers' Committee for Civil Rights and Urban Affairs. 2015. *DC Prisoners: Conditions of Confinement in the District of Columbia.*

Waters, Anita M. 1997. Conspiracy Theories as Ethnosociologies: Explanation and Intention in African American Political Culture. *Journal of Black Studies* 28(1): 112–125.

Watkins-Hayes, Celeste. 2014. Intersectionality and the Sociology of HIV/AIDS: Past, Present, and Future Research Directions. *Annual Review of Sociology* 40(1): 431–457.

Watkins-Hayes, Celeste. 2019. *Remaking a Life: How Women Living with HIV/AIDS Confront Inequality.* University of California Press.

Weber, Bret A., and Amanda Wallace. 2012. Revealing the Empowerment Revolution: A Literature Review of the Model Cities Program. *Journal of Urban History* 38(1): 173–192.

Weber, Max. 1978 (1922). *Economy and Society: An Outline of Interpretive Sociology.* Edited by Guenther Roth and Claus Wittich. University of California Press.

Wei, Rong, Robert N. Anderson, Lester R. Curtin, and Elizabeth Arias. 2012. US Decennial Life Tables for 1999–2001: State Life Tables. *National Vital Statistics Reports* 60(9).

Weitzer, Ronald. 1999. Citizens' Perceptions of Police Misconduct: Race and Neighborhood Context. *Justice Quarterly.* 16(4): 819–846.

Weitzer, Ronald. 2009. Sociology of Sex Work. *Annual Review of Sociology* 35(1): 213–234.

Weitzer, Ronald. 2010. *Sex for Sale: Prostitution, Pornography, and the Sex Industry.* Routledge.

Weitzer, Ronald, Steven A. Touch, and Wesley G. Skogan. 2008. Police-Community Relations in a Majority-Black City. *Journal of Research in Crime and Delinquency* 45(4): 398–428.

Wendland, Claire L. 2022. *Partial Stories: Maternal Death from Six Angles.* University of Chicago Press.

West, Candace, and Don H. Zimmerman. 1987. Doing Gender. *Gender and Society* 1(2): 125–151.

Westbrook, Laurel, and Kristen Schilt. 2014. Doing Gender, Determining Gender: Transgender People, Gender Panics, and the Maintenance of the Sex/Gender/Sexuality System. *Gender & Society* 28: 32–57.

Western, Bruce. 2006. *Punishment and Inequality in America.* Russell Sage.

Western, Bruce. 2018. *Homeward: Life in the Year After Prison.* Russell Sage.

Whetstone, Sarah, and Teresa Gowan. 2017. Carceral Rehab as Fuzzy Penality: Hybrid Technologies of Control in the New Temperance Crusade. *Social Justice* 44(2–3): 83–112.

Whitehead, Tony L. 1997. Urban Low-Income African American Men, HIV/AIDS, and Gender Identity. *Medical Anthropology Quarterly* 11(4): 411–447.

Wiederman, Michael W. 1997. Extramarital Sex: Prevalence and Correlates in a National Survey. *Journal of Sex Research* 34(2): 167–174.

Wildeman, Christopher. 2009. Parental Imprisonment, the Prison Boom, and the Concentration of Childhood Disadvantage. *Demography* 46: 265–280.

Wilder, Sandra. 2014. Effects of Parental Involvement on Academic Achievement: A Meta-Synthesis. *Educational Review,* 66(3): 377–397.

Wilkinson, Richard. 1996. *Unhealthy Societies: The Afflictions of Inequality.* Routledge.

Williams, Brett. 1988. *Upscaling Downtown: Stalled Gentrification in Washington D.C.* Cornell University Press.

Williams, Brett. 2001. A River Runs Through Us. *American Anthropologist* 103(2): 409–431.

Williams, David R., and Chiquita Collins. 2001. Racial Residential Segregation: A Fundamental Cause of Racial Disparities in Health. *Public Health Reports* 116(5): 404–416.

Williams, David R., and Pamela Braboy Jackson. 2005. Social Sources of Racial Disparities in Health. *Health Affairs* 24(2): 325–334.

Williams, David R., and Michelle Sternthal. 2010. Understanding Racial-Ethnic Disparities in Health: Sociological Contributions. *Journal of Health and Social Behavior* 51: S15-S27.

Williams, Terry. 1992. *Crack House: Notes From the End of a Line.* Da Capo Press.

Wilson, David, and Daniel T. Halperin. 2008. "Know Your Epidemic, Know Your Response": A Useful Approach, If We Get It Right. *The Lancet* 372(9637): 423–426.

Wilson, William Julius. 1978. *The Declining Significance of Race: Blacks and Changing American Institutions.* University of Chicago Press.

Wilson, William Julius. 1987. *The Truly Disadvantaged: The Inner City, The Underclass, and Public Policy.* University of Chicago Press.

Wilson, William J. and Kathryn Neckerman. 1987. Poverty and Family Structure: The Widening Gap between Evidence and Public Policy Issues, pp. 63–92. In William J. Wilson 1987.

Winant, Howard. 2000. Race and Race Theory. *Annual Review of Sociology* 26: 169–85.

Wingood, Gina W., and Ralph J. DiClemente. 1998. Partner Influences and Gender-Related Factors Associated with Noncondom Use among Young Adult African American Women. *American Journal of Community Psychology* 26(1): 29–51.

Winling, LaDale C., and Todd M. Michney. 2021. The Roots of Redlining: Academic, Governmental, and Professional Networks in the Making of the New Deal Lending Regime. *Journal of American History* 108(1): 42–69.

Woodson, C. G. 1949. Review of "Segregation in Washington" by The National Committee on Segregation in the Nation's Capitol. *The Journal of Negro History* 34(2): 229–231.

Wright, Jerome. 1993. African-American Male Sexual Behavior and the Risk for HIV Infection. *Human Organization* 52(4): 421–431.

Wrigley-Field, Elizabeth. 2020. US Racial Inequality may be as Deadly as COVID-19. *Proceedings of the National Academy of Sciences* 117(36): 21854–21856.

Xavier, Jessica M., Marilyn Bobbin, Ben Singer, and Earline Budd. 2005. A Needs Assessment of Transgendered People of Color Living in Washington, DC. *International Journal of Transgenderism* 8(2–3): 31–47.

Xu, Jiaquan, Sherry L. Murphy, Kenneth D. Kochanek, and Elizabeth Arias. 2022. *Mortality in the United States, 2021.* NCHS Data Brief No. 456. December 2022.

Zinberg, Norman E., and Wayne M. Harding. 1979. Control and Intoxicant Use: A Theoretical and Practical Overview. *Journal of Drug Issues.* 9(2): 121–143.

NEWSPAPERS

General

Dec 22, 1800—Woodward, Augustus. City of Washington. *National Intelligencer.*

Feb 12, 1986—Jackson, Kirk. Barry Gives High Marks to District. *Washington Informer.*

May 14, 1986—[No author.] AIDS Discrimination Bill Introduced. *Washington Informer.*

May 21, 1986—Crawford, Nicole S.—Council Passes AIDS Bill Introduced by Ray. *Washington Informer.*

Jun 4, 1986—Crawford, Nicole S. City Council Passes AIDS Insurance Bill. *Washington Informer.*

Oct 1, 1989—Massing, Michael. Crack's Destructive Sprint Across America. *New York Times*.

Sep 16, 1992—[No author.] Area Schools Take on Added Focus. *Washington Informer*.

Sep 1, 1993—[No author.] New Coalition Formed to Secure Equal Funding for AIDS. *Washington Informer*.

May 23, 1994—Nicholas Eberstadt—Washington as Infant Mortality Capital. *Washington Times*.

Mar 30, 1994—[No author.] Confab Focuses on "Who Is My Neighbor?" *Washington Informer*.

Jun 29, 1994—Peabody, Alvin. City Awards AIDS Contract to Whitman Walker Clinic: Decision Called A "Death Sentence" For City's Poor. *Washington Informer*.

Mar 24, 1995—Rosenbaum, Claudia. Bad Guys, Jailhouse Shock. *Washington City Paper*.

May 17, 1995—[No author.] Putting a Strain on City Services. *Washington Informer*.

May 1, 1996—Peabody, Alvin. Inmates to be Excluded. *Washington Informer*.

May 8, 1996—Peabody, Alvin. Fed to Take Over AIDS Payment Process. *Washington Informer*.

Aug 16, 1996—Cloud, John. Living, for the Moment. *Washington City Paper*.

Sep 4, 1996—Peabody, Alvin. Budget Cuts Force Community AIDS Service Center to Close. *Washington Informer*.

Apr 3, 1997—Olds, Dana. The Church Responds to HIV/AIDS. *Washington Informer*.

Apr 25, 1997—Cummins, Ken. Twisting Slowly in Barry's Wind. *Washington City Paper*.

Sep 26, 1997—Peterson, Chris. House of Pain. *Washington City Paper*.

Jul 17, 1998—Park, Paula. Delinquent Oversight. *Washington City Paper*.

Aug 20, 1999—Ripley, Amanda. Closing Arguments. *Washington City Paper*.

Nov 2, 2001—Summersgill, Bob. GLAA Slams Mismanagement and Unresponsiveness at HIV/AIDS Administration. *GLAA*.

Mar 6, 2002—Summersgill, Bob. GLAA Slams Mismanagement, Lack of Oversight at DC Dept of Health. *GLAA*.

Jan 27, 2003—[No author.] Washington D.C. HIV/AIDS Office Investigated in Connection with Washington Teacher's Union Scandal. *Kaiser Health News. KNH Morning Briefing*.

Jul 7, 2004—[No author.] An Election-Year Guide to Local Gay and Lesbian Issues in Washington D.C. *GLAA*.

Jan 1, 2008—Ellis, Kirsten H. HIV/AIDS Rate in Washington, D.C. Highest among U.S. Cities. *Healio. Infectious Disease News*.

Oct 20, 2009—Connolly, Katie. Why So Few D.C. Residents Are Married. *Newsweek*.

Jun 9, 2010—Chibbaro, Lou, Jr. Questions Surface over Resignation of AIDS Director; Catania Calls Loss of Hader 'Catastrophic.' *Washington Blade*.

Aug 30, 2010—Jaffe, Harry. So-Called Plan for White Supremacy Lives On in DC. *Washington Examiner.*

Sep 8, 2011—Staff Reporters. Brass Rail Reunion at Remington's Sunday. *Washington Blade.*

Jun 29, 2012—Howell, Tom, Jr. D.C. DOH Director to Request Leave of Absence. *Washington Times.*

May 21, 2013—Chibbaro, Lou, Jr. Gay DC Psychiatrist Named Head of APA. *Washington Blade.*

July 24, 2013—Chibbaro, Lou, Jr. Gray Names New Health Director. *Washington Blade.*

Jul 31, 2013—Chibbaro, Lou, Jr. Pappas 'Steps Down' As Head of DC AIDS Office. *Washington Blade.*

Nov 21, 2014—Sheir, Rebecca. Meet the Man Who Tackled D.C.'s First Heroin Epidemic. *WAMU Metro Connection.*

May 5 2015—Vinik, Danny. Washington, D.C. Has the Highest Infant Mortality Rate of 25 Rich World Capitals. *The New Republic.*

Feb 8, 2018—Jacob, Angela. DC Has Highest Maternal Mortality Rate in US; Council Wants to Learn Why. *NBC Washington.*

Oct 15, 2019—Chibbaro, Lou, Jr. Blade's 50-Year History Reflects Struggles, Advances of LGBT Community. *Washington Blade.*

May 5, 2021—Chibbaro, Lou, Jr. Activists Concerned Over Removal of D.C. AIDS Office Executive. *Washington Blade.*

July 27, 2022—WI Web Staff. Sharon Lewis Tapped as Interim D.C. Health Director. *The Washington Informer.*

Nov 16, 2022—Barnes, Denise Rolark. From 'Singing Hat Check Girl' to Journalist and Civic Leader Who Predicted 'The Plan' for D.C. *The Washington Informer.*

Dec 26, 2022—Summerhays, Anne. Inmates in Mississippi Prisons Cost over $59 per Day. *Magnolia Tribune.*

Washington Post

Feb 6, 1944—Meyer, Agnes E. Negro Housing—Capital Sets Record for U.S. in Unalleviated Wretchedness of Slums.

Jul 8, 1960—Weiss, Kenneth. D.C.-Bound Car Yields Dope Cache; 3 Arrested.

Jul 15, 1960—Lewis, Alfred E. Drug Traffic Seen Losing Ground Here.

Oct 27, 1960—[No author.] Trial Hears N.Y. Supplies Addicts Here.

Apr 1, 1961—Munsey, Everard. DC Narcotic Suspect Is Seized with $50,000 Heroin.

May 22, 1961—Dixon, George. Washington Scene.

May 23, 1961—[No author.] 24 Indicted as Heroin Smugglers.

Dec 10, 1961—Kluttz, Jerry. The Federal Diary.

Feb 28, 1964—Anderson, Jack. Diplomats Tailed in Dope Probe.

Sep 9, 1965—Downie, Leonard, Jr. Drug-Taking Spreads on Nation's Campuses.

Oct 18, 1965—Lewis, Alfred. 789 Burglaries in Month Set Record for City: Drug Addicts Blamed.

Dec 19, 1965—[No author.] 37 Public Housing Projects Are Home to 41,500 Citizens.

Jan 2, 1966—Thompson, Robert E. Mafia Still in Control of US Heroin Traffic.

Oct 20, 1966—Morgan, Dan. 5th Largest Addict Population in US Costs Many Lives.

Oct 21, 1966—Morgan, Dan. Heroin Alley.

Oct 22, 1966—Morgan, Dan. Heroin Highs Are Costly.

Oct 23, 1966—Morgan, Dan. Addicts Offered Little Help.

Jan 30, 1968—Bernstein, Carl. Heroin Traffic Flourishing.

Jun 23, 1968—Asher, Robert L. Nixon Labels D.C. A "Crime Capital."

Feb 16, 1969—Carter, Philip D. Heroin Invades Middle Class.

Feb 6, 1970—Kessler, Ronald B. Death Threats to Peddlers Cited.

Dec 18, 1970—Ungar, Sanford J. 6 Convicted on All Counts in Drug Trial.

Mar 16, 1972—Woodward, Bob. Heroin Quality Declines.

Apr 11, 1972—Claiborne, William L. Heroin Problem Peaks in D.C., to Ease in 2 years, Doctor Says.

Jul 7, 1972—Valentine, Paul W., and Bob Woodward. Heroin Supply Said to Drop in Nixon Effort.

Sep 16, 1972—Scharfenberg, Kirk. Public Housing Reforms to Be Urged.

Nov 10, 1974—Feinberg, Lawrence. Heroin Use Reported on Rise in D.C.

Nov 8, 1975—[No author.] Massive Heroin Seizure Said to Break up Ring.

Mar 17, 1976—Auerbach, Stuart. Epidemic' of Heroin Continuing.

Mar 24, 1976—Dash, Leon. 2 Charged in Heroin Smuggling.

Apr 1, 1976—Dash, Leon. DC Heroin Addicts up 43%.

Apr 18, 1976—Dash, Leon. Heroin Trail: From Mexico to Streets of DC.

Apr 20, 1976—Valentine, Paul W. Narcotic Unit Is Closed to New Patients.

May 23, 1976—Dash, Leon. DC Addicts Are Link in Mafia's Multimillion-Dollar Trade.

May 24, 1976—Dash, Leon. Part 2. Tracing DC Drug Route: White Dragon Pearl and Amsterdam Link.

Jun 30, 1976—Dash, Leon. Methadone Flayed at Heroin Hearing.

Sep 6, 1976—Dash, Leon. Seven Major Drug markets thrive in City.

Nov 14, 1976—Williams, Juan, and Lynn Darling. Potent Heroin Fatal to 4.

Aug 6, 1977—Stevens, Joann. Maple Glen Inmates Sent to Group Homes in DC.

May 26, 1978—Colen, B.D. Use of PCP in D.C. Metropolitan Area Called 'Endemic' by Drug Officials.

Jun 24, 1979—Tofani, Loretta. City Owns a Heroin 'Shooting Gallery.'

Aug 26, 1979—Valentine, Paul W. Glut of Heroin Triggers Surge in Drug Activity.

Jan 24, 1979—Shaffer, Ron and Lawrence Meyer. Alleged Heroin King, 9 Others Arrested.

Jun 24, 1979—Tofani, Loretta. City Owns a Heroin 'Shooting Gallery'.

Feb 8, 1980—Robinson, Timothy S., and Paul W. Valentine. Iranian Turmoil Fueling Surge of Heroin here.

Feb 9, 1980—Pichirallo, Joe. Customs Agents Seize 10 Pounds of Cocaine on Jet-liner at Dulles.

Feb 25, 1980—Krause, Charles A. Colombia's 'Gold' Proves Both Blessing and Curse.

May 31, 1980—Krause, Charles A. Peru in Major Campaign Against Drug Traffickers.

Jun 11, 1980—[No author.] Comedian Pryor Critically Burned as Drug Mix Explodes in His Face.

Jun 22, 1980—Anderson, Jack. 'Cocaine Cowboys.'

Oct 7, 1980—Stevens, Joann. The Boy-Whore World: Male Prostitutes Prowl D.C. Street Corners.

Feb 14, 1981—Pichirallo, Joe. FBI Targets Owners, Profits of Sex Businesses in D.C. Area.

May 21, 1981—Knight, Athelia. $2 Million in Cocaine Seized in Arlington.

May 22, 1981—Piantadosi, Roger. Heroin Overdose Deaths in May Soar to 10 Year Record Here.

Jun 25, 1981—Sargent, Edward D. Running Barry Farms.

Jul 11, 1981—Smith, Philip. 'Jaws,' Drug Laws Await Passengers From Peru.

Aug 5, 1981—Lewis, Alfred E., and Tom Sherwood. Heroin Deaths Soar here.

Sep 3, 1981—Robinson, Eugene. Service Mourns Heroin Victims.

Sep 10, 1981—Smith, Philip and Celestine Bohlen. Drug Probe Hits Ring of 'Preppies.'

Feb 25, 1982—Diehl, Jackson. Bolivia's Economic Woes Threaten New Military Government's Stability.

Jun 15, 1982—O'Toole, Thomas. Addiction Called No.1 Health Hazard.

Nov 8, 1982—Pincus, Walter. Aid to Bolivia Tied to Progress in Cocaine War.

Feb 13, 1983—Milloy, Courtland, and Milton Coleman. Prison Has Become "Rite of Passage."

Jun 13, 1983—Kessler, Ronald. Deaths from Heroin Use Increasing: Middle Class Addiction on Rise.

Sep 6, 1983—Cody, Edward. Steady Traffic Defies War on Drugs: Cocaine Flows to U.S. in Record Amounts.

Sep 22, 1983—Engel, Margaret. Private NW Clinic Has Support Plan for Victims of AIDS.

Sep 27, 1983—Kamen, Al, and Alfred E. Lewis. DC Leading Nation in Heroin Overdose.

Mar 15, 1984—Slacum, Marcia A. Barry Launches Crackdown on Drugs at Lorton.

Apr 26, 1984—Teeley, Sandra Evans. 10% at Lorton Used Drugs, Barry Reports.

Aug 7, 1984—Engel, Margaret. PCP Called 'Key to St. E's': PCP 'Epidemic' Monitored at St. Elizabeths.

Sep 28, 1984—Bredemeier, Kenneth. Record Seen in 1981 D.C. Heroin Deaths.

Oct 17, 1984—Greene, Marcia Slacum. Drug-Treatment Bill Is Introduced.

Dec 13, 1984—Bruske, Ed. Cocaine Use in D.C. Rises: Tests Positive in 22% of Criminal Suspects.

Dec 23, 1984—Mathews, Jay. Drug Abuse Takes New Form: Rock Cocaine Is Peddled to the Poor in Los Angeles.

Mar 10, 1985—Milloy, Courtland, and Linda Wheeler. District Is a Major Center of Heroin Trade.

May 15, 1985—Evans, Sandra. Recent Cocaine Use Seen in 30% of D.C. Arrestees.

Jul 4, 1985—Sargent, Edward D. Student Test Scores Released: Student Tests.

Sep 11, 1985—Evans, Sandra. D.C. Faulted on Special Education.

Nov 25, 1985—Wheeler, Linda. Gunfights Heighten Danger at Drug-Plagued Hanover Place.

Nov 27, 1985—Feinberg, Lawrence. Drug 'Kingpin' Pleads Guilty: Called Key Hanover Pl. Figure.

Dec 22, 1985—Wheeler, Linda. From Drug Mart to Great Neighborhood?

Jan 19, 1986—Feinberg, Lawrence. D.C. Population Shows First Rise Since 1963.

Jan 25, 1986—Engel, Margaret. Community Clinics in Area Face Closure.

Jan 29, 1986—Engel, Margaret. Area AIDS Cases Multiply Faster Than in Other Cities.

Feb 7, 1986—Engel, Margaret. City to Handle AIDS Bodies.

Mar 19, 1986—Thornton, Mary. Mexican Corruption Spurring Drug Trade, Says U.S. Official.

Apr 12, 1986—Anderson, John Ward. 6 Persons Are Shot in Legs: D.C. Police Fear Drug War.

Apr 23, 1986—Harris, Lyle V. Montgomery Grand Jury Probes Growing Cocaine Problem.

Apr 28, 1986—Moore, Molly, and John Ward Anderson. The Drug Fiefdom of Northern Mexico.

May 2, 1986—Lewis, Nancy. D.C. Prison Consultant Appointed.

May 7, 1986—Lewis, Nancy. New Statute Provides 30-Year Prison Terms.

May 9, 1986—Engel, Margaret. D.C. Lacks Policy on Scores of Inmates Exposed to AIDS Virus.

May 14, 1986—Berg, Paul. Cocaine's Deceit: Ring The Brain Down the Path of Addiction.

May 21, 1986—Anderson, John Ward. Six Men Arrested, Charged in Miami-D.C. Cocaine Case.

Jun 11, 1986—Evans, Sandra. Sentencing Law Would Exempt Some Addicts.

Jun 22, 1986—Melton, R. H., and Linda Wheeler. Once for Elite, Cocaine Now an Equal-Opportunity Vice.

Jun 30, 1986—LaFraniere, Sharon, and Sandra Evans. District Drug Agency's Promises Go Unfulfilled.

Jul 16, 1986—Arocha, Zita. Ex-Addict Says He Cooked Cocaine at 10 Houses.

Jul 19, 1986—Sargent, Edward D. D.C. Students Attain Mixed Scores.

Aug 5, 1986—Engel, Margaret. Top District Public Health Official Resigns.

Sep 5, 1986—Wheeler, Linda. D.C. School Board Adopts Stringent Disciplinary Rules.

Sep 6, 1986—Engel, Margaret. Full-Time Clinic to Treat AIDS Planned in D.C.

Oct 19, 1986—Musto, David F. Drugs: Crusades Always Start When Use Already Is Going Down.

Nov 5, 1986—Walsh, Elsa. Mandatory Drug Terms Are Upheld. D.C. Panel Rules on Constitutionality.

Nov 25, 1986—Walsh, Elsa. 33% of Youths Arrested in D.C. Have Used Drugs.

Dec 1, 1986—Fisher, Marc. Schools Tighten Discipline Code.

Dec 4, 1986—Wheeler, Linda. New Life for Dead-End Street.

Dec 21, 1986—Robinson, Eugene. 'Clean Sweep' Doesn't Work.

Jan 12, 1987—Boodman, Sandra O. Home for People with AIDS Prompts Concern.

Mar 4, 1987—Okie, Susan, and Linda Wheeler. D.C. Prostitutes Show a 50 Pct. AIDS Virus Rate.

Mar 5, 1987—Sherwood, Tom. DC Report on AIDS Released: Blacks Urged to Take Threat Seriously.

Mar 9, 1987—Editorial. Where Drug Dealers Prey.

Mar 18, 1987—Lewis, Nancy. Drug Arrests on Trains Rise as Couriers Switch to Tracks.

Apr 21, 1987—Barker, Karlyn. D.C. Names Substance Abuse Chief; Special Office to Coordinate AIDS Programs Also Created.

May 6, 1987—Hall, Charles W. Cocaine Seizure Is Largest Ever in Md. Suburbs.

Jul 4, 1987—Horwitz, Sari. Barry Acts to Free 350 Prisoners.

Jul 28, 1987—Lewis, Nancy. Out-of-Town Drug Dealers Invade Area: 'Mayfair Market' Is Latest Battleground.

Aug 2, 1987—Churchville, Victoria. NE Tenants Hope to Outlast Siege of Drug Violence.

Aug 4, 1987—Boodman, Sandra G. Women with AIDS Get a Place of Their Own.

Aug 10, 1987—Evans, Sandra. Crack Goes Far Afield: An Urban Drug Infiltrates Rural Md., Va.

Aug 13, 1987—Churchville, Victoria. District Drug Sweep Snares Children Drawn into Dealing.

Sep 1, 1987—[No author.] Dr. Reed Tuckson, Leading the City's AIDS War.

Sep 2, 1987—Cohn, D'Vera. Crowded, Costly Drug Programs Out of Many Fairfax Teens' Reach.

Sep 24, 1987—Wheeler, Linda. D.C. Tops Country in Drug Arrests.

Nov 8, 1987—Wheeler, Linda. Southeast's Search for a Little Understanding.

Nov 19, 1987—Wheeler, Linda, and Keith Harriston. Jamaican Gangs Wage War over Drugs.

Dec 10, 1987—Duggan, Paul. 15 Are Arrested in Crack Raids in Montgomery.

Jan 23, 1988—Yorke, Jeffrey. Area Police Execute Sweep Of 17 Cocaine Ring Suspects.

Jan 26, 1988—Wheeler, Linda, and Sari Horwitz. Operation Clean Sweep's Future Uncertain.

Jan 30, 1988—Horwitz, Sari. Crack Flooding D.C. Drug Market, Police Say.

Feb 10, 1988—Jordan, Mary. Seizures of Drugs Double in Fairfax, Montgomery.

Feb 19, 1988—Churchville, Victoria. D.C. Officers Urge Stiffer Gun Laws.

Feb 21, 1988—Abramowitz, Michael. Concern Mounts Over Lengthy Wait for Drug Treatment in D.C.

Feb 23, 1988—Churchville, Victoria. Elusive Jamaican Drug Gangs Frustrate Police.

Feb 26, 1988—Duke, Lynne. Suburban Drug Use Here Worst in U.S.

Feb 28, 1988—Jordan, Mary. Street-Level Drug Sales Invade Washington Suburbs, Police Say.

Mar 12, 1988—Lait, Matt. The Battle to Control 50,000 Gang Members on the Streets of Los Angeles.

Mar 21, 1988—Sanchez, Carlos. The Sordid World of Blagden Alley.

Apr 14, 1988—Sanchez, Rene. Hide-and-Seek With Drug Smugglers.

Apr 22, 1988—Gaines-Carter, Patrice and James Rupert. Muslims Gain Barry's Support and Find Services in Demand.

Apr 23, 1988—Rupert, James. Youths Back in the Swing of Things.

Apr 24, 1988—Horwitz, Sari. A Drug-Selling Machine That Was All Business.

May 10, 1988—Colburn, Don. AIDS in US Prisons Mirrors Outside World.

Jun 9, 1988—Hockstader, Lee. DC Urged to Move or Free Inmates.

Jun 26, 1988—Morin, Richard, and Jodie Allen. Are We Shooting Ourselves in the Foot in the War on Drugs?

Jun 29, 1988—Churchville, Victoria. Jamaican Gangs Spread Drug War.

Jun 30, 1988—Sklansky, Jeff, and Rene Sanchez. D.C. Killings Soar Toward Record High.

Jul 5, 1988—Boodman, Sandra G. D.C.'s Media Campaign Against AIDS Is Delayed.

Jul 6, 1988—Meyer, Eugene L. P.G. Crack Buyers: Everyday People.

Jul 22, 1988—Wheeler, Linda. Drug Arrests of Juveniles Soar in D.C.

Jul 27, 1988—Sanchez, Rene. DC School Scores Are a Mixed Bag.

Aug 6, 1988—Hockstader, Lee, and Nancy Lewis. Barry Blames Reagan for Prison Crisis.

Aug 8, 1988—Boodman, Sandra G. AIDS Spreading Faster Among D.C. Blacks.

Aug 9, 1988—Hockstader, Lee. Barry Defends City's Handling of Prison Crisis.

Sep 6, 1988—Hines, William, and Judith Randal. Teaching Your Kids About AIDS.

Sep 15, 1988—Harriston, Keith. 72% of New Inmates Test Positive for Drugs.

Oct 5, 1988—Boodman, Sandra G. and Eric Pianin. DC Moves to Repeal AIDS Law.

Oct 10, 1988—Jordan, Mary. Months After Drug Summit, Efforts Remain Uneven.

Oct 26, 1988—Horwitz, Sari, and Nancy Lewis. Drug Wars Push D.C. to Brink of Homicide Record.

Oct 28, 1988—Lewis, Nancy, and Sari Horwitz. Hundreds Flee Fatal Shootout Near SE Club.

Nov 13, 1988—Milloy, Courtland. Stopping the Craziness.

Nov 20, 1988—Horwitz, Sari. NE Drug Gangs' War Has Bloody Price Tag.

Dec 8, 1988—Lewis, Nancy, and Victoria Churchville. Turner Says Clean Sweep Has Failed.

Dec 11, 1988—Lewis, Nancy. As Night Falls, Guns Rule Many City Streets.

Dec 18, 1988—Hockstader, Lee. Sudden Move Severs Inmate's Ties to D.C.

Dec 27, 1988—Colburn, Don. Undoing the Damage.

Jan 13, 1989—Wye, Brad. How Drug Markets Compare with Homicide Locations in DC.

Feb 22, 1989—Boodman, Sandra G. D.C. to Get AIDS Effort Off Ground.

Feb 25, 1989—Abramowitz, Michael. DC 1990 Budget Shortfall Squeezes AIDS Programs.

Mar 9, 1989—Horwitz, Sari. D.C. Killings Top 100 With No Solution in Sight.

Mar 11, 1989—Isikoff, Michael. FBI's Drug Target List Omits Washington.

Mar 12, 1989—Boodman, Sandra, and Sari Horwitz. Night of Violence Leaves 4 Dead in D.C.

Mar 14, 1989—Isikoff, Michael, and Eric Pianin. Bennett Gives D.C. Top Priority in Drug War.

Mar 17, 1989—Lewis, Nancy. Hill Pressure Builds as Slaying Toll Soars.

Mar 19, 1989—Isikoff, Michael. Strike Force Planned in D.C. War on Drugs.

Mar 25, 1989—Pianin, Eric. Turner Says Police Can't Halt Killings.

Apr 2, 1989—Duke, Lynne, and Debbie M. Price. At the Roots of the Violence: The Agony of Potomac Gardens.

Apr 4, 1989—Price, Debbie. 'Murder Capital' Label Has Long Stalked D.C.

Apr 9, 1989—Webb, Joseph. D.C. Schools Are Failing Our Children.

Apr 11, 1989—Horwitz, Sari and Chris Spolar. Bennett Faces Inherent Hurdles in Plan to Rid D.C. of Drugs.

Apr 19, 1989—Abramowitz, Michael, and Shaon LaFraniere. D.C. Drug Treatment Clinics Behind the Times, Study Says.

Apr 22, 1989—Kurtz, Howard. Carrying Cocaine From N.Y. to Washington.

Apr 24, 1989—Abramowitz, Michael. D.C. Medical Office in Decline.

May 7, 1989—Thomas, Pierre, and Veronica T. Jennings. Drug Trade Thrives Beyond Beltway.

May 8, 1989—Spolar, Chris. City Shelters Drugs, Blight: Group Finds D.C. Owns Troubled Houses.

May 16, 1989—Abramowitz, Michael. Drug Arrests Put Squeeze on Area Treatment Programs.

May 17, 1989—Thompson, Tracy. 26 Arrested in Cartel Linked to Big Drug Shipments Here.

Jun 14, 1989—Pianin, Eric. House Votes to Add 700 D.C. Officers.

Jun 15, 1989—Abramowitz, Michael. D.C. Health System Gutted, Tuckson Says.

Jul 3, 1989—Walsh, Elsa. Drug Use at Lorton 'Disturbing': Increased Demand by Inmates Feared.

Jul 28, 1989—Sanchez, Carlos. A Fifth of Poor D.C. Youths in Study Involved with Drugs.

Jul 19, 1989—Duke, Lynne. Drugs Are a Shadowy Force in D.C. Area's Economy.

Aug 15, 1989—Isikoff, Michael. Drugs Top Problem in U.S., Poll Finds.

Aug 31, 1989—Milloy, Courtland. Insulation on the White Side of Town.

Sep 13, 1989—Abramowitz, Michael. Senate Panel Approves 1,000 New D.C. Police.

Sep 23, 1989—Torry, Saundra and Sari Horwitz. Jail Crowding Derails Massive Drug Sweeps.

Oct 23, 1989—Anderson, Jack and Dale Van Atta. Life in Lorton Is Like Life on the Street.

Nov 26, 1989—Buckley, Stephen. D.C.'s Cocaine Supply Line Withstands Police Offensive.

Dec 15, 1989—Twomey, Steve. Drug War's Forgotten Victims: The Wounded.

Jan 6, 1990—Lewis, Nancy. Drug Rate Declines Among D.C. Court Defendants.

Jan 10, 1990—Lynne Duke. D.C. Health Nominee Inherits Complex Problems.

Jan 19, 1990—Melton, R. H. and Michael Abramowitz. Barry Arrested on Cocaine Charges in Undercover FBI, Police Operation.

Feb 16, 1990—York, Michael and Elsa Walsh. Barry Indicted on Cocaine, Perjury Charges; Mayor Calls Process a 'Political Lynching'

Feb 18, 1990—Duke, Lynne. Increase in AIDS Cases Slowing Down in Area.

Mar 19, 1990—Price, Debbie. Terror Stills Drug War Victims: Area Police Hindered by Lack of Information.

Apr 20, 1990—Buckley, Stephen. NE Street's 'Invisible Wall' Keeps Drug Trade at Bay.

May 10, 1990—Walsh, Elsa. D.C. Report Blasts Focus of Drug War: More Treatment, Alternatives to Prison Urged.

Jun 10, 1990a—Dash, Leon. Drugs in the Ranks: Users in the Jail. A System Beset from Within. *Series.*

Jun 10, 1990b—Dash, Leon. Officer Slept at Key Posts: Exhaustion After Extended High Compromised Safety of Others. *Series.*

Jun 11, 1990a—Dash, Leon. Jail Officer Traded Inside Information for a Discount. *Series.*

Jun 11, 1990b—Dash, Leon. Officer Smoked Crack on the Job: Bringing in Supplies Was Easy. *Series.*

Jun 12, 1990—Dash, Leon. Contraband in a Box of Chicken: Smuggling at the DC Jail. *Series.*

Jun 13, 1990—Dash, Leon. Officer's Addiction Was No Secret: Hiring and Firing. *Series.*

Jun 17, 1990—Knight, Athelia. Drop Out Lessons: The Kids Who Didn't Graduate and What They Have to Teach Us.

Jun 23, 1990—Howe, Robert F. 7 Officers At Lorton Indicted: FBI Alleges Drugs Were Sold to Inmates.

Jul 11, 1990—Sanchez, Rene. DC Glum Over Latest Test Scores.

Sep 5, 1990—Abramowitz, Michael. Biggest D.C. Deficit in 10 Years Looms Amid Region's Economic Downtown.

Nov 4, 1990—Isikoff, Michael and Tracy Thompson. Getting Too Tough on Drugs.

Nov 24, 1990—Escobar, Gabriel. D.C. Homicides, at 436, Set 3rd Straight Record.

Dec 18, 1990—Colburn, Don. The Risky Lives of Young Black Men.

Dec 26, 1990—Melton, R.H. and Michael Abramovitz. The Barry Years: Mayor Leaves Shadow Over Achievements.

Feb 4, 1991—McCall, Nathan. AIDS Toll Rising in DC Jails.

Feb 21, 1991—Torry, Sandra. AIDS Protestors Invade DC Health Offices.

June 4, 1991—Henderson, Nell. Noted Researcher Will Head D.C. Office on AIDS Affairs.

Jun 17, 1991—Mooar, Brian. Prostitutes Fan Out as D.C. Police Crack Down on L Street Business.

Jun 30, 1991—Horwitz, Sari. The Ghosts Are Always Around a Little Bit.

Jul 28, 1991—Pressley, Sue Ann, and Richard Morin. The Long Shadow of Gun Violence.

Aug 18, 1991—Thomas, Pierre. D.C.'s Modern-Day Gunrunners.

Sep 19, 1991—Mercer, Joye. Memories Bind Tenants of Premier Black Apartment Complex.

Sep 20, 1991—Goldstein, Amy. Dixon Fills Health Job, Sources Say.

Oct 14, 1991—Greene, Marcia Slacum. Addicts Swamp City Facilities.

Dec 19, 1991—Isikoff, Michael. Cocaine Use on the Upswing.

Mar 15, 1992—Wilson, Jerry. D.C.'s Other Crime Crisis: Our Vanishing Veteran Cops.

Mar 18, 1992—Harriston, Keith. D.C. Jail Officers Accused of Buying Drugs for Inmates.

Mar 19, 1992—York, Michael. Drug Trial Testimony Links R Street Crew to L.A. Gang.

May 13, 1992—Isikoff, Michael. Hospital Data Indicate Rise in Hard-Core Drug Abuse.

May 18, 1992—Goldstein, Amy. AIDS Plan Creates Prison Paradox.

Jul 30, 1992—York, Michael. Group Accused of Violent Drug Enterprise.

Sep 17, 1992—Horwitz, Sari, and Mary Jordan. D.C. Dropout Rate Among Worst in US.

Oct 22, 1992—Howe, Robert F. 11 Lorton Employees Are Charged with Drug Smuggling.

Dec 31, 1992—Harriston, Keith A., and Paul Duggan. Across the Area, Tide of Killings Recedes in 1992.

Jan 7, 1993—York, Michael. P. Street Crew Case Ends Without Trial.

Jan 31, 1993—Mencimer, Stephanie. D.C.'s New Death Row: AIDS Is Devastating the District's Prisons and Busting Its Budget.

Apr 1, 1993—Harriston, Keith A. D.C. to Close Cedar Knoll by May 31.

Apr 18, 1993—Boo, Katherine. Stairway to Hell: Squalor and Squatters in D.C.'s Worst Project.

May 31, 1993—Gladwell, Malcolm. Crack Epidemic Appears to Wane.

May 31, 1993—Robberson, Tod. Mexican Drug Dealers Cut Pervasive Path.

Jul 7, 1993—Booth, William. Drug War Locks Up Prisons.

Jul 11, 1993—Goldstein, Amy. Where AIDS and Money Cross Paths.

Aug 31, 1993—Goldstein, Amy. The Young in D.C. Meet Drugs Early.

Oct 24, 1993—Knight, Athelia. Of 1,286 Slaying Cases, 1 in 4 Ends in Conviction.

Nov 16, 1993—Miller, Bill. Drug Use at Lorton Called 'Public Scandal.'

Nov 17, 1993—Miller, Bill, and Rene Sanchez. D.C. Prison Employees Charged in Probe of Drug Trade at Lorton.

Nov 29, 1993—Weinraub, Judith. The Politics of AIDS: Caitlin Ryan Once Led the City's Fight Against the Disease.

Nov 30, 1993—Goldstein, Amy. New York AIDS Fighter to Lead District Agency.

Dec 16, 1993—Flaherty, Mary Pat, and Keith Harriston. Corruption Due to Rush to Hire.

Feb 20, 1994—Leiby, Richard. A Crack in the System: This Small-Time Dealer Is Doing 20 Years. He Might Be Better Off if He'd Killed Somebody.

Jun 14, 1994—Vest, Jason. Fewer Americans Use More Cocaine, Study Says.

Jun 23, 1994—Goldstein, Amy. AIDS Chief in DC Quits After 6 Months.

Jun 29, 1994—Peabody, Alvin. City Awards AIDS Contract to Whitman Walker Clinic.

Aug 28, 1994—Harriston, Keith, and Mary Flaherty. District Police Are Still Paying for Forced Hiring Binge. *Series.*

Aug 30, 1994—Harriston, Keith, and Mary Flaherty. Police Credibility on Trial in D.C. Courts. *Series.*

Aug 31, 1994—Harriston, Keith, and Mary Flaherty. Delays Defeat Police Efforts to Clean House. *Series.*

Nov 20, 1994—Milloy, Courtland. Police Talk to Youth.

Dec 31, 1994—Castaneda, Ruben. Killings Drop by 11 Percent in the District.

Jan 13, 1995—Lewis, Nancy. Massive Effort Planned to Rid D.C. of Guns.

Jan 29, 1995—Loeb, Vernon. In an Ailing City, Vital Services Cease to Function.

Feb 2, 1995—Schneider, Howard and David A. Vise. Barry Says D.C. Deficit Now $722 Million.

Feb 10, 1995—Miller, Bill. Inmate Ran Prison Heroin Network from His Lorton Cell, Indictment Says.

Mar 3, 1995—Loeb, Vernon and Lorraine Adams. In a System Laden with Security, the Toughest Job Is Cutting a Job.

Mar 26, 1995—McGee, Jim. Drug Smuggling Industry Is Built on Franchises.

May 8, 1995—Miller, Bill. Addicts Get a Hand Up from D.C.'s Drug Court.

May 12, 1995—Goldstein, Amy. Staff Found to Fill Gaps at AIDS Clinic.

Jun 18, 1995—Goldstein, Amy. Advocate to Head D.C. AIDS Agency.

Jul 12, 1995—Locy, Toni. U.S. Judge Seizes Control of D.C. Jail Medical Care.

Aug 13, 1995—Moore, Margaret A. A Prison in Dire Need of Corrections.

Aug 16, 1995—Loeb, Vernon. A Miserable Place to Call Home.

Sep 5, 1995—Bowles, Scott. D.C. Police Probe Link in 20 Deaths.

Sep 17, 1995—Reding, Andrew. The Fall and Rise of the Drug Cartels.

Sep 28, 1995—Hall, Charles W. Inmate Gets Life for Role as Kingpin.

Dec 6, 1995—Locy, Toni. Occoquan Called District's Most Violent Prison.

Jan 12, 1996—Smith, R. Jeffrey. Cocaine Flow Not Slowed, General Says.

Jan 25, 1996—Hall, Charles W. Lorton Guard Charged in Prison Drug Ring Probe.

Apr 28, 1996—Moore, Molly and John Ward Anderson. The Drug Fiefdom of Northern Mexico.

Sep 23, 1996—Goldstein, Amy. Little Room for Recovery: Deep Cuts in Local Funding Hurt Drug, Alcohol Treatment Programs in D.C., PG.

Sep 29, 1996—Harris, Hamil. Better Days at D.C. Morgue.

Oct 9, 1996—Flaherty, Mary Pat, and William Casey. Judges Hand Blacks Longer Prison Times.

Oct 18, 1996—Boo, Katherine. Misery's New Landlord.

Feb 4, 1997—Miller, Bill, and Mary Pat Flaherty. D.C. Criminals Would Face Harder Time Under Clinton's Aid Plan.

Feb 10, 1997—Williams, Vanessa. Barry Puts His Money on Southeast.

Feb 17, 1997—Williams, Vanessa. "I'm Not the Problem," Barry Insists.

Mar 30, 1997—Farah, Douglas, and Molly Moore. Mexican Drug Traffickers Eclipse Colombian Cartels.

May 5, 1997—Brown, DeNeen L. Death Rates for Children Rise in D.C.

Jun 8, 1997—Frankel, Glenn. U.S. War on Drugs Yields Few Victories.

Jul 12, 1997—Thompson, Cheryl W. Drug Use Appears Rife Among D.C. Prisoners.

Jul 15, 1997—Editorial. Jails Without Walls.

Jul 16, 1997—Amy Goldstein. After Describing Job Frustrations, D.C. Health Chief Is Ordered to Vacate Office.

Aug 17, 1997—Burleigh, Nina. Death and Life in a Neighborhood No One Really Sees.

Sep 7, 1997—David Simon and Edward Burns. Too Much Is Not Enough: In the Endless War on Drugs We're Filling the Jails but Losing the Streets.

Sep 25, 1997—Harris, Hamil. Success, One Addict at a Time.

Oct 19, 1997—Opinion. Round Two: Harvey Sloane Deserved the Ax.

Oct 28, 1997—Goldstein, Avram. Head of DC AIDS Agency Removed.

Nov 18, 1997—Faiola, Anthony. As Coca Market Goes, So Shall They Reap.

Dec 14, 1997—Davis, Patricia, and Pierre Thomas. Suburban High: In Affluent Suburbs, Young Users and Sellers Abound.

Dec 15, 1997—Davis, Patricia, and Pierre Thomas. A Business That Knows No Boundaries: Drugs Flow From Adult Organizations.

Apr 11, 1998—Horwitz, Sari. Metro in Brief.

Apr 29, 1998—Mann, Judy. Playing Politics With the Public's Health.

May 24, 1998—Slevin, Peter. At Lorton, New Math Holds Prisoners Back.

May 26, 1998—Goldstein, Amy. Hank Carde, the Ardent AIDS Activist.

Aug 25, 1998—Slevin, Peter. In D.C., Many Addicts and Few Services.

Sep 3, 1998—Matthews, Jay. Lives of D.C. Children Improve, Study Finds.

Sep 11, 1998—Slevin, Peter. Receivership Sought for DC Youth Prison.

Sept 23, 1998—Vise, David A. Barnett Fills Key Health Post.

Sept 27, 1998—Vise, David A. Ga. Physician Declines D.C. Health Post.

Nov 15, 1998—Leen, Jeff, Jo Craven, David Jackson, and Sari Horwitz. District Police Lead Nation in Shootings.

Apr 17, 1999—Horwitz, Sari. Study Finds Drug Abuse at Heart of City's Ills.

Aug 20, 1999—Horwitz, Sari. District to Pay Top Dollar for Incoming Public Health Director.

Sep 23, 1999—Strauss, Valerie. One-Third of District Students Drop Out.

Dec 3, 2000—Thompson, Cheryl, Ira Chinoy and Barbara Vobejda. Unsolved Killings Plague District. *Series.*

Dec 5, 2000—Vobejda, Barbara, and Ira Chinoy. As D.C. Police Falter, Revenge Fills the Void. *Series.*

Dec 6, 2000—Vobejda, Barbara, and Ira Chinoy. A Deadly Past Repeats Itself. *Series.*

Feb 11, 2001—Lotke, Eric. Lorton Closing Opens a Door for Reform.

Mar 14, 2002—Goldstein, Avram. No Plan Yet on Replacing Walks.

Mar 21, 2002—Santana, Arthur. Families Lamenting Life After Lorton.

May 16, 2003—Goldstein, Avram. HIV/AIDS Director Defends Leadership Before D.C. Council.

Nov 11, 2003—Rosenzweig, Dan, and Andrea Salcedo. The 'D.C. Madam' Riveted Washington Long Before This Week's Brothel Case.

Aug 5, 2004—Wilgoren, Debbi. D.C. Picks ER Doctor to Head Health Dept.

Jun 8, 2005—Schwartzman, Paul. D.C. Gay Clubs' Vanishing Turf.

Aug 25, 2005—Montgomery, Lori. Advocate Named as D.C. AIDS Administrator.

Aug 17, 2005—Labbe, Theola. District's HIV-AIDS Director Is Fired.

Mar 25, 2006—Vargas, Jose Antonio. Once a Pioneer in AIDS Battle, District Is Now Fighting Blind.

Dec 30, 2006—Vargas, Jose Antonio. An Overwhelmed DC Agency Loses Count of AIDS Cases.

Jan 4, 2007—Levine, Susan. Fenty Declines to Reappoint HIV-AIDS Agency Director.

Jan 4, 2007—Blanks, Raymond S. District Continues to Fail Public on HIV-AIDS.

Apr 28, 2007—Kessler, Glenn. Rice Deputy Quits After Query Over Escort Service.

Jul 10, 2007—Murray, Shailagh. Senator's Number on 'Madam' Phone List.

Aug 9, 2007—Holley, Joe. Mayor Makes Choice to Run AIDS Agency.

Oct 20, 2007—Nakamura, David and Yolanda Woodlee. Health Chief Fired As Mayor Seeks More Forceful Tack.

Mar 1, 2008—Nakamura, David. Fenty Taps Md. Official to Direct Health Dept.

Apr 25, 2008—Levine, Susan. Needle Swap Programs to Receive D.C. Funds.

Jun 14, 2008—Stein, Rob. AIDS Cases Missed in D.C.; Hundreds of Deaths Unreported Over 6 Years, Study Says.

Mar 14, 2009—Vargas, Jose Antonio, and Darryl Fears. HIV/AIDS Rate in DC Hits 3%.

Oct 18, 2009—Cenziper, Debbie. Staggering Need, Striking Neglect. *Series.*

Nov 12, 2009—Cenziper, Debbie. HUD Threatens to Cut Off DC AIDS Funding Next Year. *Series.*

Dec 13, 2009—Cenziper, Debbie. D.C. AIDS Funding Shifted from Needy Neighborhoods. *Series.*

Dec 24, 2009—Cenziper, Debbie. DC's Largest Needle-Exchange Program Running Out of Cash. *Series.*

Jan 8, 2011—Stewart, Nikita. Gray Names Choices for Key Health Jobs.

Feb 5, 2011—Stewart, Nikita. D.C. Mayor Picks His HHS Deputy, 5 Other Directors.

Jul 23, 2012—Sun, Lena H. A Shift in Strategy to Treatment as Prevention for HIV/AIDS.

Dec 30, 2014—DeBonis, Mike. Bowser Nominates 3 with Fenty Ties.

Jan 23, 2015—Brown, DeNeen L. Prince George's Neighborhoods Make 'Top 10 List of Richest Black Communities in America.'

Mar 17, 2016—Shaver, Katherine, and Dana Hedgpeth. D.C.'s Decade-Old Problem of Lead in Water Gets New Attention During Flint Crisis.

Mar 14, 2018—Nirappil, Fenit. D.C. Has a High Maternal Mortality Rate. Lawmakers Want to Know Why.

Jun 29, 2022—Van Dam, Andrew. Is Prince George's Still the Richest Majority-Black County in America?

Jun 8, 2023—Portnoy, Jenna. Mayor Bowser Names New D.C. Health Director After Year-Long Search.

Nov 11, 2023—Rosenzweig-Ziff, Dan and Andrea Salcedo. The 'D.C. Madam' Riveted Washington Long Before This Week's Brothel Case.

INDEX

Page numbers in italics denote figures. Page numbers followed by *n* denote notes.

laws, 169; purity, 158; trafficking, 250; Urban Institute report, 228–29. *See also* cocaine epidemic; crack-homicide syndemic in DC; heroin epidemic; heroin-homicide syndemic; HIV/AIDS; PCP (phenylcyclohexyl piperidine)

drug distribution: global cocaine supply chain to DC, 174–75; turf wars for, 175, 176, 179, 199–200, 201, 250; global heroin supply chain to DC, 157–58, 163, 165–66

drug networks, racially homogamous, 167. *See also* HIV/AIDS

Du Bois, W. E. B., 13, 40

Duneier, Mitch, 22

Dunlap, Eloise, 183

DuPont, Robert, 158, 160, 161, 162

Dupont Circle, 109–10, 119–20

Eason, John, 238

economic incentives vs. health protection, 194–96

Edin, Kathy, 12

education: in DC, 206, 221, 226–27; out-comes and dropping out of school, 227, 232. *See also* school, dropping out of; school-to-prison pipeline

Education Watch, 227

Ely, Richard, 65

Emancipation Act, 40

embodiment of history, 19–20

employment: occupational discrimination, 16, 38, 49, 51; racial differences in, 50, 56, 69, 76, 131, 300. *See also* unemployment

Fair Housing Act, 76

Fair Sentencing Act, 213

faith, personal, 277–78. *See also* churches; religion

family(ies): alcoholism, 141; disease vulner-abilities cluster among, 10–11; entangle-ments, 183–85; formation patterns, racial divergence in, 125–33; and HIV/AIDS epidemics, 102–3, 275–77

Family Planning and Counseling, 290

Fauntroy, Walter, 80

Feagin, Joe, 18

Federal-Aid Highway Act of 1956, 85

Federal Home Loan Bank Act, 65

Federal Housing Administration (FHA), 55, 65

Fenty, Adrian, 89, 171, 226

First Era (1790–1890): death in a syndemic zone, 48–51; health consequences, 40–48; housing and health problems, 46–48; migration and the growth of Black population in DC, 37–40; spatial racial and class containment, 40–45

First Step Act, 213

Forman, James, Jr., 205, 218, 221, 222

Frazier, E. Franklin, 56

freebasing, 173

French Connection, 157, 162

Freudenberg, Nicholas, 241–42

Friedman, Sam, 101, 164

Friesema, H. Paul, 81

Fuchs, Victor, 7

Fullilove, Mindy, 69

Fulwood, Isaac, Jr., 202

Gaffney-Bey, Keith, 251

Galster, George, 227–28

Gatewood, Willard, 44

gay and bisexual men: activism, 114, 281–83, 297, 301; AIDS deaths, 120–21, 271, 281–82; Black sexual integration, 112–14; "gay White man's disease," 118, 134, 280–83, 291, 305; HIV rates, 104, 114; intimate Black life in a syndemic zone, 115–19; sexual containment in the late 1800s–1960s, 107–11; White sexual containment, 119–21. *See also* homosexuality

Gay and Lesbian Activists Alliance, 197, 301

gayborhoods, 109, 111, 119–20

gay clubs: Black, 120, 284; closing of, 119, 120; interracial, 110, 120; White, 111

"gay ghettos," 109

gender: differences in death rates, 16; disparities and life expectancy, 5, 7; gendered sexuality in prison, 252–55; inequality, 10; minority status, 9; and opiate addiction, 155–56; and power dynamics, 132, 194–96; and sexuality, intersecting system of, 15–17

Operation Clean Sweep, 217, 218, 219, 229, 237

opioid overdose death rates, 155–56. *See also* addiction; heroin-related deaths

opportunity structures: Black youth, 227–28; and racial containment, 227–28; sexual, 254

Oppression Under Target, 297

OraSure Technologies, 306

Oster, Alexandra, 98, 117

out-migration, 76, 80, 337n51, 350n14

overdose deaths, 156, 165, 166, 172, 173–74, 242

Pager, Devah, 214–15

Pane, Gregg, 306

Papachristos, Andrew, 201

Pappas, Gregory, 289, 307

parental neglect, 141, 143

partner shortage: for heterosexual women, 130–32; for transgender women, 131, 145–46. *See also* male marriageable pool index

Passow, A. Harry, 224–25

Pattillo, Mary, 221

PAUSE (Providing Alternative Unique School Environment), 231, 236

Payne-Jackson, Arvilla, 192

PCP (phenylcyclohexyl piperidine), 174. *See also* angel dust; love boat

people who injected drugs (PWID), 167–68, 169, 171

perinatal exposure and HIV infection, 104

personal faith, 277–78. *See also* churches; religion

personal safety nets, HIV/AIDS epidemics and, 275–78

PG County (Prince George's County, Maryland), 77, 82, 83, 93, 115

The Philadelphia Negro: A Social Study (Dubois, W. E. B.), 13

Pierce, Todd, 167–68

Pinderhughes, Elaine B., 131

Place, Hanover, 178

place-based interventions, 318–19

policies: crime, 213–15, 217–20, 222–23, 230–32, 234, 235, 237; drug, 155, 161–62, 168–71, 174–75, 178–79, 180, 196–98, 234;

drug testing, 174, 248–49; educational, 224–25, 226, 230–32, 235–36; health, 20, 50, 72, 278–80, 287–93, 296, 299, 304, 306–8, 314; housing, 10, 13, 21, 29, 42, 47–48, 51, 53, 57–65, 66–67, 82–84, 85–88; land, 20, 54, 59, 60–62, 64–65, 84–85, 314; prison, 222, 242, 243–47; taxation, 39, 40, 79–82, 89, 94, 225, 239, 294, 295; transportation, 20, 84–5, 178, 315

policing practices in Black neighborhoods, 217–21

post-AIDS discourse and White community recovery, 119–21

post-slavery Reconstruction era (1862–80), 39

powder cocaine, 173, 222; economy, 175–80. *See also* cocaine epidemic

pre-criminal status, 219, 231

PrEP (pre-exposure prophylaxis) awareness, 101, 348n54, 374n78

pretext policing, 218

Prince, Sabihya, 83

prison(s): community syndemic amplification in, 260–63; consensual relationships, 255, 256; drug abuse in, 161, 241–42; drug economy in, 248–52; harm reduction in, 241, 243–44; HIV testing and segregation in, 244, 247–48; mortality rate in, 242–43; protective pairings, 257; rape in, 256–57; as sex-segregated institutions, 252; sexual economy and HIV risk, 252–60; zip codes, 219. *See also* HIV/AIDS; mass Black incarceration in DC

prison- and political-industrial complexes, 236–40; commercial demand, 239; commoditization, 236–37; symbiotic nature, 238

Promise Neighborhoods, 318

property valuation, race and, 64–65

Public Education Reform Amendment Act, 226

public housing: construction in second era, 62–63; deterioration, 84–86; as drug infrastructure, 177–80

public schools in DC (DCPS): poor conditions, 225–26; poor funding for, 224–26; segregation, 226

Pure Food and Drug Act, 172

Founded in 1893,
UNIVERSITY OF CALIFORNIA PRESS
publishes bold, progressive books and journals
on topics in the arts, humanities, social sciences,
and natural sciences—with a focus on social
justice issues—that inspire thought and action
among readers worldwide.

The UC PRESS FOUNDATION
raises funds to uphold the press's vital role
as an independent, nonprofit publisher, and
receives philanthropic support from a wide
range of individuals and institutions—and from
committed readers like you. To learn more, visit
ucpress.edu/supportus.

www.ingramcontent.com/pod-product-compliance
Lightning Source LLC
Chambersburg PA
CBHW032337280326
41935CB00008B/360